Genetic Toxicology Testing

Genetic Toxicology Testing

A Laboratory Manual

Edited by

Ray Proudlock, MPhil, BSc

Boone, North Carolina, USA

AMSTERDAM • BOSTON • HEIDELBERG • LONDON
NEW YORK • OXFORD • PARIS • SAN DIEGO
SAN FRANCISCO • SINGAPORE • SYDNEY • TOKYO

Academic Press is an imprint of Elsevier

Academic Press is an imprint of Elsevier
125 London Wall, London EC2Y 5AS, UK
525 B Street, Suite 1800, San Diego, CA 92101-4495, USA
50 Hampshire Street, 5th Floor, Cambridge, MA 02139, USA
The Boulevard, Langford Lane, Kidlington, Oxford OX5 1GB, UK

Notices

Knowledge and best practice in this field are constantly changing. As new research and experience broaden our understanding, changes in research methods, professional practices, or medical treatment may become necessary.

Practitioners and researchers must always rely on their own experience and knowledge in evaluating and using any information, methods, compounds, or experiments described herein. In using such information or methods they should be mindful of their own safety and the safety of others, including parties for whom they have a professional responsibility.

To the fullest extent of the law, neither the Publisher nor the authors, contributors, or editors, assume any liability for any injury and/or damage to persons or property as a matter of products liability, negligence or otherwise, or from any use or operation of any methods, products, instructions, or ideas contained in the material herein.

British Library Cataloguing-in-Publication Data
A catalogue record for this book is available from the British Library

Library of Congress Cataloging-in-Publication Data
A catalog record for this book is available from the Library of Congress

ISBN: 978-0-12-800764-8

For Information on all Academic Press publications
visit our website at http://www.elsevier.com/

  Working together
to grow libraries in
developing countries

www.elsevier.com • www.bookaid.org

Publisher: Mica Haley
Acquisition Editor: Erin Hill-Parks
Editorial Project Manager: Molly McLaughlin
Production Project Manager: Karen East and Kirsty Halterman
Designer: Victoria Pearson Esse

Typeset by MPS Limited, Chennai, India

Contents

List of Contributors... *xvii*

Foreword .... *xix*

Preface .... *xxi*

Chapter 1: A Practical Guide to Genetic Toxicology Testing 1

Ray Proudlock

1.1 Introduction 1

References 3

Chapter 2: General Recommendations 5

Ray Proudlock

2.1 Establishing a New Assay... 6

    2.1.1 Method Set-Up 6

    2.1.2 Method Validation... 8

2.2 Spreadsheets and Manipulation of Results.. 10

2.3 Laboratory Historical Control Databases 11

    2.3.1 Vehicle/Negative Control Database 11

    2.3.2 Positive Control Database... 13

    2.3.3 Spreadsheet Calculations 13

2.4 Use of Computer Systems... 13

2.5 Study Design 15

2.6 Evaluation Criteria 17

    2.6.1 Valid Assay 17

    2.6.2 Criteria for Interpretation of Results 18

    2.6.3 Statistical Analysis 19

2.7 Organization of SOPs... 20

2.8   Planning a Study 22

2.9   Preparing a Protocol Complying with GLP 23

         2.9.1   Standardized Boilerplate Protocols 28

2.10   Collecting Results 29

         2.10.1 Data Tabulation 30

         2.10.2 Presentation of Report Tables.. 30

2.11   Reports.. 31

2.12   Training 36

2.13   Improving Quality and Efficiency 37

         2.13.1 Improving Quality 38

         2.13.2 Minimizing the Potential Problems on Studies 38

         2.13.3 Reducing the Need for Repetition of Parts of the Study 39

         2.13.4 Accommodating Repeat or Supplementary Tests........................... 40

         2.13.5 Running More Studies in a Given Timeframe 40

         2.13.6 Timeframe for Routine Studies... 41

         2.13.7 Reducing the Effort Needed to Prepare Protocols, Tables,
                    and Reports.. 43

         2.13.8 Reducing the Effort Needed to Perform the Study........................ 43

         2.13.9 Reducing Costs or Labor Requirement 44

2.14   QA 45

2.15   Qualifying a Contract Laboratory.. 47

2.16   Responsibilities of the Study Monitor... 48

References 49

Chapter 3: Formulation of Test Articles **51**

Annie Hamel and Ray Proudlock

3.1   Introduction 52

         3.1.1   Safety 52

         3.1.2   Selecting an Appropriate Formulation 52

3.2   Formulation Laboratories... 53

         3.2.1   Designing and Equipping a Genetic Toxicology Formulation
                    Area.. 53

         3.2.2   Personal Protective Clothing.. 56

3.3   Safety Data Sheets 57

3.4   Receipt of the Test Article... 59

3.5   Formulation Types and Planning.. 59

3.6   Solubility and *In Vitro* Compatibility Testing 60

         3.6.1   Introduction 60

3.6.2   Choice of Solvent 61
3.6.3   Solubility Testing 62
3.6.4   Calculations and Checking: Small-Volume (*In Vitro*) Assays 64
3.6.5   Compatibility of Formulation with Culture Medium 65
3.7   Formulation of Dose Solutions 68
3.8   Formulation of Bulk Formulations 71
3.9   Formulation of Suspensions 71
3.9.1   Aqueous Suspending Agents 71
3.9.2   Large Volume Suspensions 73
3.9.3   Small Volume Suspensions 74
3.10   Chemical Analysis and Stability 74
References 77

Chapter 4: The Bacterial Reverse Mutation Test 79

Annie Hamel, Marise Roy and Ray Proudlock

4.1   Introduction 80
4.2   History 80
4.3   Fundamentals 83
4.4   Equipment 84
4.5   Consumables 85
4.6   Reagents and Recipes 86
4.6.1   Ampicillin 2 µg/disc 87
4.6.2   Biotin 0.37 mg/mL 87
4.6.3   Crystal Violet 5 µg/disc 87
4.6.4   Glucose 0.4 g/mL 87
4.6.5   *G6P 1M*: Glucose-6-Phosphate 88
4.6.6   *HBT*: 500 µM Histidine, 500 µM Biotin, 500 µM Tryptophan Solution .. 88
4.6.7   Histidine HCl.H$_2$O 5 mg/mL 88
4.6.8   KMg 88
4.6.9   MGA Plates 88
4.6.10 Minimal Glucose Master (MGM, MGMA and MGMAT) Plates 89
4.6.11 NADP 0.1 M 90
4.6.12 Nutrient Agar Plates 90
4.6.13 Nutrient Broth 90
4.6.14 Phosphate Buffer 0.2 M pH 7.4 90
4.6.15 Positive Control and Diagnostic Mutagen Solutions 90
4.6.16 S9 Fraction 91
4.6.17 S9 Mix 91
4.6.18 Tetracycline 1 µg/disc 92
4.6.19 Top Agar Incomplete: TAI 92

	4.6.20	Top Agar Complete: TAC	92
	4.6.21	Tryptophan 5 mg/mL	93
	4.6.22	VB Salts 50×: Vogel-Bonner Salts	93
4.7	Suggested Phases in Development of the Test		93
4.8	The Bacterial Strains		94
	4.8.1	Genotypes of Routinely Used Strains	95
	4.8.2	Obtaining the Tester Strains	95
	4.8.3	Receipt of Bacterial Strains	96
	4.8.4	Phenotyping of New Isolates	98
	4.8.5	Freezing of Selected Isolates	100
	4.8.6	Diagnostic Mutagen Test	101
4.9	Routine Testing		105
	4.9.1	Designing a Study	105
	4.9.2	Test Article Considerations	106
	4.9.3	Positive Controls	113
4.10	Standard Test Procedures		114
	4.10.1	Plate Incorporation Method	114
	4.10.2	Preincubation Method	115
	4.10.3	Standard Study Design	116
	4.10.4	Examination of the Plates	118
	4.10.5	Interpretation of Results	119
	4.10.6	Presentation of Results	121
	4.10.7	Testing of Volatile and Gaseous Compounds	125
4.11	Screening Tests		126
	4.11.1	Simplified Test Systems	126
	4.11.2	Screening Tests Using Standard Tester Strains	127
	4.11.3	Reduced Format Tests Using Standard Tester Strains	129
4.12	Appendix 1: Growing and Monitoring Suspension Cultures		130
References			134

Chapter 5: The Mouse Lymphoma TK Assay **139**

Mick Fellows and Melvyn Lloyd

5.1	Introduction		139
5.2	History		141
5.3	Provenance of the Cells		143
5.4	Spontaneous Mutation Frequency		144
5.5	Materials		145
	5.5.1	Safety	145
	5.5.2	Growth Medium	145
	5.5.3	Cell Culture	146

	5.5.4	Metabolic Activation	147
	5.5.5	Test Item	148
	5.5.6	Vehicle	148
	5.5.7	Positive Controls	148
5.6	Study Design		148
	5.6.1	General Test Conditions	148
	5.6.2	Preliminary Toxicity Test	150
	5.6.3	Main Mutation Test	151
5.7	Evaluation Criteria		155
5.8	Predictivity of the MLA		156
	References		158

Chapter 6: The In Vitro Micronucleus Assay 161

Ann Doherty, Steven M. Bryce and Jeffrey C. Bemis

6.1	Introduction		163
6.2	Practical Considerations		165
	6.2.1	Regulatory Guidelines	165
	6.2.2	Good Laboratory Practice (GLP)	165
	6.2.3	Cell Types	166
	6.2.4	Laboratory Proficiency	166
	6.2.5	Controls	166
	6.2.6	Metabolic Activation	167
	6.2.7	S9 Rat Liver Homogenate	167
	6.2.8	Experimental Design	167
	6.2.9	Cytotoxicity Measures	167
	6.2.10	Historical Controls	169
6.3	Methods		169
	6.3.1	Mononuclear Assay	169
	6.3.2	Binuclear Assay	169
	6.3.3	Centromeric Labeling	169
	6.3.4	Nondisjunction Assay	170
6.4	Materials		171
	6.4.1	Mononuclear Assay	171
	6.4.2	Binuclear Assay	172
	6.4.3	Centromeric Labeling	172
	6.4.4	Nondisjunction Assay	172
6.5	Protocols		172
	6.5.1	S9 Mix	172
	6.5.2	Mononuclear Assay	173
	6.5.3	Binuclear Assay	177

        6.5.4   Centromeric Labeling 181
        6.5.5   Nondisjunction Assay 183
    6.6   Flow Cytometric Method 184
        6.6.1   Equipment 184
        6.6.2   Consumables 185
        6.6.3   Reagents and Recipes 185
        6.6.4   Suspension Cell Protocol 187
        6.6.5   Attachment Cell Protocol 188
        6.6.6   Flow Cytometric Data Acquisition 189
        6.6.7   Flow Cytometric Data Analysis 193
        6.6.8   Creating an Analysis Template 195
        6.6.9   Example Plate Layout 198
        6.6.10   Example Results Table 199
        6.6.11   Advice for Test Article Exposure 200
        6.6.12   Use of Multichannel Aspirator with Bridge 202
        6.6.13   Plate Placement During Nucleic Acid Dye B Photoactivation 203
        6.6.14   Updates and Future Work 203
    References 203

Chapter 7: The In Vitro Chromosome Aberration Test 207

Marilyn Registre and Ray Proudlock

    7.1   Introduction 208
    7.2   History 209
    7.3   Fundamentals 211
    7.4   Equipment 212
    7.5   Consumables and Reagents 214
    7.6   Reagents and Recipes 215
        7.6.1   Colcemid 10 µg/mL in PBS 216
        7.6.2   Fix 216
        7.6.3   F-12 Complete 216
        7.6.4   Freezing Medium 10% (CHO Cells) 216
        7.6.5   Hypotonic Solution (0.075 M KCl) 217
        7.6.6   Heparin Sodium 1000 U/mL 217
        7.6.7   G6P 1 M: Glucose-6-Phosphate 217
        7.6.8   KMg 217
        7.6.9   NADP 0.1 M 217
        7.6.10   PHA M Form (Phytohemagglutinin) 217
        7.6.11   Phosphate Buffer 0.2 M, pH 7.4 218
        7.6.12   Positive Control Solutions 218
        7.6.13   RPMI Complete 218
        7.6.14   S9 Fraction 218
        7.6.15   S9 Mix 219

7.7   Phases in Development of the Test 219

7.8   Cell Characterization 221

    7.8.1   Modal Chromosome Number 222

    7.8.2   Mycoplasma 224

    7.8.3   Cell-Cycle Time 224

7.9   Routine Testing 225

    7.9.1   General Considerations 225

    7.9.2   Dose Regimens 225

    7.9.3   Metabolic Activation System 226

    7.9.4   Test Substance Considerations 226

    7.9.5   Vehicle Selection and Dose Volume 227

    7.9.6   Dose Level Selection 227

    7.9.7   Positive Controls 230

7.10   Standard Test Procedures 230

    7.10.1   Experimental Design Spreadsheet 231

    7.10.2   CHO Cells: Test Procedures 233

    7.10.3   HPBL Test Procedures 238

    7.10.4   Slide Staining: All Cell Types 241

    7.10.5   Selection of Slides for Detailed Examination 242

    7.10.6   Slide Coding 243

    7.10.7   Preliminary Slide Reading 243

    7.10.8   Slide Scoring 244

7.11   Interpretation of Results 253

    7.11.1   Evaluation of Toxicity 253

    7.11.2   Validity of the Study 253

    7.11.3   Criteria for Negative/Positive/Equivocal Outcome 253

    7.11.4   Interpretation of Numerical Aberrations 257

    7.11.5   Unexpected and Borderline Results 257

    7.11.6   Follow-up *In Vivo* Testing 257

    7.11.7   Reporting 258

    7.11.8   Historical Control Results 262

    7.11.9   Testing of Volatile and Gaseous Compounds 262

7.12   Screening Versions of the Test 263

7.13   Automation 264

References 264

Chapter 8: The *In Vivo Rodent Micronucleus Assay* 269

Laura Custer, Ann Doherty, Jeffrey C. Bemis and Ray Proudlock

8.1   Introduction 270

8.2   History 271

8.3 Fundamentals 271

8.4 Test Substance Considerations 273

8.5 Study Design 273

    8.5.1 Animal Source, Housing, Maintenance, and Identification.................. 274

    8.5.2 Animal Species, Strain, Age, and Sex.. 275

    8.5.3 Historical Negative/Vehicle and Positive Control Data........................ 276

    8.5.4 Number and Size of Treatment Groups... 277

    8.5.5 Acute and Repeat-Dose Schedules.. 278

    8.5.6 Dose Level Selection 279

    8.5.7 Dose Range-Finding Experiment 280

    8.5.8 Dose Administration 281

    8.5.9 Dose Volume 281

8.6 Manual Methods... 282

    8.6.1 Equipment and Consumables.. 282

    8.6.2 Reagent Preparation.. 282

    8.6.3 Sample Preparation 283

    8.6.4 Microscopic Methods.. 283

    8.6.5 Records... 290

    8.6.6 Identification of Aneugenic Agents 291

    8.6.7 Centromeric Staining Using FISH 292

    8.6.8 Kinetochore Labeling 294

8.7 Automated Analysis and Flow Cytometry 297

    8.7.1 Individual Reagents 297

    8.7.2 Solution and Material Preparation 297

    8.7.3 Flow Cytometry Method.. 299

    8.7.4 Blood Collection.. 299

    8.7.5 Bone Marrow Collection and Processing 299

    8.7.6 Collect and Fractionate Bone Marrow Samples 300

    8.7.7 Fixation of Blood and Bone Marrow Samples 300

    8.7.8 Storage of Fixed Samples 303

    8.7.9 Transfer Samples to LTSS... 304

    8.7.10 Label Washed Samples for Flow Analysis.. 305

    8.7.11 Flow Cytometric Analysis 306

    8.7.12 Analysis of Experimental Samples 311

    8.7.13 Template Preparation for Flow Cytometric Analyses............................ 312

8.8 Study Validity 314

8.9 Interpretation of Results and Statistical Analysis 315

    8.9.1 MIE Values 315

    8.9.2 Proportion of Immature Erythrocytes.. 316

8.10 Nongenotoxic Mechanisms of Induction of Micronucleated Erythrocytes 317

    8.10.1 Causes 317

    8.10.2 Avoiding and Recognizing Irrelevant Positives 317

8.11   Limitations of the Rodent Erythrocyte Micronucleus Test........................ 318

References... 319

Chapter 9: The Rodent Bone Marrow Chromosomal Aberration Test.....................323

Ray Proudlock

9.1   Introduction 324
9.2   History 324
9.3   Related Methods... 325
9.4   Study Design and Performance.. 326
  9.4.1   Vehicle/Negative Control and Formulation........................ 326
  9.4.2   Positive Control Group 327
  9.4.3   Sex and Group Size 327
  9.4.4   Number of Groups.. 327
  9.4.5   Evidence of Target Organ Exposure 328
  9.4.6   Dose Selection... 328
  9.4.7   Dose Administration.. 328
  9.4.8   Treatment Schedule 329
  9.4.9   Animal Observations 329
  9.4.10 Animal Euthanasia... 329
9.5   Terminal Procedures 330
  9.5.1   Equipment 330
  9.5.2   Consumables 331
  9.5.3   Advance Preparation.. 331
  9.5.4   Bone Marrow Collection 332
  9.5.5   Slide Preparation 333
  9.5.6   Slide Staining 333
  9.5.7   Slide Examination 334
  9.5.8   Calculations and Reporting of Results 334
  9.5.9   Acceptability of the Study 335
  9.5.10 Evaluation and Interpretation of Results............................. 335
  9.5.11 Test Report.. 337
  9.5.12 Integration into Other Studies.. 339
  9.5.13 Cytonucleus Test 339
Appendix... 340
References... 341

Chapter 10: The In Vivo *Comet Assay Test* 345

Marie Z. Vasquez and Roland Frötschl

10.1   Introduction 346

10.2   The *In Vivo* Comet Assay in Regulatory Safety Testing...................... 348
        10.2.1   Follow-Up of Positive *In Vitro* Standard Battery Tests...................... 350
        10.2.2   Follow-Up of Negative *In Vitro* Standard Battery Tests 351
10.3   Fundamentals 351
10.4   Equipment and Nondisposable Supplies 352
10.5   Consumables 354
10.6   Reagents and Solutions.. 354
        10.6.1   Reagents 354
        10.6.2   Solutions.. 355
10.7   Test System 356
10.8   Study Design Considerations... 357
        10.8.1   Test Article.. 357
        10.8.2   Vehicle Selection 357
        10.8.3   Positive Control 359
        10.8.4   Number of Animals 359
        10.8.5   Route of Exposure 359
        10.8.6   Treatment Schedule/Sample Time 360
        10.8.7   Dose Selection and Cytotoxicity.. 361
        10.8.8   Tissue Selection 361
10.9   Standard Test Procedures... 362
        10.9.1   Preliminary Procedures 362
        10.9.2   Sample Collection... 363
        10.9.3   Comet Slide Preparation 364
        10.9.4   Alkaline Electrophoresis 365
        10.9.5   Slide Staining 367
        10.9.6   Image Analysis Scoring 367
10.10 Data and Reporting 369
        10.10.1 Statistical Analysis 369
        10.10.2 Validity of a Test.. 372
        10.10.3 Positive Response Criteria 372
        10.10.4 Cytotoxicity.. 373
        10.10.5 Reporting results.. 376
10.11 Evaluating Unclear Results.. 378
        10.11.1 Equivocal Results 379
        10.11.2 Positive Results 379
        10.11.3 Negative Results... 380
Acknowledgments... 381
References... 381

Chapter 11: The Pig-a Endogenous Gene Mutation Assay *383*

Jeffrey C. Bemis, Svetlana L. Avlasevich and Stephen D. Dertinger

11.1   Introduction 384

11.2   History 384

11.3   Fundamentals.. 385

11.4   Study Design 389

    11.4.1   Animal Species/Strain/Sex/Age............................... 389

    11.4.2   Number of Animals Per Experimental Group 390

    11.4.3   Group Selection/Identification 390

    11.4.4   Negative and Positive Controls 390

    11.4.5   Acute or Integrated Repeat-Dose Studies................... 390

11.5   Equipment... 392

11.6   Consumables... 393

11.7   Reagents and Recipes... 393

    11.7.1   Solution and Materials Preparation 393

11.8   Method Overview.. 395

11.9   Blood Collection 396

11.10 Leukodepletion and Platelet Removal................................. 397

11.11 Sample Labeling... 397

11.12 Column Separation and Sample Staining 400

11.13 Flow Cytometric Analysis: 96-Well Plate-Based Protocol...... 403

11.14 Tabulating and Summarizing Results................................... 409

11.15 Evaluation and Interpretation of Results 410

    11.15.1 Statistics 410

    11.15.2 Criteria for a Valid Assay 411

    11.15.3 Comparison to Historical Controls........................... 411

    11.15.4 Biological Relevance 411

11.16 Flow Cytometric Template Preparation................................ 412

11.17 Example Plots... 414

11.18 Storage and Shipment of Blood Samples............................. 414

11.19 Aspiration of Postcolumn Samples...................................... 416

References... 416

Index.. *419*

List of Contributors

Svetlana L. Avlasevich   Litron Laboratories, Rochester, NY, USA

Jeffrey C. Bemis   Litron Laboratories, Rochester, NY, USA

Steven M. Bryce   Litron Laboratories, Rochester, NY, USA

Laura Custer   Bristol-Myers Squibb, New Brunswick, NJ, USA

Stephen D. Dertinger   Litron Laboratories, Rochester, NY, USA

Ann Doherty   AstraZeneca Innovative Medicines and Early Development, Cambridge, UK

Mick Fellows   AstraZeneca Innovative Medicines and Early Development, Cambridge, UK

Roland Frötschl   Genetic and Reproductive Toxicology, Federal Institute for Drugs and Medical Devices (BfArM), Bonn, Germany

Annie Hamel   Department of Genetic Toxicology, Charles River Laboratories, Montreal, ULC, Canada

Melvyn Lloyd   Covance Laboratories Ltd, North Yorkshire, UK

Ray Proudlock   Boone, North Carolina, USA

Marilyn Registre   Department of Genetic Toxicology, Charles River Laboratories, Montreal, ULC, Canada

Marise Roy   Department of Genetic Toxicology, Charles River Laboratories, Montreal, ULC, Canada

Marie Z. Vasquez   Helix3 Inc, Morrisville, NC, USA

Foreword

The first works indicating that chemicals were mutagenic were published during the mid-1940s. Soon after those publications, the study of chemical mutagenesis and the possible relationship between mutagenicity and carcinogenicity started to become areas of interest and research. The field currently known as Genetic Toxicology got its start in 1969 with a series of interconnected events: the formation of the Environmental Mutagen Society in the United States, the release of a report from the US Department of Health Education and Welfare recommending mutagenicity testing for pesticides and suggesting tests that could be used, and, later that year, the establishment of the Genetic Toxicology Branch within the Toxicology Division of the US FDA. The publications by Ames and his group in 1973–1975 indicating that mutagenicity in salmonella bacteria was highly predictive of carcinogenicity in mammals energized the scientific and regulatory communities, and all types of *in vitro* and *in vivo* genetic tests and endpoints began to be proposed to identify carcinogens. National and international validation studies were started to validate or justify the various tests.

At the same time, the US Toxic Substances Control Act was passed, which specified genetic toxicity testing for newly developed industrial chemicals and chemicals already in commerce. Other countries followed suit, and the initial years saw many efforts by test advocates to validate and accept their tests for routine testing, although not necessarily in that order. One unexpected consequence of the Ames group publications was a shift away from the previous concern about using short-term genetic toxicity tests to identify germ cell mutations, the risks to future generations, to their use for the identification of carcinogens.

By the late 1970s, regulatory authorities in many countries were requiring genetic toxicity testing of chemicals, including drugs, food additives, and agrochemicals, prior to marketing approval. Positive responses in any of these required tests were considered to indicate a presumptive carcinogen and therefore were not likely to be approved for use without proof or evidence of their noncarcinogenicity. The general consensus at that time was that tests were needed to identify chemicals that induced gene mutations, as were tests for chromosome-damaging agents. The initial test requirements were that chemicals would be first tested *in vitro*, and then positive chemicals would be tested *in vivo* to "confirm" the initial positive response and provide data that might be relevant to the effect of concern, cancer, or germ cell mutation. It is notable that although these tests were widely used at this time and were used to support industrial and regulatory decisions, there were relatively little data regarding their performance.

Although some of the regulations also acknowledged the importance of germ cell mutagenicity, it was clear that the decisions would be made on the basis of carcinogenicity. The time since the late 1980s has seen a general homogenization of genetic toxicity test requirements across countries and among regulatory authorities, which has been assisted by the development of formal OECD test guidelines for chemicals and pesticides and ICH guidelines for pharmaceuticals. These test requirements are evolving with science and the recognition of relevant biological endpoints that were not addressed by traditional tests.

The tests described in this volume are the *in vitro* and *in vivo* genetic toxicity tests most commonly required by regulatory authorities for new substances and also other tests used as supplemental tests or that will be potentially useful in the future. They are described by the people who are performing and evaluating the tests on a routine basis. They reflect the most recent formal international test guidelines, which are recommended reading for anyone considering starting to perform the tests and for the experienced laboratories that want to stay current with old and new tests.

Errol Zeiger, PhD, JD, ATS
Errol Zeiger Consulting, North Carolina, USA

March 2016

Preface

Throughout the world there are perhaps 100 commercial laboratories performing genetic toxicology tests on a routine basis. In addition, there are at least as many laboratories performing studies for investigative or basic research purposes. However, only a small proportion of those laboratories obtain high-quality results on a consistent basis without needing to repeat part or all of the individual experiments. In certain situations, there is an inclination to report or publish results from experiments that do not meet acceptable standards. A major purpose in compiling this book is to help laboratories produce high-quality experiments on a efficiently, and in a timeframe, according to standards that are acceptable to the scientific community and regulatory bodies. The contents of this book also allow study monitors to identify those facilities and individuals that follow best practices.

There is an art to genetic toxicology that is best learned from reading, practice, and consistently following established procedures. In addition, insight and in-depth knowledge of practical aspects of the field are sometimes needed to design a study that will provide meaningful results. Each chapter in this book is written by scientists who have a great deal of technical experience in study performance. The practical aspects of method development, routine testing, and reporting of each of the tests are covered in depth. Whether you are a newcomer to an individual test method or have decades of experience with it, I am sure you will find much of use here. When describing the methods, it is easy to overlook important aspects that might seem obvious to experienced workers in a particular laboratory. I recommend you follow the procedures exactly; sometimes, apparently minor deviations can have an adverse effect on the quality of results (e.g., in chromosome and micronucleus slide preparations).

The present guide focuses only on those tests currently in routine use for regulatory submission and can therefore afford to include many important details that may have been overlooked in previous, more general, genetic toxicology texts. However, several previous guides on specific tests, including those written by originators of the techniques (e.g., Refs [1] and [2]), provide an excellent introduction to the methods and should still be considered essential reading because they include many of the aspects of testing that have been overlooked elsewhere.

A chapter by Werner Schmid (the originator of the rodent micronucleus test) was included in the first edition of the *Handbook of Mutagenicity Test Procedures* published by Elsevier in 1977, whereas the Maron and Ames chapter describing technical aspects of the bacterial mutation test in excellent detail was reprinted in the second edition of the same handbook published in 1984. Time marches on, and while the procedures for the plate incorporation version of the Ames bacterial mutation test remain largely unchanged, many options and refinements have been made to the standard test systems described in these early editions. The procedures described here follow the updated recommendations of OECD and, in the case of pharmaceuticals, ICH (most of the relevant guidelines have been revised in the past 4 years). In addition, we describe several more recently developed tests, including the *in vitro* micronucleus, comet, and *Pig-a*, that are already or are becoming widely used. Where appropriate, we have also included details of automated methodologies that have only recently been adopted.

Ray Proudlock
Boone, North Carolina, USA

References

[1] Maron DM, Ames BN. Revised methods for the Salmonella mutagenicity test. Mutat Res 1983;113 (3−4):173−215.
[2] Schmid W. The micronucleus test. Mutat Res 1975;31(1):9−15.

CHAPTER 1

A Practical Guide to Genetic Toxicology Testing

Ray Proudlock

Boone, North Carolina, USA

Chapter Outline
1.1 Introduction 1
References 3

1.1 Introduction

As a result of public concern over chemically-induced heritable effects and carcinogenicity, genetic toxicology testing has become a regulatory requirement for all new chemicals and many other materials in virtually every developed country in the world. Regulations exist for testing pharmaceuticals, pharmaceutical degradants/impurities, unique human metabolites of pharmaceuticals, medical devices, agrochemicals, industrial chemicals and intermediates, household chemicals, food additives, unintentional/indirect food additives, and environmental media, such as air and water. In practice, this means that genetic toxicity testing is mandatory for virtually any new chemical where significant human exposure is expected.

The purpose of this book is not to describe testing requirements or test strategies for these materials but rather to describe how these genetic toxicology studies can be performed to appropriately high standards on a routine basis in an efficient manner, while producing reliable results. Ideally, study design and performance should be standardized and optimized to minimize risk of failure (and subsequent repeats) while providing results and the draft report in a minimum timeframe. These principles apply equally to formal Good Laboratory Practice (GLP) studies for regulatory submission and to non-GLP tests for screening or investigative purposes. In the latter case, the documentation requirements are generally reduced and there is no QA involvement.

I first started work in the field of genetic toxicology testing in the United Kingdom in 1978, when each industry and country had different testing requirements or expectations. In those days, many of the current test methods were in their infancy and there were no internationally agreed test method guidelines, so we generally followed the recommendations of the innovators of the test methods, particularly as described in a series of volumes edited by Alexander Hollaender and, later, with Frederick de Serres [1] over the period 1971 to 1986 [1]. The first comprehensive handbook of mutagenicity testing procedures [2] covered several of the test systems still in common use today in a single volume. Other practical guides followed, including a second edition of the Kilbey handbook [3] and several compilations coordinated largely through the UK Environmental Mutagenesis Society [4–7], including a consensus on the application of statistical methods for interpretation of results in the major test systems [8].

In the UK in the late 1970s, studies did not follow any standardized protocol or procedure, and records were incomplete, consisting in some cases, of little more than the results and a summary protocol. Staff did not work to any formal instruction or SOPs, and it soon became apparent to me that the quality of much of the work was inadequate. One of my main responsibilities became to improve technical aspects of various study types, primarily the bacterial mutation, *in vitro* and *in vivo* cytogenetics, and UDS tests. I took the opportunity to formally document standardized instructions, which allowed entry of specific details and results. GLPs subsequently became a regulatory requirement for all studies and, consequently, these documents became formally incorporated into SOPs. Complete formal instructions and records minimize the chance of errors on a study and facilitate any retrospective investigation of problems or unexpected results.

Experience has repeatedly shown that the effort spent in setting up an assay properly so it produces reliable results will be rewarded many times over when performing routine studies. These characteristics are clearly of paramount importance when test results are often pivotal, either allowing a chemical to proceed to market, or being dropped from further development. My background and technical expertise in a wide range of test types were essential in designing and establishing the Genetic Toxicology Department at Charles River Laboratories (then CTBR) in Montreal in 1999, the largest CRO toxicology facility in the world. Subsequently, I have assisted several test facilities in trouble-shooting or setting up these tests in-house. This experience forms the basis for my recommendation in this and the subsequent chapter titled General Recommendations on Assay Performance.

Although this book is not intended to cover testing strategy, the reader must consider the appropriateness of any test system(s) used when evaluating a test material. It is important to obtain chemical and physical information on the test material, including solubility, volatility, stability, functional groups, and potential metabolites. Much of this information will be available from the chemist responsible for developing the material or, in the case of contract research, will be obtainable from the study monitor. In the case of medical devices and similar "inert" materials, the study director should obtain information on potential leachables and extractables (i.e., amounts and chemical nature). Consideration of these factors and information on related chemicals, will allow the study director to make a preliminary assessment of the relevance of the test and whether there is a need for modifications to the standard test methods, e.g., for volatile materials, sealed systems might be considered for *in vitro* testing, and the pre-incubation procedure would be preferred over the plate incorporation bacterial mutation test for reasons of sensitivity e.g., [9,10]. For *in vivo* systems, especially when following up *in vitro* results, consider the relevance of the endpoint (is it expected to be sensitive to the effect seen *in vitro*). It particularly important to consider the likely exposure levels (concentration over time) of the target organ to the active chemical and, in the case of genotoxins that require metabolic activation *in vitro*, any active metabolites. In this case the extrapolated target exposure levels should be compared to the *in vitro* system where exposure levels can be much higher. Conversely, *in vivo* systems can be more sensitive to some genotoxins with very low aqueous solubility that require metabolic activation (e.g., some polyaromatic hydrocarbons). Other examples where *in vivo* systems are more sensitive or can give more relevant results have been discussed by the IWGT (InternationalWorkshop on Genotoxicity Testing) [11].

References

[1] Hollaender A., de Serres F.J., editors. Chemical mutagens: principles and methods for their detection, vols. 1−10. New York, NY: Plenum Press; 1971−86.

[2] Kilbey BJ, Legator M, Nichols W, Ramel C, editors. Handbook of mutagenicity test procedures. Amsterdam: Elsevier; 1977.

[3] Kilbey BJ, Legator M, Nichols W, Ramel C, editors. Handbook of mutagenicity test procedures. 2nd edition. Amsterdam: Elsevier; 1984.

[4] Venitt S, Parry JM, editors. Mutagenicity testing: a practical approach. Washington, DC: IRL Press; 1984.

[5] Kirkland DJ, editor. Basic mutagenicity tests: UKEMS Recommended Procedures. Cambridge: Cambridge University Press; 1990.

[6] Kirkland DJ, Fox M, editors. Supplementary mutagenicity tests: UKEMS recommended procedures. Cambridge: Cambridge University Press; 1993.

[7] Parry JM, Parry EM, editors. Genetic toxicology: principles and methods. New York: Humana Press (Springer); 2012.

[8] Kirkland DJ, editor. Statistical evaluation of mutagenicity test data. Cambridge: Cambridge University Press; 1990.

[9] Araki A, Kamigaito N, Sasaki T, Matsushima T. Mutagenicity of carbon tetrachloride and chloroform in Salmonella typhimurium TA98, TA100, TA1535, and TA1537, and Escherichia coli WP2uvrA/pKM101 and WP2/pKM101, using a gas exposure method. Environ Mol Mutagen 2004;43(2):128−33.

[10] O'Donovan MR, Mee CD. Formaldehyde is a bacterial mutagen in a range of Salmonella and Escherichia indicator strains. Mutagenesis 1993;8(6):577−81.

[11] Tweats DJ, Blakey D, Heflich RH, Jacobs A, Jacobsen SD, Morita T, et al. IWGT Working Group. Report of the IWGT working group on strategy/interpretation for regulatory in vivo tests II. Identification of in vivo-only positive compounds in the bone marrow micronucleus test. Mutat Res 2007;627 (1):92−105.

CHAPTER 2

General Recommendations

Ray Proudlock

Boone, North Carolina, USA

Chapter Outline

2.1 **Establishing a New Assay** 6
  2.1.1 Method Set-Up 6
  2.1.2 Method Validation 8
2.2 **Spreadsheets and Manipulation of Results** 10
2.3 **Laboratory Historical Control Databases** 11
  2.3.1 Vehicle/Negative Control Database 11
  2.3.2 Positive Control Database 13
  2.3.3 Spreadsheet Calculations 13
2.4 **Use of Computer Systems** 13
2.5 **Study Design** 15
2.6 **Evaluation Criteria** 17
  2.6.1 Valid Assay 17
  2.6.2 Criteria for Interpretation of Results 18
  2.6.3 Statistical Analysis 19
2.7 **Organization of SOPs** 20
2.8 **Planning a Study** 22
2.9 **Preparing a Protocol Complying with GLP** 23
  2.9.1 Standardized Boilerplate Protocols 28
2.10 **Collecting Results** 29
  2.10.1 Data Tabulation 30
  2.10.2 Presentation of Report Tables 30
2.11 **Reports** 31
2.12 **Training** 36
2.13 **Improving Quality and Efficiency** 37
  2.13.1 Improving Quality 38
  2.13.2 Minimizing the Potential Problems on Studies 38
  2.13.3 Reducing the Need for Repetition of Parts of the Study 39
  2.13.4 Accommodating Repeat or Supplementary Tests 40
  2.13.5 Running More Studies in a Given Timeframe 40
  2.13.6 Timeframe for Routine Studies 41
  2.13.7 Reducing the Effort Needed to Prepare Protocols, Tables, and Reports 43

Genetic Toxicology Testing.
DOI: http://dx.doi.org/10.1016/B978-0-12-800764-8.00002-1

2.13.8 Reducing the Effort Needed to Perform the Study   43
2.13.9 Reducing Costs or Labor Requirement   44
2.14 QA   45
2.15 Qualifying a Contract Laboratory   47
2.16 Responsibilities of the Study Monitor   48
References   49

2.1 Establishing a New Assay

When developing and optimizing an assay that is new to your facility, the test should ideally:

1. Operate according to sound scientific principles in accordance with established methodology, including, when appropriate, specific guidelines published by OECD (Organisation for Economic Cooperation and Development), ICH (International Council for Harmonisation of Technical Requirements for Pharmaceuticals for Human Use), and regulatory bodies, including the FDA.
2. Produce results in a minimum timeframe.
3. Be standardized with a minimum number of variables and show little variation in results when performed using the same standardized methods. Results should be recorded and presented in a format to allow assessment of inter-test variability and of how control results might vary with time.
4. Be robust. The methods should produce good results on a consistent basis without requiring repetition of part or all of the study.
5. Be appropriately sensitive to weak genotoxic agents or low doses of potent genotoxic agents.
6. Be sensitive to reference genotoxic agents with a variety of mechanisms of action.
7. Be cost-efficient and require minimal effort to monitor, set-up, perform, report, audit, and review.

In addition, when developing *in vitro* systems, it is useful to establish the limitations of the test in terms of the volume of a range of solvents that can be added or the pH swing that is acceptable before interfering with parameters measured in the assay. For *in vivo* assays, maximal volumes of aqueous formulations should be based on local regulations (e.g., as determined by the Institutional Animal Care and Use Committee) and as published in relevant guidance documents [1,2].

2.1.1 Method Set-Up

The set-up phase establishes procedures that give good quality results on a routine basis. It involves a series of small experiments looking at optimizing individual aspects of the procedure. In terms of slide production, establishing a method that standardizes cell density and ensures quality is particularly important and worth spending extra effort on because it will improve the reliability of results and greatly reduce slide reading time and operator fatigue in subsequent routine experiments.

The design of each experiment will often depend on results of the previous experiments. Because the experiments will not necessarily follow formal SOPs and a study (termed *study plan* by OECD GLP) protocol (synonymous with *study plan* in OECD GLP terms), study set-up is necessarily non-GLP.

The responsible scientist should read the relevant OECD and other associated procedural guidelines, including papers written by the originators of the method and the relevant chapter in this manual. In addition, it will be helpful to enlist the help of an external scientist who has recognized technical expertise in the specific test system—he/she may even furnish you with example slides that you can use as a quality control standard. The scientist should then list a series of components of the procedure that need to be evaluated to establish the assay in the laboratory and then place those steps in a logical series. For example, in the case of a chromosome aberration test using a cell line, the list might include:

1. Obtain the cells from a reputable source and establish them in culture in the recommended medium. At this point, a formal *test system maintenance log* should be established indicating when and from where the cells were obtained, the details of characterization experiments, and records of culturing and subculturing (including passage number) and purification.
2. Confirm that the cells have the appropriate characteristics. Determine the doubling time and confirm that the procedures for growing the cells and subculturing them do not inhibit growth. Details should be recorded in the maintenance log. Note that cell lines should always be maintained in log phase and never grown to confluence to avoid selection of inappropriate characteristics. Similarly, bacteria should never be grown beyond the late log phase.
3. Establish frozen stocks of the cells and confirm absence of mycoplasma. It may also be useful to karyotype the cells (e.g., by G-banding) for reference purposes and to check for potential genetic drift later. Details should be recorded in the maintenance log.
4. Establish procedures for harvesting cells from the culture vessel that will be used for exposure to the test materials.
5. Establish procedures for quantifying viable cells.
6. Determine the cell cycle time for the cell line under standardized growth conditions, as will be used for exposure to test materials. For cell lines (as opposed to mitogen-stimulated lymphocytes), this is expected to be very similar to the population doubling time.
7. Evaluate mitotic arrest, hypotonic, and fixation procedures.
8. Optimize slide preparation ("dropping") procedures so that chromosomes are well spread but still associated (not floating off) with a clear outline (e.g., determine a target humidity level).

9. Optimize the staining procedure so that chromosomes are well-defined against the background.
10. Check that standard amounts of DMSO, positive control, and S9 mix are not excessively toxic. Note that it may be useful to prequalify a particular batch of S9 fraction by confirming low toxicity, and then reserve that batch for upcoming experiments.
11. Test a range of dose levels of the chosen positive controls in the absence and presence of S9.

Many of these steps may be omitted if the laboratory has worked with the cell line before. In addition, several steps will usually be incorporated into a single experiment. For each experiment, in turn, the scientist should number the experiment, document its purpose, and list the procedural steps as instructions in an electronic document that will eventually evolve into the SOP. These procedural steps should allow insertion of appropriate details (e.g., time of addition of the mitotic arresting agent, reagent batch numbers) and have columns for date and initials of the person performing the test. This document should also include a data collection form for capturing the results and any associated comments. If necessary, the person performing the test can make changes to the form as a result of accidental or intended changes at the time of the experiment to facilitate subsequent revision. Once the experiment is complete, the scientist should summarize the results together with conclusions and recommendations going forward and retain the information in a binder and in an electronic folder. The effort involved in this documentation is small but will produce a very useful record in the near future. The electronic procedural documents and forms can then be used as the basis for the procedural records for the next experiment in the series.

During method set-up, validation, and even in routine testing, you should check the cells at each step of the way (e.g., check cell lines at harvesting under the inverted microscope before and after trypsin treatment). In addition, a well-trained technician will always check things like the temperature and carbon dioxide levels of the incubator before opening it. In this way, if you do end up with a lot of dead cells at the completion of an experiment, you will have a good idea of which step(s) resulted in the problem. These checks do not require formal documentation unless the scientist decides they are critical.

During the set-up phase, the scientist should organize a presentation of the test method to interested staff members, including the technicians who will be performing the test and, in a GLP facility, the QA unit. The presentation should describe the principles of the test as well as the procedures and outline those aspects considered critical.

2.1.2 Method Validation

Once the method is established and gives good quality results (e.g., reasonable mitotic index and good quality metaphase preparations in these example), the scientist will want to proceed with an internal formal validation of the system. The scientist should prepare a formal SOP that explains the basics of the test and the training needed to perform the associated tasks. The SOP should include procedural and results forms as appendices and should be reviewed by management, technical staff, and QA before being finalized. Minor amendments to the SOP will probably be required during the validation phase.

Method validation involves a series of studies to establish reliability, robustness, and sensitivity of the test. In addition, this phase will confirm that results are consistent with those obtained in other reliable laboratories (usually by comparison with published results). This phase of testing should also be designed to provide an adequate laboratory historical positive and (particularly important) negative control database. If the test may be used for regulatory submission, then method validation should be performed under GLP. If the test is a variation of a method that is already established in the laboratory, then only a limited (cross) validation may be needed to confirm that results are as expected and consistent with the original method.

The scientist should prepare a study plan/protocol for each phase of the validation that includes the scientific rationale and regulatory purpose of the test method. It should include the study design, the purpose of the study, endpoint(s) assessed, measurements taken, and criteria for acceptability and evaluation of results, including a full description of calculations and statistical methods, if appropriate. The plan should include a list of relevant guidelines and reference methodological publications. In this case, the sponsor will be listed as the test facility in the protocol.

Typically, the validation might involve at least three or four phases, with each including at least one vehicle control group:

1. *Demonstration of an appropriate response with standard positive control agents.* Choose appropriate positive control agents from those listed in the relevant OECD guideline that will be routinely included in future tests guidelines. For *in vitro* studies, this should include at least one direct-acting and one indirect-acting (requiring metabolic activation) agent, such as mitomycin C and cyclophosphamide monohydrate in the case of the mammalian cell tests. Each should be tested at a range of dose levels from a low dose that is expected to show no clear effect to that expected to show a substantial response based on published information. Water-soluble positive controls may be preferable because of ease of formulation in the case of *in vivo* systems, whereas precipitation of compounds with limited aqueous solubility in the culture medium will limit exposure and can lead to odd dose-response curves in the case of *in vitro* systems.

2. *Demonstration of ability to detect weak mutagens and relatively low doses of potent mutagens.* Choose chemicals with various modes of action (e.g., spindle poisons and antimetabolites in the case of rodent micronucleus test). Dose levels should be chosen on the basis of published information. Use a range of dose levels to establish the dose-response curve and the lowest limit of detection; *in vivo* studies need to use only three dose levels, including one expected to produce only a moderate response. This and all subsequent experiments should also use standard positive controls at dose levels established in the first validation. Because of the size of the experiment, it will usually be necessary to break-down this phase of the validation into two or more studies.

3. *Demonstration of robustness and reliability.* This phase is intended to demonstrate the reproducibility of results obtained for the negative controls and moderate doses of appropriate positive controls. *In vitro* testing might also examine limitations on dose volume for common solvents (e.g., DMSO) and pH before excessive toxicity occurs.
4. Additional (ancillary) validation work might be considered at this point or later to accommodate specialist methodologies (e.g., comparison of sizing and centromere-staining methods to distinguish clastogens and aneugens in *in vitro* and *in vivo* micronucleus tests).

A major purpose of the validation work is to establish an adequate laboratory historical control database. This is particularly important in the case of the negative control database, which gives a very good idea of the expected spontaneous aberration/mutation/reversion rates. To accelerate validation and gain experience, an untreated group should be included at each sampling/exposure time used and consideration should be given to inclusion of more than one solvent/vehicle control group in each experiment. The minimum size historical control database that can generally be considered acceptable in a GLP environment consists of at least 10 and preferably 20 independent groups once the method is standardized [3]. Outlier values in the historical negative control database or big shifts imply that there is a problem with the test method that should be addressed before the method is considered validated.

After acceptable results are obtained in each phase of the validation and the historical database is considered adequate, the test can be used on a routine basis once the reports have been audited and finalized.

2.2 Spreadsheets and Manipulation of Results

Spreadsheets are used at many points of the study for things such as allocation of animals to groups, calculations in preparation of formulations, as well as analysis and presentation of study results and historical control data. In some cases they may need to be printed out, signed/initialed, and dated, and then saved as raw data. Standard calculations of means, standard deviations, and other statistical parameters can be performed automatically within spreadsheets or data management systems, allowing report tables including calculated values to be produced with little need for editing.

As mentioned later in the historical control section, blank or completed spreadsheets should be subject to version control; appropriate checks (including double data entry) should be incorporated into their use and appropriate parts of the sheet (e.g., formulae) should be locked to prevent accidental change. It is useful to include version/change history and instructions in the sheet itself. Adopting the spreadsheet as an SOP may be a useful way of controlling access and preventing accidental changes, although historical control databases need to be continually updated to ensure they contain the most relevant results. Because of the nature of spreadsheets, it is not practical or possible to validate them fully, but you should ensure that they comply with any of your facility SOPs on their design or use.

2.3 Laboratory Historical Control Databases

In the context of this discussion, I have used the phrase "negative control" to describe groups that are either untreated or treated with the vehicle, solvent, or a placebo. Once the methodology is established and standardized, results from the validation and subsequent studies should be included in the historical negative and positive control databases. All individual and group mean results should be included in the databases, unless there is a good scientific reason for their exclusion, such as error in formulation or dosing, failure of cells to grow normally, or obvious outliers caused by suspected dosing error (e.g., not dosed in the case of the positive control). The reason for exclusion should be documented and approved by the responsible scientist.

Because of the importance of databases in confirming the proficiency of a laboratory's ability and acceptability of individual studies, historical control databases were the subject of deliberations by the International Workshop on Genotoxicity Testing (IWGT) in Basel, Switzerland in 2009. The outcome of these deliberations was published 2 years later [3] and taken into account in those OECD guidelines that have been introduced or updated since. Although the OECD decided that the 1997 bacterial mutation test guideline [4] did not require updating, the same principles apply equally to that test. These databases are important because:

1. Criteria for assay acceptability will be included in each study protocol and should include a comparison of current negative and positive control values with expected values based on the laboratory historical control results. (During assay validation phases and particularly when the laboratory has limited experience, results for the negative control are expected to be similar to those obtained by reliable laboratories, as described in the literature and in individual chapters in this handbook.)
2. The historical control information is used to confirm that there has not been any excessive shift in results over time due to unintentional changes in the methodology, the evaluation methods, or the test system (bacteria, cells, or animals). It is used to confirm that the system is under control.
3. Negative control data are useful for designing experiments and assessing the applicability of statistical methods.
4. Finally, and perhaps most importantly, during the course of routine testing, historical negative control results are used to determine whether apparently increased values for individual treatment groups are within normal limits.

2.3.1 Vehicle/Negative Control Database

Although the concurrent vehicle control group results are very important within an individual experiment, apparent increases in genetic damage in individual test substance treatment groups can occur as a result of chance variation. This is especially true when comparing many groups with the concurrent control or when the value obtained for the control group is somewhat lower than normal. In these cases, it is important to know whether the value obtained for the treated group is within normal (i.e., negative control) limits, based primarily on the laboratory vehicle/negative control database.

The database should be established at the outset of the validation experiments and continually updated and maintained. The best approach is to create a template spreadsheet for each system that can be used to assess the impact of all the factors that might influence the results. It is important to make the spreadsheet comprehensive (i.e., include all these factors) at the outset because retrospective changes to the spreadsheet can be extremely laborious and subject to error. Given the importance of the spreadsheet, appropriate version control and checks (including double data entry) should be included. In addition, calculations in the sheet should be locked to prevent accidental damage. The sheet is considered a controlled document and, because the information present will usually be summarized in individual study reports, is subject to QA audit.

Where differences in results between strains, species, cell types, or test methods (e.g., preincubation and plate incorporation methods in the Ames test) are known or suspected, they should be listed on separate spreadsheets; other factors of potential interest should be listed individually under separate column headings including (where relevant):

- Study reference number
- Date of dosing
- Vehicle
- Dose volume
- Sampling or exposure time
- S9 (%, type, absent or present)
- Slide reader

Inclusion of additional factors should be considered depending on the test system, including age, source, breed, mean weight (for animal studies), passage number, donor reference number (in the case of human lymphocytes), S9 fraction batch number, and FCS batch number. In general, these factors are expected to have little or no effect on results; therefore, they can be pooled for consideration and reporting. Even so, the information may be useful for internal quality control purposes, such as to determine whether low mitotic indices in the *in vitro* chromosome aberration test are associated with a particular batch of S9.

The results for individual cultures/animals should be listed in the adjacent columns and then calculations of mean values and sample standard deviations should be included in the final columns. The mean value for each experimental point in the spreadsheet should be confirmed against the reported value as a quick check of the accuracy of the entries.

Entries in the spreadsheet should be made in a consistent manner to facilitate sorting and grouping, with standard format for dates and standard abbreviations. Normally, the results are ordered by date, with the latest experiment being entered on the bottom row. The spreadsheet should cover at least the main parameter measured in the test (e.g., percent cells with chromosome aberrations) but may include ancillary results (e.g., mitotic index) in subsequent columns. As mentioned in the previous paragraph, if there are no apparent differences in the measured parameter over time or between vehicles, then the historical control results can be grouped and considered in their entirety.

2.3.2 Positive Control Database

A positive control spreadsheet should be constructed in the same way as the negative control sheet. In this case, there will usually be fewer columns because the dose level/ volume will be standardized; however, results for each sampling time and associated calculations (mean and standard deviation) should be listed in separate columns.

2.3.3 Spreadsheet Calculations

Each row of the spreadsheet should have a column to include calculation of mean and sample standard deviation values. At the top of each group mean value, you should include grand mean and sample standard deviation values. The spreadsheet should also be used to calculate the upper and lower expected limits (quantiles) of the distribution; using Microsoft Excel, the formulae = PERCENTILE (A1:A200,0.025) and = PERCENTILE (A1:A200,0.0975) in two adjacent cells will show the upper and lower limits of a range containing 95% of values in cells A1−A200. Similar confidence or tolerance limits can be calculated based on the assumption that results follow a Gaussian (normal) distribution; however, in this case, especially if absolute values are low, they may need an appropriate transformation so they more closely fit a normal distribution.

The frequency of each mean value should be calculated and presented in graphical form in each study report. The 95% limits, grand mean values, total number of mean values, and standard deviation of the mean values should be presented within or below the chart together with the time period covered by the experiments. This allows the scientist and any reviewer to determine whether values obtained in the study are within normal limits and facilitates evaluation of results. Note that the historical control values presented in a report should not include results for the study being reported.

2.4 Use of Computer Systems

Although raw data were traditionally recorded on paper, records and results from a study can be typed directly into a computer data management system that uses an electronic signature—a process referred to as *direct data entry*. Results can also be saved directly from digital electronic instruments in a process referred to as *direct data capture*, particularly (in the case of genetic toxicology testing) image analysis systems (used for automatic colony counting in mutation tests and for analyzing slides in the comet assay). Although the information may subsequently be printed, the original electronic file is considered to contain the raw data. Finally, statistical analysis of results is usually performed using a computer program.

Use of computer systems to capture and assess results in a GLP environment is covered by regulations and guidance of the FDA [5,6] and the OECD [7]. A draft update to the OECD guidance was issued in 2014 [8]. The FDA "e-rule" or "Part 11" applies to records in electronic form that are created, modified, maintained, archived, retrieved, or transmitted to the FDA. OECD guidance states "All computerized systems used for the generation, measurement, or assessment of data intended for regulatory submission should be developed, validated, operated, and maintained in ways which are compliant with the GLP Principles." This guidance applies to both hardware and software components of the system. The FDA and OECD requirements for systems and their validation are open to interpretation, which results in wide differences in requirements between facilities. If you intend to make use of data capture systems, then I recommend you consult your QA department and your internal validation specialists well in advance, particularly to ensure that a disproportionate effort will not be needed to validate the system. Depending on the complexity of the system and its potential impact, you will need to perform a formal system validation that includes generation of a study plan/protocol, testing performance, and reporting results. Less extensive validation may be needed if captured information is not subject to potential change/alteration. Validation of a commercial system in widespread use may require less effort than validation of an internally developed system; in addition, the supplier will probably be able to help you with development of a reasonable validation plan. Neither FDA nor OECD provides detailed recommendations on system set-up, validation, operation, maintenance, or retiring.

OECD indicates risk assessment is needed before deciding what extent of validation is needed, and data integrity controls should be based on a justified and documented risk assessment. Therefore, key points that need to be addressed before implementing a computerized system that is considered to fall under regulatory and OECD e-rule requirements include:

- Risk assessment.
- Vendor qualification in the case of commercial systems to ensure user requirements and quality standards are achievable.
- Development and validation strategy; designate personnel with specific responsibility for the development, validation, operation, and maintenance of computerized systems including a responsible scientist (often the study director of the validation), QA, computer information technologist, and a validation specialist.
- Access controls and hierarchy; prevention of unauthorized changes or access.

- Results/record control—changes to raw data should be identifiable, justified, and traceable in the same way as paper records. It may greatly simplify validation and implementation if changes to the raw data cannot be made by operational personnel once the results are captured.
- System change control (closely linked to system maintenance).
- Validation plan including acceptance criteria, procedures should confirm that facilities, equipment, and data handling procedures produce reliable records/results of an adequate standard. The plan should indicate which functions of the system will not be used or influence results and, therefore, do not need to be evaluated.
- Design and development history file.
- Preliminary testing and records (system set-up, non-GLP).
- Validation testing including formal acceptance testing, records, and report.
- System maintenance log.
- System operation and maintenance SOP—system layout/design, systems checks and audits, responsibilities, training, and training records need to be addressed. The SOP should also cover data back-up, disaster control, and maintenance.
- Designation of a System Manager.

Electronic signature and management systems can also be useful in maintaining controlled documents (including templates, spreadsheets, standard templates). Similar document management systems with version control are often used to store SOPs, drafts, and final study protocols and reports. These systems do not necessarily fall under the auspices of the e-rule but should be covered by facility SOPs and validated accordingly.

2.5 Study Design

Normally, each test substance is tested at a range of dose levels up to the maximum level proscribed in the relevant OECD or, in the case of intended pharmaceuticals, the ICH guideline [9]. The doses are generally separated by a standard geometric dose-interval (often twofold in the case of *in vivo* studies), with the highest dose usually being the lowest of the following:

- The standard limit dose described in the guideline
- The maximum practical dose based on compatibility of the solvent with the test system
- The limit of solubility in the chosen solvent (*in vitro* systems only)
- A level that causes visible precipitation in the test system (*in vitro* systems only)
- The limit of toxicity of the test substance in the test system. For *in vivo* systems, this would be termed the maximum tolerated dose (MTD) and is defined as a level just below that expected to cause death or evidence of pain, excessive body weight loss, or suffering/distress that would necessitate euthanasia for humane reason, or a level that causes severe interference with the parameters being measured.

Table 2.1: Dose level selection for standard genotoxicity tests

OECD TG[a]	Test[b]	Limit Dose OECD[c]	Limit Dose ICH[c]	Max Dose[d]	No. Dose Levels[e]	Dose Interval[f]
471	BMT	5 mg or 5 µL/plate	Per OECD	MTD	5	$\sqrt{10}$
487	IVM	10 mM, 2 µL, or 2 mg/mL	1 mM, 0.5 mg/mL	55 ± 5% or ppt	3	2−3
473	CAT	10 mM, 2 µL, or 2 mg/mL	1 mM, 0.5 mg/mL	55 ± 5% or ppt	3	2−3
490	MLA	10 mM, 2 µL, or 2 mg/mL	1 mM, 0.5 mg/mL	80−90% or ppt	4	2−3
474	RMT	2000 mg/kg/day (1000 mg/kg/day, ≥14 days)	Per OECD	MTD	3	2−4 (2−3 per ICH)
475	RCA	2000 mg/kg/day (1000 mg/kg/day, >14 days)	2000 mg/kg/day (1000 mg/kg/day, ≥14 days)	MTD	3	2−4 (2−3 per ICH)
489	COMET	2000 mg/kg/day (1000 mg/kg/day, ≥14 days)	Per OECD	MTD	3	2−4 (2−3 per ICH)
486	UDS	2000 mg/kg	Per OECD	MTD	2	2−4 (2−3 per ICH)
None	Pig-A	Regulatory guidance not yet available, suggest same dose levels as for RMT for shorter-term studies, or as justified in the study plan for subchronic or chronic studies				

[a]Relevant OECD Test Guideline.
[b]BMT, bacterial mutation; IVM, *in vitro* micronucleus; CAT, *in vitro* chromosome aberration; MCM, mammalian cell mutation TK locus; RMT, rodent micronucleus; RCA, rodent chromosome aberration; COMET, *in vivo* comet; UDS, *in vivo* rodent liver UDS.
[c]When not limited by practical considerations, toxicity or (in the case of *in vitro* mammalian cell tests) precipitation.
[d]If lower than the limit dose: % toxicity or (ppt) precipitating concentration (*in vitro*), whichever is lower.
[e]Minimum number dose levels assessed.
[f]Unless justified based on toxicity parameters.

This guidance is summarized in Table 2.1, but readers should refer to the appropriate chapters in this book and the guidelines for more complete information.

On occasion, higher dose levels than those listed here may be justified, such as when testing mixtures of materials or complex mixtures, or when qualifying an impurity within a pharmaceutical. From Table 2.1, it will be evident that there are slight differences in dose selection between ICH and OECD for the mammalian cell tests. Although there are no differences for the bacterial mutation test, ICH does not require a confirmatory test in cases where the main bacterial mutation test is clearly negative.

For *in vivo* systems, it will normally be necessary to perform a preliminary toxicity test to approximate the MTD or to confirm the standard limit or maximum practical dose is tolerable. The main test usually involves the high dose and two additional dose levels separated by a standard dose interval (conventionally twofold rather than fourfold because genotoxic effects are usually more evident at higher dose levels). If the purpose of the test is to establish a dose-response curve or a no observable effect level, then additional dose levels and a different dose interval may be appropriate. If the test substance is nontoxic, then it may be permissible to test only the limit dose (refer to the specific guideline) at one or more sampling times in the case of *in vivo* studies.

For *in vitro* studies, a preliminary solubility assessment will normally be required to establish the maximum dose in the dose system; please refer to the Formulation chapter for details. For the bacterial mutation, it is usually most efficient to go straight into the main test using eight dose levels separated by the half $\log_{10}$ ($\sqrt{10}$) dose interval, which will almost always produce five analyzable (i.e., not overtly toxic) dose levels. If, however, it is known or expected that the test material will be toxic in the test system, then it will be necessary to perform a preliminary toxicity test (e.g., using a fivefold dose interval and only one replicate at each point) to establish a suitable maximum for use in the main test. Even so, it might still be appropriate to use eight dose levels so that at least the top one shows toxicity in the main test. For the *in vitro* mammalian cell tests, a similar approach can be taken using a narrower dose interval (e.g., twofold), especially if it is known or expected that the test material will be nontoxic. However, for the mammalian cell mutation test, it is usually necessary to perform a preliminary dose range—finding test because the target for toxicity (80—90%) is narrow and more stringent.

Although most of the guidelines for *in vitro* studies mention potential use of single cultures at each experimental point, this is not recommended in case of a technical problem with an individual culture. For the bacterial mutation test, I recommend using at least three plates at each experimental point, because then loss of an individual plate (e.g., due to microbial contamination) does not raise questions about the validity of the test.

2.6 Evaluation Criteria

2.6.1 Valid Assay

Criteria for a valid test should be presented in the study plan/protocol and discussed in the report. Where part or all of a study does not meet acceptance criteria, the study director may decide that all or part of the study is invalid, in which case it will normally need to be repeated. If part of the study does not meet acceptance criteria but results are still considered acceptable, then appropriate justification should be given by the scientist in the report, usually after discussion with the study monitor. If the scientist is unsure whether additional work is needed, then it will normally help to consider the wording in the report for justifying not repeating the affected part of the study. Typically, the study protocol would indicate that vehicle control values should fall within or close to the expected range based on the 95% limits of the historical control range. The positive control is expected to cause a substantial (statistically significant if statistics are used) genotoxic effect compared to the relevant vehicle control group. Although values for the positive control normally fall within the limits of the laboratory historical positive control distribution, positive control values tend to be more variable and, therefore, although comparable, do not necessarily need to fall within that range. The criteria for substantial or statistically significant in this case should match those defined for interpretation of results for the test substance as outlined in the next section.

2.6.2 Criteria for Interpretation of Results

Criteria for interpretation of results should also be presented in the study protocol and discussed in the report. Usually it is appropriate to describe criteria for clear "negative" (no indication of genotoxicity) and "positive" (clear evidence of genotoxicity). The protocol should also describe potential ways of addressing borderline results, such as when results are not clearly negative or positive. Example criteria that you might consider adapting to individual assays and that are in agreement with OECD criteria (see next section) are listed here

A test substance is considered to have shown no evidence of genotoxicity and is considered negative if:

- None of the treatment groups exhibits a substantial increase in the level of damage compared with the concurrent vehicle control; in this case, substantial would be defined for each assay in the protocol based on the experience of the individual laboratory using that test. *Substantial increase* is normally defined in terms of a fold and/or absolute increase compared with the concurrent control but may be replaced by the term *statistically significant increase* if statistical testing is used, such as when evaluated by an appropriate trend test (using three dose groups plus the vehicle/negative control) or an intergroup comparison (single dose group versus the concurrent vehicle negative).

AND

- Mean values for the test article groups are below the upper limit (97.5 percentile) of the distribution of the historical negative control data.

A test substance is considered to have shown genotoxic potential and is considered positive if:

- More than one of the treatment groups shows a substantial increase or at least one dose level shows a substantial and reproducible increase in genetic damage with mean values above the upper limit (97.5 percentile) of the distribution of the laboratory historical negative control data and there is evidence of a dose response. Again, the term *substantial* should be replaced by *statistically significant* if formal statistical analysis is performed.

A test substance is considered to have shown unclear or equivocal results if it does not meet either of these criteria. In this case, additional slide reading and/or experimentation may be considered to resolve the final conclusion.

Most guidelines specify that indications of genotoxicity only seen close to the limits of toxicity in *in vitro* mammalian cells should be interpreted with caution. In cases where borderline results are seen, the study director should review the raw data and then check the plates (in the case of the bacterial mutation test, it is important for the scientist to review results before plates are discarded) or the slides (in the case of cytogenetic tests) for quality and artifacts. To facilitate review, it is useful to routinely record vernier readings of aberrations scored in the case of cytogenetic studies. Provided that slide quality is adequate and there was not a problem with the training of the original reader, the scientist may decide that the borderline result can be resolved by reading additional cells, or the scientist can have the slides read by a second technician before combining results from both analyses. In other cases (particularly in the bacterial mutation test), a supplementary test may be needed to clarify the affected part of the study. The scientist should document their review and any relevant comments in the raw data. Any additional testing will almost always use a narrower dose interval and a dose range that covers at least the range of affected values in the original test. Additional slide reading or supplementary testing should be described in a protocol amendment that, in the case of a contract laboratory, will have been discussed in advance with the study monitor. Repetition of an invalid part of a study does not necessarily require a protocol amendment provided that scenario is covered in the original protocol.

2.6.3 Statistical Analysis

There has been much debate over choice of appropriate statistical methods for interpretation of genotoxicity tests, and recently this was the subject of a detailed discussion by an OECD working group [10]. Genetic toxicology studies are generally designed to meet OECD specifications and practical considerations, which limit the applicability and power of statistical analysis. Care should be taken to avoid indicating statistical significance in tables (particularly use of asterisks) when values are within normal limits and apparent increases in damage are not biologically meaningful. In particular, the following points should be noted (most of which were discussed by the OECD working group):

1. Genotoxicity assays involve multiple comparisons of treatment groups with concurrent controls, which greatly increases the likelihood of a false-positive claim (i.e., when the apparently increased value is within normal limits). Corrections for multiple comparisons can be included in the statistical test but can result in a result probability estimate that is too conservative, missing a real treatment-related increase. In most assays, genetic damage usually increases with dose, so a test for trend not only is more powerful (especially for *in vivo* tests where the group size is limited) but also reduces the chance of a false-positive claim. Any groups showing excessive toxicity should be excluded from the analysis because there is often a down-turn in response at doses

approaching the limit of toxicity. In particular, nonparametric methods have low statistical power when performing intergroup comparisons of *in vivo* tests when the group size is generally small and, in such cases, are inappropriate.

2. Toxicity tests are not fully randomized and are therefore prone to systematic effects. For example, all animals within a specific cage receive the same treatment (so they are not truly randomized). In addition, cages are not usually assigned to random positions on a rack. These factors could theoretically have a slight effect on the parameter being measured. Animals are generally stratified (assigned to groups) based on body weight but, in view of the increased effort and chance of errors, if animals were randomized for dosing or sampling, then further "randomization" is not recommended.

3. *In vitro* tests generally consider the cell to be the unit of variance, although cells at each experimental point are usually sampled from two (or occasionally one) cultures. This ignores the potential impact of culture-to-culture variations. In this case, small differences between cultures can lead to inference of statistical significance that is due to culture-to-culture variation rather than the effect of the test substance.

4. In most assays (with the possible exception of the comet assay), we are interested only in increases in a particular parameter. In that case, any probability values quoted should be one-sided (i.e., based on the upper tail of the distribution).

Provided that the study is well-designed with an adequate group size and that appropriate cautions are taken to minimize any important systemic effects, the outcome of the statistical analysis should reflect an experienced scientist's own interpretation [11]. Any critical probability levels identified in the protocol should be sufficiently conservative to avoid false-positive calls (particularly * in tables), e.g., 0.01 rather than 0.05 may be chosen before statistical significance is assigned to allow for the effect of multiple comparisons. In addition, an overall trend test is generally easier to interpret and less prone to inappropriate indications of genotoxicity. Before adopting any statistical method or evaluation criteria, the scientist should explore the performance of the test using typical results arranged into borderline cases, such as real increases and chance variation, to evaluate the limitations of the methods and set appropriate probability levels for defining negative and positive results.

Perhaps the most appropriate and practical approach would be to indicate that no statistical analysis will be performed if there is no evidence of the test substance causing any substantial increase in genetic damage (see previous section for definitions of substantial).

2.7 Organization of SOPs

SOPs on use and maintenance of equipment will normally apply to the whole facility; this avoids any conflict if staff work in more than one area. However, many of the SOPs

Table 2.2: Typical list of SOPS found in a genetic toxicology laboratory

EQ	Automatic colony counter*
EQ	Coulter counter*
EQ	Electrophoresis system*
EQ	Image analysis and data capture systems*
EQ	Laminar flow cabinets*
EQ	Liquid nitrogen cell store*
EQ	Metered dispensing pumps*
GP	Animal receipt, husbandry, clinical signs, and euthanasia
GP	Approved suppliers list
GP	Aseptic technique
GP	Bacterial culture, strain verification, and maintenance
GP	Cell culture and maintenance
GP	Disposal of bacteria and cells
GP	Historical control databases
GP	Medium and reagent preparation and records to be maintained
GP	Monitoring visual and viable growth of bacterial cultures
GP	Slide randomization and coding
GP	Solubility testing and preparation of formulations for *in vitro* assays
GP	Statistical analysis packages
GP	Template protocols and reports
SP	Bacterial mutation test
SP	Chromosome aberration test
SP	Cytotoxicity testing
SP	*In vitro* micronucleus test
SP	*In vivo* comet assay
SP	Mammalian cell mutation test
SP	Rodent chromosome aberration test
SP	Rodent liver UDS test
SP	Rodent micronucleus test

EQ, equipment; GP, general procedure; SP, study-specific procedure.
*Describes operation, cleaning, maintenance, and (where applicable) calibration.

used in genetic toxicology will apply only to that department. These should be organized in a logical manner at the outset to avoid issues later and can be conveniently organized into three groups: equipment, general procedures, and test procedures. An example list of SOPs that you might consider relevant is given in Table 2.2.

A suggested approach is to use the main SOP to include approval signatures, purpose, scope, responsibilities, definitions/abbreviations, required materials/equipment/reagents, revision history, and training implications (of the most recent revision). Appendices attached to each SOP would include detailed procedures and results collection forms associated with each SOP. The main SOP would also explain the use of any procedural and results collection forms attached to the SOP. For example, recipes for each reagent, positive control, or buffer prepared during the course of routine testing would be included as appendices to the SOP on media and reagents. Staff training would cover the main SOP and, as a minimum, the procedures detailed in each of the appendices applicable to their role. All nonstudy-specific maintenance details of equipment, bacteria, and cells should be recorded in the maintenance log associated with the appropriate SOP; details of any failure and their resolution should also be recorded in the log. Characterization of bacteria (e.g., strain verification) and cells (e.g., determination of cell cycle time, karyotype, absence of mycoplasma) should also be recorded in the log; when that characterization is performed routinely, the procedures should be covered within the appropriate SOP.

SOPs, like other controlled documents, should be available for use by appropriate staff in read-only folders and are subject to version control. Instruction manuals associated with equipment should be readily available if necessary in the laboratory (in a central location or adjacent to equipment) or the general office area. It may be most convenient to maintain copies of manuals electronically. Other details will be as dictated by the Facility Management and national GLPs.

2.8 Planning a Study

Very early in the planning process, it is appropriate to consider what studies are required on a particular test substance and their relative timing. Solubility testing should be coordinated for all the *in vitro* toxicology tests, including *in vitro* HERG. The dose levels and therefore the timing for the *in vivo* micronucleus test will often depend on results of an acute toxicology test. The vehicle will be determined for the *in vivo* studies and, when chemical analysis of formulations is planned, the relevant scientists will be able to advise the chemist about the nature of the formulations and the concentration ranges that need to be covered by their analytical method. Any planned chemical analysis or bioanalysis set-up and validation work should be designed to cover the formulations and concentration ranges for all the planned toxicology tests to avoid additional work and costs later. It may be appropriate to combine formulation and subsequent chemical analysis from two studies or phases of a test to minimize internal costs, especially if formulation stability data are available to support formulation and analysis ahead of dosing. An inhalation genotoxicity test might be performed adjacent to another inhalation test on the same compound to reduce analytical and set-up costs Finally, some *in vitro* tests require both an initial test and a confirmatory test; combining those into a single test will save substantial labor (and chemical analysis, if performed) costs while reducing the overall duration of the study. For example, formulations of a test substance could be prepared in the chosen solvent on Monday, analyzed overnight to confirm the achieved concentration, and then dosed in the plate incorporation and preincubation versions of the bacterial mutation test on Tuesday and in the short and prolonged exposure arms of the accompanying mammalian cell test on Wednesday.

2.9 Preparing a Protocol Complying with GLP

The following recommendations apply to GLP study protocols, although there is no reason why the same principles should not apply to non-GLP studies. In the case of non-GLP studies, the protocol and any amendments do not need to be sent to the QA unit, although appropriate details may need to be entered into the facility's master schedule.

Preliminary work will usually be necessary to develop an appropriate formulation and determine appropriate dose levels based on formulation constraints (e.g., viscosity, solubility, etc.) or toxicity. This work is investigational in nature and subject to continual changes. In addition, the results may apply to several studies. Although procedures should be covered by appropriate SOPs, because it is not normally practical to perform them as per a detailed protocol, they cannot comply with GLP. In this case, they can be performed under an internal study number and any formal procedures, raw data collected, and associated notes (or exact copies thereof) attached to the raw data files of subsequent linked studies. Potential non-GLP preliminary work can be mentioned in the protocol; methods and results obtained can be used to justify appropriate aspects of study design in the study report under the heading Non-GLP Preliminary Work.

Each study to be performed should be accompanied by a study protocol (termed *study plan* by OECD GLP). The protocol must be approved by the study director, facility management, and the study monitor in advance of the test and will often require input from scientific staff responsible for specific aspects of the test (e.g., formulation analysis chemist or an inhalation specialist), although most GLPs indicate that only the study director needs to sign and date the protocol. Some of the details in the protocol are specified by GLP, and others are used to confirm details with the study monitor/sponsor and to advise staff of any particular considerations.

Obtaining relevant information on the test substance is particularly important when designing a study and may even determine whether the test method is appropriate (e.g., the preincubation version of the bacterial mutation test is not appropriate for bactericides). Important things to know, where applicable, are: structural formula, molecular weight, physical nature, stability, compatibility/solubility/suitability in vehicles compatible with the test system, results of any acute toxicity testing, results of any previous genetic toxicology test, planned route of exposure and vehicle for other toxicology studies, route of maximal human exposure (often oral for nonpharmaceuticals) or intended route of human administration, biological mode of action for pharmaceuticals, and whether closely related to other chemicals. If an *in vivo* micronucleus test is planned, then you should also ascertain whether the test substance is likely to interfere with hematopoiesis or cause hemolysis (e.g., as a result of methemaglobinemia) or prolonged departure from normal body temperature. You should also ascertain whether a certificate of analysis (COA) and a safety data sheet are available. A copy of the COA will normally be included in the study report; if the material is re-analyzed after the biological test, then the new COA should also be included in the report as confirmation of stability. Some of this information may also be useful in performing any internal safety assessment to define appropriate precautions although, normally, it is convenient to handle test chemicals in a manner similar to that of positive controls. If you are working in a contract laboratory and your sponsor feels that any of this information cannot be given to you for confidentiality reasons, then any subsequent testing that is required as a result of lack of knowledge will not be your responsibility (Table 2.3).

Table 2.3: Suggested inclusions in a standard protocol

A	*A unique identifying study number*
B	*Descriptive title (e.g., Compound X: Bacterial Mutation Test)*
	The address of the testing facility where the study is being conducted
	The name and address of the sponsor
C	*Name and role of responsible personnel including:*
	Name and contact details for the study monitor
	Name and contact details for the study director
	Identification of any aspects of the study that will be conducted remotely, in which case the name and address of the test site(s) and name and contact details of the principal investigators should be stated
	The proposed experimental starting date, target approximate experimental completion date, and draft report date
	Method/route/duration/number of dose administrations and justification
	Identification of the test and any reference articles by trivial name, chemical name, and/or structural formula, chemical abstract number, or code number
	Lot number, expiry or reanalysis date, physical nature, and appearance of the test substance
	Storage conditions and stability of the test substance and formulation, if known
	Test substance composition/characterization and whether any correction for content/purity will be applied. The protocol should mention that the method of production of this lot of the test substance is available from the sponsor if requested by the regulatory agency
	Method of formulation, including description and specification of solvents, emulsifiers, etc., used to solubilize or suspend the test substance. Details of atmosphere generation and any monitoring should be given in the case of gaseous, vapor, or inhalation studies. Reference should be made to the analytical report(s) of the suitability of the analytical method and stability of the formulation under conditions and over the concentration range to be used in the present study
	Details of any formulation samples that will be taken for confirmation of homogeneity and/or achieved concentration, including concentration, volume, storage, and transfer as well as acceptability criteria. Note that chemical analysis is normally performed on test substance formulations rather than their dilutions in the culture medium/agar for practical reasons. Positive controls are not considered in the same way as other reference substances and best not referred to as reference substances; positive control formulations are not subjected to chemical analysis for safety and economic reasons because the response of the test system is considered to be an appropriate measure of their acceptability. (OECD guidance indicates that the extent to which negative and positive controls should be analytically characterized may, however, be different from the requirements of reference items)
	Procedures for dealing with out-of-specification results in the case of chemical analysis
	Details of any bioanalytical samples that will be taken, including sampling times, volume, storage, and transfer

(Continued)

Table 2.3: (Continued)

D	GLP compliance including the national body complied with
	QA monitoring details
	Reference to the appropriate OECD test guideline and any other relevant guidelines or methods
	Statement of the purpose/objectives of the study
	The justification for selection of the test system
	Introduction to the test method, basis of the test, parameters measured, implications of results, bibliography of formative papers, and nonregulatory test guidelines. Although this section is not required by GLP, it will help many study monitors and give a professional appearance to the protocol and subsequent report
	Full description of the test methods, materials and conditions, type and frequency of analysis, measurements, observations, and examinations to be performed, including:
	• The number, body weight range, sex, source of supply, species, strain or breed age, and disease status (e.g., specific pathogen-free) of the test system[a]
	• Housing, husbandry, and acclimation period[a]
	• Frequency of recording clinical signs during acclimation and after dosing[a]
	• Animal allocation procedure[a]
	• Food and water supply and specifications, frequency of tests used to ensure levels of contaminants expected to be present do not interfere with the study (i.e., do not exceed established specifications)[a]
	• The procedure for identification of the test system (e.g., tail-marking or labeling)
	• Procedures for dealing with animals outside acceptable weight limits, showing signs of disease, signs of mis-dosing, or severe clinical signs[a]
	• Strain/cell line characteristics including any checks for mycoplasma[b]
	• Details of the origin (e.g., date and source) of the test system and its subsequent maintenance, including, if applied, acceptable passage number limits[b]
	• Culture medium and conditions, culture vessel, and cell density[b]
	• Details of the metabolic activation system, usually S9 fraction and S9 mix composition[b]
	• Details of positive control articles, including full chemical name, chemical abstract number, supplier vehicle, formulation (e.g., solution or suspension), appearance, formulation concentration (specify whether in terms of material as supplied or otherwise), dose volume, and dose level
	• Study design table
	• Criteria used for dose selection
	• A description of the chronological procedures involved in the study, including:
	  ◦ Methods to control bias, including stratification, randomization, and coding of slides
	  ◦ Criteria or justification for selection of the vehicle
	  ◦ Concentrations, dose levels, and dose volumes of the test, control, and reference articles
	  ◦ Detailed description of statistical methods to be used (if any)
	  ◦ Method, frequency, duration, and timing of administration
	  ◦ The type and frequency of tests, analyses, and measurements to be made
	  ◦ Details of any procedural checks (e.g., for sterility)
	  ◦ Criteria for parameters being measured (e.g., identification of micronuclei) and methods used to avoid artifacts
	  ◦ Ancillary observations, including assessments of toxicity and precipitation
	  ◦ A statement of the proposed statistical methods to be used, including calculations made for results obtained
	  ◦ Description of any direct data entry capture systems and GLP compliance
	  ◦ Description of computer systems used to allocate animals, process results, or other procedure
	  ◦ Criteria for a valid/acceptable test
	  ◦ Criteria for evaluation of results
	• List of contents of the report (usually based on the relevant OECD guideline)

(Continued)

Table 2.3: (Continued)

	Archiving: Lists of samples and records that will be maintained, location, conditions (e.g., for samples), duration, and subsequent disposition Procedures to be followed for issuing a protocol amendment Procedures for assessing the impact of and dealing with deviations to GLP, the protocol, or SOPs
E	*The date of approval of the protocol by the sponsor and the dated signature of the study director* Some authorities or companies may also require signed and dated approval of the protocol by test facility management, the sponsor, and any principal investigators

Note that items that are likely to vary between protocols are indicated in italics in this table.
[a]*In vivo* studies.
[b]*In vitro* studies.

Any intentional changes to the final protocol should be by formal amendment, copies of which (like the original protocol) should be sent to all appropriate personnel, including QA, principal investigators, and contributing scientists. Amendments should be retained along with the original protocol. If changes to the protocol have any impact on the procedures being performed, then the study director must ensure that the appropriate persons are informed. Where practical, the study director should discuss the draft amendment with the study monitor before signing the final version. Each facility will have its own procedures for monitoring work flow using a master schedule system: it is the responsibility of management to assign the study director and ensure adequate trained staff, equipment, materials, and facilities are available to perform the planned studies. Depending on the local GLP regulations, QA and/or facility management are responsible for maintaining and monitoring the master schedule, which is, essentially, a summary of the planned studies and work flow.

Up-to-date versions of all US FDA GLP documents can be found at http://www.ecfr.gov under Title 21, along with related guidance. Many of the national and international regulations relevant to genetic toxicology and related short-term studies are listed in Table 2.4. The reader should also be aware of the responsibilities, requirements, and practical guidance described in the OECD documents listed in the Table. There are minor differences in wording and requirements between different GLPs. It is generally best to be aware of the requirements of all the GLP regulations and guidance that your laboratory may be asked to comply with and adjust your standard procedures accordingly to facilitate future submissions; however, your generic protocols should only list the regulations that your facility usually complies with.

Medical devices are often subjected to genetic toxicology and cell toxicity tests depending on the nature of the material, degree of contact, duration, and potential for absorption. In this case, the user should refer to appropriate national and ISO guidelines to prepare the protocol and design the study. In some cases, the tests required and methods differ (most

Table 2.4: GLP regulations, guidelines, and related documents*

Good Laboratory Practice (GLP) Guidelines for the Validation of Computerized Systems Working Group on Information Technology (AGIT) Release Date: December 14, 2007 Version: 02 http://www.bag.admin.ch/anmeldestelle/12828/12832/index.html?lang = de&download = NHzLpZeg7t, Inp6I0NTU042I2Z6In1acy4Zn4Z2qZpnO2Yuq2Z6gpJCFfYB3fWym162epYbg2c_JjKbNoKSn6A

Huntsinger DW (2008) OECD and USA GLP applications. Ann 1st Super Sanita 2008; 12: 403–406

Japanese Ministry of Health, Labor and Welfare (1997) No. 21—Good Laboratory Practice Standards for Nonclinical Safety Studies on Drugs (GLP)

OECD Series on Principles of Good Laboratory Practice and Compliance Monitoring:
- No. 1, January 26, 1998, OECD Principles on Good Laboratory Practice
- No. 2, June 14, 1995, Revised Guides for Compliance Monitoring Procedures for Good Laboratory Practice
- No. 4, October 26, 1999, Quality Assurance and GLP
- No. 5, September 28, 2000, Compliance of Laboratory Suppliers with GLP Principles
- No. 7, February 13, 2003, The Application of the GLP Principles to Short-Term Studies
- No. 8, September 15, 1999, The Role and Responsibilities of the Study Director in GLP Studies
- No. 10, October 05, 1995, The Application of the Principles of GLP to Computerized Systems
- No. 11, January 22, 1998, The Role and Responsibility of the Sponsor in the Application of the Principles of GLP
- No. 13, February 25, 2002, The Application of the OECD Principles of GLP to the Organization and Management of Multi-site Studies
- No. 14, December 01, 2004, The Application of the Principles of GLP to *in vitro* Studies

OECD Series on Testing and Assessment Number 34, Guidance Document on the Validation and International Acceptance of New or Updated Test Methods for Hazard Assessment

UK (Department of) Health and Safety—The Good Laboratory Practice Regulations 1999. No. 3106 http://www.legislation.gov.uk/uksi/1999/3106/contents/made

UK Medicines and Healthcare Products Regulatory Agency (MHRA) webpage link to related documents. https://www.gov.uk/guidance/good-laboratory-practice-glp-for-safety-tests-on-chemicals

US Environmental Protection Agency—TOSCA (2007) 40 CFR 792—Good Laboratory Practice Standards. https://www.gpo.gov/fdsys/

US Environmental Protection Agency—FIFRA (2007) 40 CFR 160—Good Laboratory Practice Standards. https://www.gpo.gov/fdsys/

US FDA (2004) Comparison Chart of FDA and EPA Good Laboratory Practice (GLP) Regulations and the OECD Principles of GLP. US Department of Health and Human Services, Food and Drug Administration, Office of Regulatory Affairs

US FDA (2007) Guidance for Industry, Good Laboratory Practices Questions and Answers. US Department of Health and Human Services, Food and Drug Administration, Office of Regulatory Affairs

US FDA (2010) 21CFR Part 58 [Docket No. FDA-2010-N-0548]—Good Laboratory Practice for Nonclinical Laboratory Studies. Federal Register 75: 80011–8013. http://www.ecfr.gov

US FDA, Electronic Records; Electronic Signatures, Final Rule, 21 CFR 11 (1997, Revised April 1, 2015). http://www.ecfr.gov

Whitmire M, Ross R, Mwalimu J, Porter L, Whitsel M (2011). A Global GLP Approach to Formulation Analysis Method Validation and Sample Analysis. Pharm Anal Acta S2:001. http://www.omicsonline.org/a-global-glp-approach-to-formulation-analysis-method-validation-and%20sample-analysis-2153-2435.S2-001.php?aid=1830

World Health Organization (2009) Handbook: Good Laboratory Practice (GLP): Quality practices for regulated nonclinical research and development (2nd ed.)

*Please check the official website of the relevant organization for potentially more recent versions of these documents before using them. Check the appropriate website for GLPS of regulatory bodies not listed here.

notably between Japan, United States, and Europe). Note that ISO standards can be purchased directly from ISO at http://www.iso.org. Some of the most relevant guidelines that should be consulted in this case are:

Use of International Standard ISO-110993, "Biological Evaluation of Medical Devices Part 1: Evaluation and Testing" Draft Guidance for Industry and Food and Drug Administration Staff April 23, 2013 http://www.fda.gov/downloads/MedicalDevices/DeviceRegulationandGuidance/GuidanceDocuments/UCM348890.pdf
ISO 10993-1:2009 Biological evaluation of medical devices Part 1: Evaluation and testing in the risk management process
ISO 10993-2:2006 Biological evaluation of medical devices Part 2: Animal welfare requirements
ISO 10993-3:2014 Biological evaluation of medical devices Part 3: Tests for genotoxicity, carcinogenicity, and reproductive toxicity
ISO 10993-5:2009 Biological evaluation of medical devices Part 5: Tests for *in vitro* cytotoxicity
ISO 10993-12:2012 Biological evaluation of medical devices Part 12: Sample preparation and reference materials
Japanese Ministry of Health and Welfare. Japanese Guidelines for Basic Biological Tests for Medical Devices and Materials, Notification no. 99 (1995)
Japanese Ministry of Health, Labour, and Welfare, Pharmaceutical and Food Safety Bureau, Testing Methods to Evaluate Biological Safety of Medical Devices, Notice from the Office Medical Devices Evaluation, Number 36, March 19, 2003

2.9.1 Standardized Boilerplate Protocols

The study director will put considerable effort into writing the first protocol of a particular study type. Subsequently, scientists, technicians, QA staff, and the study monitor will need to read and understand the protocol; they will likely ask for corrections and clarifications before or even after it is finalized. Subsequent studies will likely be very similar (e.g., 90%) to previous studies with differences primarily in terms of the sponsor, the test substance, and the planned start date (other dates can be given relative to start date or receiving the study monitor's comments on the draft report, although, of course, individual studies might need insertion of specific dates to meet target deadlines).

It seems unreasonable to expect personnel to plow through each protocol when 90% of it will be repetition; they will not usually have the time or patience. In addition, hidden in the routine details there may be important information unique to that study that could get overlooked. My recommended approach is to use boilerplate (template) protocols for each study type as mentioned by OECD "For short-term studies, a general study plan accompanied by a study-specific supplement may be used" [12]. You should check with your QA unit before considering this approach.

The layout of a boilerplate protocol should follow the standard style of the test facility as far as practical but would normally be expected to include the following:

A. Study reference number included in the header of each page; pagination on each page (e.g., in the format Page 1 of 12 in the footer of each page).
B. Title page with study title, address of the testing facility, name and address of the sponsor (i.e., all the items mentioned in section B of Table 2.3).
C. Study-specific details (i.e., all the items mentioned in section C of Table 2.3), plus an indication of any changes to laboratory standard procedures described in the General Procedures section. All staff involved in the study are expected to be aware of the contents of this section, which is reasonable given that it normally fits on a single page.
D. General procedures section that includes all the information indicated in Table 2.3 and that includes an identifying version number or date.
E. The dated signed approval of the final protocol by the study director plus a list of any other approvals/signatures required as listed in section E of Table 2.3.

Once the layout of the boilerplate protocol has been established and reviewed by QA and management, it should be saved as a controlled document with appropriate version control measures. This can be performed by converting the document to a form in Word with appropriate parts of the document (including the General Procedures section) being locked to prevent accidental changes. The boilerplate protocol should be saved in a folder that has read-only access to all but approved staff. Any revision to the standard would require an update to the version number in the general procedures section and authorization or acknowledgment by QA and management. A version history folder may also be of use with tracked changes for older versions of the standard protocol. If use of a boilerplate protocol is not acceptable to your facility, then a similar approach should be taken to developing a standard template protocol for each study type. In this case, the latest version of the template should be maintained internally and should be the only version used to prepare study protocols. Changes to the template will be made continually by scientific staff as a result of guideline changes, client comments, and QA comments.

Assuming staff and the study monitor are familiar with the generic template, they would normally need to only review the title page and the study-specific details, making special note of any changes to standard procedures mentioned there.

2.10 Collecting Results

Results should be collected directly onto raw data forms (SOP appendices). Each page of the form should include entries by the technician/scientist showing the study number, the date of the entries (in standard unambiguous format) or date of completion of the entries, and their initials. Dates (and time) may be needed for specific entries if they are time-critical. Direct data entry or collection systems should include the same information but should include the electronic signature of the operative in place of the initials. The layout of data collection forms (e.g., slide reading) should match that used for presentation in the final report as closely as practical to facilitate subsequent checking of tabulated results against the raw data.

The study director should review the results as soon as possible after collection to ensure details are accurate. He/she should review any results that appear anomalous (e.g., by checking the original culture plates or microscope slides). The study director should also check some individual results on occasion to confirm their accuracy. The study director should document any review directly in the raw data. If any changes are needed, then the study director should justify them by an appropriate note in the raw data. The study director should also check the raw data for completeness just after the end of the in-life phase of the study and document any checks/reviews.

2.10.1 Data Tabulation

Critical results (e.g., colony counts, slide reading) should be tabulated as soon as practical after collection to facilitate review. Often, results will be entered or captured in a spreadsheet that is then used to order or re-order results (in the case of decoding of randomized slides) and perform calculations (typically mean values and sample standard deviations) that are linked to a summary table. Individual culture/animal and summary results can then be directly pasted into a Word template or directly linked to the template. Templates with completed entries are then used to populate the report. Direct data capture systems usually handle information in the same way, with results being saved into a database (rather than a spreadsheet) and report tables being prepared automatically. The study director should review these results as soon as practical. Whatever system is used should minimize the chance of transcription errors; if results are transcribed (e.g., from handwritten form into an electronic form and then decoded), then the best way of checking may involve a double entry system with appropriate cross-checks (e.g., results are entered twice and calculated mean values are cross-checked).

2.10.2 Presentation of Report Tables

Summary and individual results tables should be presented in a consistent format (e.g., columns in the same order with the same units used in both) with related values (e.g., mean % aberrations) arranged in columns that are decimally aligned—whole numbers rather than derived percent values are easier to read and compare. Tables should contain minimal ruling—usually above and below the column heading and at the bottom of the table is adequate. Wider spacing can be used to separate exposure times and groups. Ideally, all critical results should be summarized in a single table on one page to facilitate report review by the study monitor and the regulatory agency. Results should be presented to only a meaningful number of significant figures (ideally with the same number of decimal places or to the nearest whole number) to facilitate review and interpretation—usually two significant figures are adequate. Standard deviations of small samples should usually be calculated as sample standard deviations (e.g., using the STDEV or STDEVA function in Excel) and, because individual experiments usually involve only a limited number of replicates, are not particularly accurate or useful (e.g., the highest individual values are generally the most important in terms of looking for effects in the rodent micronucleus test). The SD values are calculated as a square root, so they should not be quoted as $\pm$ values because they are absolute.

Examples of well-presented tables may be found in individual journals and many of the individual chapters of this book (e.g., Chapter 9, the rodent bone marrow chromosomal aberration test).

2.11 Reports

A screening study report may be limited to a title page, a summary page describing any deviation to the standard method (usually included in a standard protocol and appended to the report), a study director signature page, and tabulated results including summary of any statistical evaluations performed. Direct data entry, use of a simple electronic signature, and conversion of the draft report to a final PDF (e.g., using the capabilities of Microsoft Word) greatly facilitate report finalization and allow the report to be e-mailed directly to the study monitor in fully searchable electronic format. In this way, most short-term screening tests can be performed and reports finalized within a week or 10 days of test substance receipt.

Reports for GLP studies are more extensive and require review by the study monitor; the QA unit will also need to audit the draft report at some time and review the final version before it can be signed as final by the study director. The following text in this section describes details necessary to produce a high-quality, GLP-compliant report.

A well-written report will allow the reader to understand the methods and results in adequate detail to allow them to repeat the experiment, obtain similar results, and come to the same conclusions as in the original study. Inadequate descriptions of evaluation criteria and statistical methods can lead regulatory reviewers to reanalyze results and reach different conclusions leading to rejection of the study. You (the investigator) will usually have the advantage of having an experienced statistician on site who can help with experimental design, statistical analysis, and presentation of methods and results (the regulator may not have that luxury)—you should make use of them, especially for optimizing appropriate basic study designs, for interpretation/reporting purposes, and, finally, to make sure a comprehensive description of any statistical methods is included in the protocol and report [13,14]. If the test has several phases, then avoid overlong or inconsistent descriptions of each phase, that is, match the description to the study details and results tables, for example, preliminary test, main test, supplemental test, and confirmatory test are all useful descriptions. If part of a test is considered invalid, then details of that part of the study and any results do not need to be reported provided that the report gives adequate justification—this will avoid unnecessarily confusing the reviewer.

The minimal contents of the study report are listed by GLP regulations and by the OECD guideline related to the test used. The order and actual layout of the report will depend largely on the test facility (each tends to have their own template). The test report should include all the items covered by the protocol and listed in the Report section of that document as well as any additional details of methodology not specified originally (e.g., batch number and supplier, the solvent used to formulate the test substance). Some authorities (e.g., US EPA) have additional requirements or recommendations related to layout, font, and summary tables that the study director needs to be aware of, such as a tabulated summary report [15]. The following list follows a logical order and includes the items mentioned by EPA, FDA, and OECD GLPs [16] and items included in the specific OECD guideline for the tests.

Section	Contents
All pages	The unique study number indicated in the protocol
	Pagination and total number of pages (e.g., Page 1 of 52)
Title page	Report status (e.g., draft unaudited)
	Descriptive title (e.g., Compound X: Bacterial Mutation Test)
	The address of the testing facility where the study is being conducted
	The name and address of the sponsor
	Date of issue
Table of contents	Can be generated automatically based on styles in Word
Study director compliance page	Indicates GLPs complied with and any deviations. Statement that the report is an accurate reflection of the procedures used and the results obtained. The study director's dated signature on this page is considered to be the date of issue of the final report unless otherwise indicated. The wording on this page will generally reflect the test facility's standard report format/template
QA statement page	Tabulated summary of critical phases and/or processes inspected with dates, stating when findings were reported to the study director, scientific and facility management
	Statement signed and dated by the QA report auditor confirming the accuracy of the report
Responsible personnel page	Includes (as a minimum) the name of any scientists who contributed reports (e.g., chemist, pathologist), scientists, professionals and all supervisory personnel involved in the study. Identification of any aspects of the study that were conducted remotely, including name and address of the test site(s) and the principal investigators. Include role and qualifications of each
Summary	Usually a single-page executive summary including objective, name of the test substance, summary of procedure, study design, dose route, and reason for dose level selection
	Incidental observations, including observations of toxicity, precipitation, and evidence of exposure
	Results
	Single-paragraph conclusion—this should match the conclusion in the main body of the report
	The summary may also include a tabulated summary report (this may be needed in any case either separately or in the report by individual companies or regulatory agency), for example, as per the ICH eCTD [15]

(Continued)

(Continued)

Section	Contents
Introduction	Introduction to the test method, basis of the test, parameters measured, implications of results, bibliography of formative papers, and nonregulatory test guidelines. Although this section is not required by GLP, it will help many study monitors and give a professional appearance to the protocol and subsequent report
Test guidelines	List of official guidelines complied with, such as FDA Redbook 2000, EPA, OECD, and ICH
Objectives	As per protocol
Critical dates	Dates of animal arrival, formulation, and dosing for each phase of the study. Date of completion
Test substance:	Source, CAS, or other reference number (if assigned), lot number, stability, and/or limit date for use (specify if expiry date or reanalysis date), storage, homogeneity (if applicable), purity, composition, and analysis (refer to certificates of analysis and reanalysis after dosing is complete) if applicable and include in appendices. Date of arrival (indicate phases when each aliquot was used if more than one shipment was received). Chain of custody, monitoring of usage, and final disposition. The report should indicate if the method of production of the lot(s) of test substance used in the study is available from the sponsor if requested by the regulatory agency
Vehicle	Reason for selection based on OECD guideline and any preliminary work. Details of composition and formulation if a mixture, batch number, expiry date, supplier and product number, and physical characteristics. Whether anhydrous (as specified by OECD) in the case of organic solvents. Dose volume and, for *in vitro* studies, level present in the test system
Formulation	Method of formulation and justification Stability and homogeneity of formulation under conditions of storage and use and over the concentration range used in the present study; cross-reference to the appropriate analytical chemistry stability report(s) Time between preparation and completion of dosing Final disposition of any unused formulations
Formulation sampling and analysis	If performed, assessment of achieved concentration and, in the case of suspensions, physical stability and homogeneity. Cross-reference the relevant analytical chemistry method validation report(s) Final disposition of any unused samples
Positive controls	Full chemical name (use same format as OECD guideline where appropriate), CAS number, supplier, product number, lot number, expiry date, physical description, storage conditions, purity and whether any correction for purity, salt form or water applied, vehicle, nature of formulation, concentration, dose volume, and dose level. Time between preparation and use of formulations and storage conditions
Test system details	Include details described in the protocol, including (in the case of animals and for each phase of the study) age, body weight range, number of animals received and allocated, husbandry, and diet Details of S9 fraction including species, breed of animal, inducing agent and dose, expiry date, storage. Details of S9 mix composition and time and conditions of storage before use Details of buffer dosed in absence of S9 mix, if appropriate (usually 0.1 M phosphate in the case of the bacterial mutation test). Levels of S9 and buffer present in the test system after dosing

(*Continued*)

(Continued)

Section	Contents
Confirmation of sterility Test methods	Methods of assessing sterility of vehicle and formulations, if performed
	Include appropriate details of any preliminary work not included under justification
	Other methods should be described as per protocol
Dose regimen	Exposure route, duration, number, and spacing of exposures; justification based on OECD specifications including cell cycle time in the case of *in vitro* cytogenetic tests. Details of atmosphere generation and any monitoring should be given in the case of gaseous, vapor, or inhalation studies
Study design	Table indicating formulation concentration, dose volume, dose level, number of replicates, exposure time (if variable) and strains dosed (for the bacterial test), and (for *in vitro* tests) absence or presence of S9. Include tables for each phase of the study, including initial, confirmatory, repeat, and supplementary tests, if applicable
	Justification for selection of dose levels of the test substance
Computer systems	Include details of any systems used to allocate animals, randomize slides, capture or record or process results, including direct data entry or capture systems and statistical programs
Evaluation of results	Details of methods used and observations performed, including number of cells analyzed. Method of assessment and criteria for:
	■ assessment of toxicity
	■ examination for precipitate
	■ any pH observations
	■ identification of micronuclei
	■ classification of aberrations
	■ details of statistical methods
Criteria for a valid test	As per protocol
Archiving	As per protocol: lists of samples and records that will be maintained, location, conditions (e.g., for samples), duration, and subsequent disposition
Deviations	A list of deviations, if any, from the protocol and assessment of their impact by the study director. A description of all circumstances that may have affected the quality or integrity of the data
Results	The results section should cross-reference appropriate Tables, Appendices, and Addenda that appear later in the report
	Summary of results from any supporting or preliminary work, including formulation analysis or bioanalysis. Discussion of whether analytical results match protocol criteria; justification for use if they do not match
	Incidental observations, such as assessment of sterility, toxicity, precipitation, clinical signs, and mortality, and how that supports dose selection. Discuss absence or presence of any signs of mis-dosing and associated postmortem examinations; indicate whether any deaths are considered to be test substance—related or procedural
	Description of results for each phase of the study and description of how they meet acceptability criteria. Include mention of any evidence that supports systemic exposure or exposure of the target cells to the test substance and/or metabolites. Discussion of how results meet evaluation criteria described in the protocol and earlier in the report in terms of absence or presence of evidence of genotoxicity

(Continued)

(Continued)

Section	Contents
Conclusion	Overall conclusion including the last paragraph of the Summary section, such as: "It is concluded that Test Substance X did not show any evidence of genotoxic activity in this *in vitro* mutagenicity assay when tested in accordance with regulatory guidelines"
References	As per protocol plus any additional ones mentioned in the discussion. Include any relevant analytical and bioanalytical validations
Summary Table	A table similar to the study design table but summarizing group mean values for important parameters measured in the test as well as statistical analysis results
Appendices	Certificate of analysis Ancillary results: tabulated clinical signs, mortalities, and (if required by regulatory authority) body weight tables Detailed results for individual plates/cultures or animals Historical negative/vehicle and positive control results—distribution showing mean values, tolerance limits (in the case of negative controls), number of experiments or groups, and period covered
Addenda	The signed and dated reports of each of the individual contributing scientists or other professionals involved in the study, including those prepared by the principal investigator(s) (e.g., analytical chemistry, bioanalysis)
Protocol	Some test facilities or sponsors require a copy of the protocol and any amendments to be included as an appendix or addendum to the report

The report should also take into account the contents of any protocol amendments produced, so you should always review any amendments when writing or reviewing the report. Some departments will use a more junior scientist or technical writer to compile the report. Whatever the situation, the responsibility for the contents and accuracy of the report is with the study director. However, it is a good idea for a second scientist (e.g., another study director or the departmental head) to peer review the draft report before it is issued. The second scientist will likely pick up most or all of any ambiguities, grammatical errors, and obvious mistakes that can otherwise creep into a report.

In the case of a CRO, the report (like the protocol) should never use a previous report for a different client as a template because there is a strong possibility of carrying over erroneous or confidential information. Instead, as for protocols, a template report should be developed and maintained by staff. Use of boilerplate reports (as described for protocols) may also be an appropriate and acceptable approach (e.g., using forms in Word). However, reports contain more detailed and varied content, although this approach is well-suited to screening study reports.

Protocols and reports for each study type should be laid out, formatted, and contain the same wording as far as possible to facilitate review. If any standard wording in a document needs updating, then consideration should be given to making similar updates in other templates and boilerplates.

2.12 Training

Presentation of any new assay should be organized by those responsible for developing the methods and presented to departmental staff. Appropriate QA personnel should also be invited and attend so that they understand the technical aspects of the study and interpretation of results. This will also help them to identify those components of the assay that are critical so they can arrange inspections accordingly. Scientific management should be present at any presentation so they can correct any misunderstandings and answer or research any questions that the presenters cannot. It may also be useful to invite an external expert to present or train staff in specific techniques (e.g., slide analysis for the chromosome aberration test or use of a new image analysis system in the comet assay). Staff should retain records of any internal or external training courses and related certificates within their training record file. Attendance and a list of presentations given at external meetings should also be included in the training file.

Routine training and competence must be documented in staff training records. Template training records should include major items in all relevant SOPs because any training given should be oriented toward signing staff off against those SOPs. New staff should be introduced to tests gradually, focusing on one area or technique at a time.

A set of training slides for each cytogenetic assay should be available. These can be prepared by mixing cells from negative and positive controls from a routine study in a range of proportions from 0% to 100% before slide making and staining in the usual way. In this way, for example, 10 or 20 rodent micronucleus slides can be made for each "dose level." An appropriate number of slides are then randomized and encoded. The trained scientist/technician should sit alongside the pupil and explain key features using negative and positive controls explaining protocol criteria, what represents a readable slide/metaphase, criteria for identification of aberrations, artifacts, and assessment of toxicity. It is useful to have a library of photographs to demonstrate examples of each that the student can help develop further if a photomicroscope is used. Then, the "student" should examine one field (or metaphase) at a time in conjunction with the trainer to ensure they can identify each aspect appropriately. Once the trainer feels comfortable with the interpretation and quantitation of events by the student, the student should be given a set of the training slides to read. Parameters (e.g., aberrations and mitotic index) assessed in this examination should show a close correlation to expected values. It is useful during this examination to record vernier locations of key events recorded by the student so that they can be confirmed by the trainer. It will usually be necessary for the student to examine more than one set of slides before they can be assessed as competent unless they have already been trained in a similar assay. The trainer should also help with or confirm proper use and set-up of the microscope as well as the scanning method (one field at time to avoid fatigue or travel sickness). If your laboratory is new to a technique, then it is a good idea to obtain a set of example slides from an experienced laboratory for quality comparison and training purposes.

Many national and international societies specialize in genetic toxicology; a link to most of them can be found at http://www.emgs-us.org. You should consider joining those relevant to your location and attending their meetings, partly to obtain the latest information on test methods and strategy, and partly to network with experts in the individual test methods who may be able to help you with assay development, training, or trouble shooting. I found the following groups of particular interest:

- Environmental Mutagenesis and Genomics Society (http://www.emgs-us.org/). EMGS holds an annual meeting in the United States. Members have free access to the journal *Environmental and Molecular Mutagenesis* (EMM), which publishes many articles relevant to genetic toxicology test methods and regulatory affairs. Their website contains links to many related groups.
- United Kingdom Environmental Mutagenesis Society (http://ukems.org.uk/). UKEMS holds an annual meeting in the United Kingdom (sometimes in conjunction with the European Environmental Mutagenesis Society). Members have free access to the journal *Mutagenesis*, which publishes a range of articles similar to EMM but tends to be more focused on technical topics relevant to genetox testing.
- Genetic Toxicology Association (http://gta-us.org/). GTA holds a 2-day scientific meeting every spring at the University of Delaware (Newark, Delaware, USA). The meeting usually covers topics that are highly relevant to genetox testing.
- The Japanese Environmental Mutagenesis Society (http://www.j-ems.org/eng/). JEMS publishes its own journal, has an annual meeting, and is very active in interlaboratory validation of assays.
- Other (generally less active) discussion groups can be reached via LinkedIn, including the Genetic Toxicology Group and the Industrial Genotoxicology Group (IGG), which organizes technical meetings approximately twice per year in the United Kingdom.

You will find it useful to keep a reference list of relevant publications and maintain copies of these and appropriate text books in a departmental library.

2.13 Improving Quality and Efficiency

Very early in the process of development and continually later on, you will (or should) be considering improvements in each study type. I have outlined some suggestions in the following sections that should be considered as examples only.

2.13.1 Improving Quality

Although quality is a major consideration during the set-up phase of an assay type, it is relatively easy to investigate potential improvements subsequently by running small non-GLP exploratory investigations along with ongoing studies, for example, by preparing and using additional cultures to investigate the effect of different slide making conditions in the chromosome aberration test. In this case, even slight improvements in the quality of slides will have a very beneficial effect in the long-term and are something you are liable to think about while actually reading slides. Your aim should be for every slide to be perfect, with (in the case of chromosome aberration slides) a high proportion of readable metaphases—perfectly spread, stained, and clear. In the case of the *in vivo* micronucleus test, cells should show good morphology with no evidence of lysis and excellent staining differentiation. Cell density should be consistent between slides and optimized to minimize scanning while avoiding overlapping.

Purification and appropriate characterization of bacteria and cells are essential to confirm their utility. Bacteria and cells should never be grown beyond the exponential phase during maintenance or when grown for testing; otherwise, they can accumulate undesirable phenotype traits, will be less sensitive to mutagens, and, in cytogenetic tests, show low mitotic indices making slide reading more laborious.

2.13.2 Minimizing the Potential Problems on Studies

Each test involves a large number of steps that can potentially go wrong; frustratingly, mistakes on a study may not be evident until the results are obtained. A little effort at the time of the test performance can greatly reduce the chance of problems arising or minimize their impact. A few suggestions (golden rules) are given here and in the individual chapters within this book:

1. Your test substance may be valuable or difficult to replace on short notice. Always transport it in a secondary container that helps prevent breakage if dropped. Never leave an open bottle of the test substance on the work surface. Help prevent spillage by placing it in a rack and immediately replacing the lid after usage.
2. It is easy to lose your place when performing dilutions or dosing a long series of cultures, particularly if interrupted. Physically move the culture/plate/bottle/animal from one area to another after the addition, for example, when adding S9 mix to a series of bottles in a rack, dose them in a consistent order (e.g., working from the top left) and move each bottle one place to the left as it is dosed while using the nondosing hand to help keep your place. Move bacterial mutation plates from the right to the left as they are plated with top agar. Move animals from their holding cage to a labeled cage with fresh bedding as each is dosed. Ask QA staff or any observers to keep any questions

or comments until you have come to a logical break in the procedures unless, of course, the scientist/technician has made an obvious error, and leave your cell phone in the office. For *in vitro* studies, keep an adequate number of spare cultures, spare racks of bottles, and spare plates to act as immediate replacements in case of an immediately obvious dosing error; make sufficient S9 mix to accommodate a few mis-dosings.

3. Do not rely solely on labeling to distinguish cultures or doses. They should be placed in order and in blocks in a consistent manner. Check that you have not gotten out of step after each block of tubes/cultures. Some laboratories use color coding to distinguish dose levels of formulations and media, in accordance with their SOPs.

4. Perform informal visual checks at each step of the test. For example, unexpected levels of liquid in bottles or in the micropipette tip will help highlight any obvious errors at an early stage. Check the temperature (and CO_2 level if appropriate) of the incubator before opening the door. Check the morphology of cells under the inverted microscope each time you remove cultures from the incubator to confirm they are healthy. Other checks are more formal and should be documented (as required by the SOP), for example, the condition of the background lawn should be noted if unexpected colony counts are obtained in the bacterial mutation test.

5. Maintain a list of supplies, suppliers, and catalog numbers that you can refer to for reordering.

6. Staff should be trained in aseptic techniques to minimize potential microbial contamination of test systems. Additional precautions include regular thorough cleaning of laminar flow cabinets and the laboratory area. Disposable protective clothing helps minimize the chance of potential microbial contamination.

7. To minimize potential chemical contamination when formulating, the vehicle should be prepared and aliquoted first before formulation of the test substance, including amounts used for diluting the stock test substance formulation and any samples taken for chemical analysis. Positive control substances should be prepared (or aliquoted from stock) separately and usually after test substance formulation. Positive control substances should, as far as is practical, be held separately from other test and reference substances. Please see the Formulation section (Chapter 3) for other precautions needed to ensure the safety of staff and minimize potential contamination of the facility.

2.13.3 Reducing the Need for Repetition of Parts of the Study

Obtaining all information on the test substance at the protocol preparation stage will help identify whether the test system and method are appropriate, for example, compounds expected to cause anemia should not be tested in the rodent micronucleus test; volatile compounds should normally be tested in the preincubation version of the bacterial mutation test, but that method is inappropriate for bactericidal compounds. This information may also tell you whether special considerations are needed (e.g., in selection of the solvent) and dose levels to be tested; a preliminary dose range—finding test will be needed to establish an appropriate dose range for the main test if compounds are suspected of being unusually toxic.

To a large extent, the checks mentioned in the previous section will reduce the need to repeat part of the study, but appropriate study design may also reduce the need for repeat testing. For example, although preliminary work in an *in vitro* study may give you a good idea of dose levels to use in the main test, toxicity tends to vary between test occasions; therefore, it is a good idea to include a slightly wider dose range by including an extra high and low dose level, for example, at least five dose levels in case of the chromosome aberration test, and then only those dose levels that achieve the targeted level of toxicity need to be subjected to detailed examination for aberrations. Similarly, *in vitro* mammalian cell tests will often include three dose levels of each positive control, with only that level showing the targeted level of toxicity being used for collection of results.

Stock reagents added to culture medium are liable to microbial contamination if opened on multiple occasions and will themselves often support microbial growth; some organisms can even use antibiotics as a carbon source. All additions to bulk media should be added via a sterile filter after a visual check of the addition for signs of contamination (e.g., turbidity).

Incubators (even cell culture ones) can develop very drying atmospheres. A stainless steel tray containing water should be placed in the bottom of the incubator to humidify the atmosphere. Small-volume cultures should be placed in a partially sealed food-grade bag or plastic box to reduce loss of volume during incubation.

Some laboratories experience issues with compatibility of certain batches of S9 fraction or serum with their test system. Consider qualifying a particular batch of these for specific tests and reserve adequate bulk amounts if found to be suitable. This is especially appropriate if the company manufacturing the product has not tested it for compatibility in an analogous system. Any performance testing or related quality control information for these and other reagents including culture medium provided by the product supplier should be retained by the laboratory.

2.13.4 Accommodating Repeat or Supplementary Tests

These can usually be run along with the next study on the next occasion of testing. Residual formulations (if known to be stable) may be stored until results of the test are available.

2.13.5 Running More Studies in a Given Timeframe

Scheduling of studies is an important aspect of planning. Usually two or three studies of the same type can be run simultaneously, and it may even be possible to use the same positive and negative control cultures/animals for each if acceptable to your QA unit, provided that appropriate samples are taken for each and precautions are taken to ensure anonymity. For example, test substances can be identified by a code letter that is related to the test substance only in that particular study file while exact copies of the encoded results are held in each file. This is less of a problem if all the test substances belong to the same sponsor, in which case it may be acceptable (or even desirable for comparative purposes) to perform the study under a single protocol with a single report. This approach not only greatly reduces the overall workload but also reduces the number of animals used for scientific research.

To simplify scheduling and reduce overtime requirements, it is often easier to always run studies of a particular type on the same day, for example, if bacterial mutation tests are performed on Tuesday and Friday, the plates can be removed on Friday and Monday morning and scored on the same day. Other procedures like maintenance, preparation of reagents, slide reading, preparation of reports, which are necessary but not time-critical, can be organized to fit around the scheduled testing.

2.13.6 Timeframe for Routine Studies

An important question that study monitors or program managers often ask is, "When can you start a study?" What they are usually most interested in is when they can get the results and the report. Clearly, it does not help with efficiency if each study is planned to start as soon as the test substance arrives without taking into account scheduling of other tests (as described). Template protocols should be prepared showing standard timeframes rather than actual dates, for example, study start within 2 weeks of approval of the final protocol and test substance arrival, results within 3–4 weeks of study start, draft unaudited report 2 weeks after final results, final report 4 weeks after draft report or 2 weeks after receipt of final principal investigators' contributing reports (if any) and 2 weeks after study monitor's comments (whichever is later). These default dates can then be used for the draft protocol that will be sent to the study monitor. Clearly, the study schedule needs to take into account any necessary preliminary genetic toxicology and analytical work, time taken for the study monitor to get the test substance to you together with information needed to finalize the protocol, your own QA unit's standard timings (you should seek their agreement for standard timings for routine testing), timings for any contributing work (e.g., analytical chemistry), and the time it takes the study monitor to agree to contents of the final report. At this point, outline dates can be agreed for the final protocol, but these should either be provisional and approximate (e.g., start date should be specified) or left as relative except under exceptional circumstances, in which case they can be specified but should include appropriate provisions.

In an ideal world, the default results timeline indicated in the template should be fairly pessimistic (e.g., to allow repeat of part of a test that failed) while still being realistic and reasonable (i.e., competitive or better than other laboratories in the case of a CRO). This can be achieved by having everything in place in advance to run studies at short notice, including template protocols and reports, stock reagents, adequate supplies, and default QA timelines. Even if the laboratory's schedule is already apparently full, it will usually be practical to add another study at short notice by running several studies in parallel (as mentioned) and by use of overtime for study set-up and slide reading. A laboratory that is operating close to capacity should allow for reasonable (e.g., 10%) overtime in its budget to maximize efficiency and throughput. Hopefully, you will soon reach a point where this overtime limit is exceeded; at that point, you will need to consider hiring additional staff or equipment to automate certain tasks.

A simple and very effective way of reducing the overall in-life phase of a study and at the same time reduce labor is to perform multiple aspects of a project in tandem. For example, you may be asked to perform Ames, chromosome aberration, and a rat micronucleus test on a single test substance with supporting formulation analysis. In this case, the relevant considerations are outlined in Table 2.5.

Table 2.5: Coordinating phases of multiple studies

Phase	Suggested Approach
Formulation development	Preliminary testing should cover all the planned studies and assess the suitability of appropriate vehicles. If the substance shows good aqueous solubility, then usually the same solvent can be used for each test; otherwise, and more typically, an organic solvent will be chosen for the *in vitro* studies and an aqueous suspending agent will be used for the *in vivo* studies as in the example in the following paragraph *Example.* In this case, DMSO was chosen as the best solvent for the *in vitro* studies and 1% methylcellulose was chosen as an appropriate suspending agent for *in vivo* studies. The solubility of the substance should be assessed in DMSO at a level that allows the highest limit dose required by the appropriate ICH or OECD guidelines. A range of dilutions should then be made and tested for compatibility with the culture medium used in the chromosome aberration test. The test substance should be suspended in 1% methylcellulose at a concentration that allows the limit dose level for the micronucleus test to be achieved using an acceptable dose volume before assessing doseability, i.e., ability to pass into a syringe and through a suitable dosing needle or cannula
Validation of the analytical method and formulation stability	The analytical work should cover the vehicles and the concentration range established during formulation development. The low concentration evaluated will be close to the limit of quantitation or based on the planned lowest dose for appropriate assay(s)

(Continued)

Table 2.5: (Continued)

Phase	Suggested Approach
Formulation and analysis for the *in vitro* studies	Chemical stability should be evaluated over a similar concentration range for a period that allows chemical analysis prior to dosing (e.g., analyzed at day 0 and day 5). Homogeneity should also be established under the same conditions in the case of suspensions Formulations for the two *in vitro* tests should be made together and analyzed in the same run. All formulations should be stored under conditions that were previously confirmed as suitable until analysis confirms acceptability
In vitro studies	Often tests are divided into main and confirmatory tests. In this case, the two phases should be performed on the same day using the same formulation. In that way, results will be available much earlier and the costs of formulation analysis will be greatly reduced

2.13.7 Reducing the Effort Needed to Prepare Protocols, Tables, and Reports

Routine protocols, reports, and tables should all be prepared from standard templates. In the case of tables and graphs prepared using a spreadsheet program (e.g., Excel), the calculations in these should automatically update as the results are entered. Conditional formatting can be used in Excel to highlight values that are outside expected limits. Links from Word to Excel files are useful but should be broken once the Word document has been updated to avoid inadvertent updates later. Note that if graphs are copied from Excel into Word, they should be pasted as *Pictures* (paste special) to avoid carryover of spreadsheet information and larger file sizes.

Slide code labels should be generated in Excel using the random function and the code should be saved electronically. Information from the electronic file can be imported into the results spreadsheet and then the table should be ordered logically (e.g., by group and animal number) using the *sort* function.

Commercial packages can handle certain aspects of tabulation and historical control information semiautomatically (e.g., Perceptive Instruments, http://www.perceptive.co.uk/).

2.13.8 Reducing the Effort Needed to Perform the Study

Labeling requirements under GLP are quite extensive and, at first sight, seem unnecessarily laborious. The requirement is that each plate, culture, animal, formulation slide, or specimen from a study should be uniquely identifiable and traceable. When any of these items will be transferred to another location, these principles should be applied rigorously: formulation samples should be labeled with study number, test item (chemical or vehicle name as appropriate), concentration, and sampling date as a minimum and accompanied by an appropriate form showing sampling details that are also used for acknowledgment of receipt; in this way the form is used to document chain of custody. In other cases, it is more convenient and appropriate to generate an alpha-numeric code within a study design spreadsheet. The spreadsheet should contain details of the contents and additions or doses administered to the plate/culture (see Fig. 4.1 for an example) and can be populated semiautomatically if linked to an input sheet. If more than one experiment is being handled in an area at any one time and there is a potential for overlap or confusion, then a prefix may be used to distinguish between experiments. For example, if Ames tests are being performed on several days of the week and the same numbering system (1, 2, 3, etc.) is used for each, then the plates dosed on Mondays, Tuesdays, and Wednesdays could be prefixed A, B, C, and so on, either individually or, if they will not be placed in the same incubator, with the prefix indicated on the top plate in each stack. Note that plates and bottles should be labeled on the side rather than on the lid if there is any chance that the lids will become mixed.

Note that several short-term *in vivo* experiments may be housed in a single room to reduce costs and save on space requirements. In this case, animals should be physically separated (e.g., housed in cages on different racks). Note that individual facilities are likely to have their own numbering systems for animals that may, for example, help distinguish between groups. The test facility SOP should be followed regarding cage labeling. Even so, the prefix system may still be used if there is any overlap in numbering of individual animals in the same room. Animals for short-term studies can be identified by tail-marking using an indelible marker (rather than tattooing), although the number may need to be reapplied after a few days.

For reference purposes, the study design spreadsheet is held in the laboratory throughout the dosing process.

2.13.9 Reducing Costs or Labor Requirement

As the volume of studies increases, continual thought should be given to improving production methods. Some examples are given:

1. Multidose micropipettes for repetitive dosing of small volumes. For example, Integra Biosciences Viaflow makes high-quality single and multichannel repeat dose pipettes (see http://www.integra-biosciences.com/sites/viaflo_pipettes.html).
2. Stock solutions of positive controls and other reagents formulated on one occasion should be batched out. Most stock positive control solutions are sufficiently stable for 6 months if stored at approximately $-20°C$ in darkness. When thawing reagents, it is important to thaw the entire contents of the vial and ensure they are completely in solution before use. Alternatively, many positive controls can be dissolved in acetone, batched out, and then dried in a fume hood before storage and reconstitution. Note that DMSO should also be batched out into dry sterile bottles with only a small air-gap to minimize chance of contamination and development of degradents.

3. For particular expensive chemicals that you use in large quantities (e.g., NADP), ask for quotes from more than one supplier and consider savings when placing a bulk order or reserving a stock at a particular supplier.

4. Metered agar pump for use in the Ames test can be piston or peristaltic. Other autoclavable repeat bottle-top dispensers are suitable for dispensing S9 mix (Socorex http://www.socorex.com/low-profile-dispensers-acurex-compact-en-1-1-11-25.html).

5. Use stainless steel slide staining racks with glass or stainless steel troughs for processing large numbers of slides simultaneously.

6. Although metal cabinets are often used by pathologists to store slides, cardboard storage boxes are much less expensive and cause less breakage to slides.

7. If you have limited labor resources, then you might consider buying reagents or poured plates from a commercial supplier (e.g., Moltox). Poured plates are liable to develop contamination during shipping, so they should be checked during the labeling process.

   If you perform a large number of studies, you might also consider:

8. Petri plate pourer and labeler (for high-volume Ames work).

9. Slide labeling/etching machine.

2.14 QA

The main function of QA is to ensure studies are performed in compliance with GLP and that the test facility complies with GLP. The unit will need to audit all GLP protocols, reports, studies, and critical processes to ensure they are compliant and that documentation accurately reflects what was done and is complete; they will also need to audit the test facility. From a business point of view, a major responsibility of the (genetic) toxicology group and QA units is to cooperate to minimize the number of checks that are needed to ensure compliance. Staff should take into account the implications of "OECD guidance documents on Application of the GLP Principles to Short-term Studies" and "The Application of the Principles of GLP to *in vitro* Studies." Many of the ways to facilitate the QA function are described elsewhere in this and other chapters but are listed here for clarity and completeness:

1. Protocols and reports: Use of standard templates will reduce the checks that QA need to do. They will have already confirmed that the standard documents are compliant with GLP and consistent between one another. When reviewing individual protocols, they should only need to read the nonstandard sections. Similarly, review of the report will be facilitated because they already know that the standard text is consistent with the protocol.

2. OECD GLP indicates that when a high number of similar routine studies are run in a facility, the in-life phase of each study does not need to be inspected. Instead, in a *process-based scheme*, each critical phase of that study type should be inspected on

a regular basis. The frequency of inspection should be stated within QA's SOPs and based on the frequency and complexity of the study type. Because it is impossible to quantify complexity and because the frequency of studies varies, I would suggest that a default 3-month cycle is reasonable and allow 1-month leeway on either side. In some cases, the processes for individual study types overlap, further reducing the number of inspections required; examples of relevant processes include formulation, dosing, and plate and slide reading. The dates of the most recent inspection of each relevant process and reporting should be indicated in the QA statement page of the report together with the protocol and report audit and reporting dates. As part of the allied facility inspection, QA should consider the list of processes used to maintain the facility and the test system (e.g., cell line) provided by OECD in their guidance on GLP aspects of *in vitro* studies. In this case, it may be convenient to have a joint schedule for process and facility inspections.

3. Genetic toxicology staff are responsible for checking information supplied in the report. In an entirely manual system, this may involve double data entry in the case of tables, appendices, and historical control information. Particular attention should be given to accuracy of any units used (e.g., mg or μg). Note that rounding of numbers for presentation will often result in an apparent rounding error if calculation checks are based on figures that have already been rounded. It is normally best to base all calculated values on the original unrounded results with an appropriate footnote in the relevant report tables.

4. It is not reasonable to expect QA staff to routinely check large numbers of entries in tables. Automated tabulation using spreadsheets as well as direct data entry or capture greatly reduces the chance of errors in tables. In this case, where reports of this study type have continually been found to show a low number of errors, the QA unit are justified in adopting a sample-based audit system for report tables. This system was originally developed for quality control in manufacturing large lots of machined components (e.g., ball bearings) where it is not practical to check each individual unit in a large batch. This is particularly applicable if the results are of an ancillary nature and any deviation will not affect the conclusion of the study (e.g., body weight tables). Sampling is based on sound statistical methods and involves taking a few numbers from representative rows and columns in a table and checking their accuracy against the raw data. If no significant number of errors is found, then the table is considered accurate; if a single error is found, then sampling is continued until the auditor is confident the table is generally acceptable. If a significant number of errors is found, then the table (and possibly the report) is rejected and returned to the study director. More information on the theory behind the method and associated tables can be found at https://www.sqconline.com/. The auditor should consider additional checks of column headings and units if these vary between reports.

2.15 Qualifying a Contract Laboratory

Before contracting routine studies to a laboratory, you should qualify it to ensure it has the right expertise and is of an appropriate standard. Recommendations on genetox laboratories can come from your peers in the field, such as project managers and genetic toxicologists at other pharmaceutical, chemical, or medical device companies, or from talking to scientists at a meeting. Key points to consider are:

- Responsiveness (difficult to quantify but probably one of the biggest concerns): Can you get through to the study director and get answers immediately? Are there alternate scientists who you can get answers from if the study director is not available?
- Timeliness: Are their lead-in times reasonable? Do they get results and reports out on time? What is QA audit turnaround time?
- Expertise: How good is the laboratory at running routine assays? How well do they cope with issues on studies?
- Capabilities: Can they handle special techniques and follow-up tests?
- Reports: Are their reports clear, well presented, and consistent between assay types?
- Flexibility: Can they run studies at short notice or to nonstandard designs?

Having established that a laboratory has a good reputation, you should contact their responsible scientist (e.g., head of department), perhaps via a conference call involving several staff at both ends. This is used to confirm these points in more detail and establish whether the laboratory is amenable for inspection at short notice and open to routine visits. You should also take into account location (accessibility to the laboratory), potential problems in transfer of samples, and possible language/communication issues. The scientist(s) should be able to assure you on these points. Ask for copies of the laboratory's standard protocols and historical control databases. Do these meet standard guideline (and your company) requirements, and do control results fall within acceptable limits?

If you feel comfortable with the laboratory, then you should consider whether to inspect the facility. Inspections can either focus on the facility's capabilities as a whole or focus on a particular area of interest (e.g., IND packages). Alternately, or at the same time, you might consider running a few trial studies (e.g., a standard genetox "package" of three studies) at the facility to get a good idea of how they perform bearing in mind that *in vitro* and *in vivo* studies might be handled differently or via different functional groups.

Under ideal circumstances, a qualifying inspection should involve both scientific and QA staff from your company and scientific QA and technical staff at the laboratory. QA will focus on documentation aspects: test system and equipment maintenance, training records, SOPs, GLP compliance, master schedule awareness and maintenance by QA and management, procedural records, and archiving. The scientist should focus on the competence of staff in dealing with routine studies and handling difficult test substances or problems that occur during study conduct. Do they discuss issues that arise on a study directly and as soon as practical with the study monitor? Ask for some examples and outline any difficult situations that you have encountered in the past to get their point of view. Your inspection should also cover the laboratory's formulation area and animal rooms. If possible, ask to view procedures that are currently being performed in the laboratory, especially if they are being performed for your company. Inspect the raw data from any studies that you have in the laboratory and discuss them with the responsible scientists. Ask to chat informally with one or two of the technicians about things like training and criteria used to identify aberrations, micronuclei, and artifacts when slide reading or examining plates. Most importantly, *ask to examine some slides chosen at random from ongoing studies*. Do not be put off with example or training slides. The laboratory should produce excellent slides on a routine basis; otherwise, they can never be expected to produce reliable results. The audit should be scheduled around an outline agenda to see several key in-life phases of the relevant tests.

Pricing may be part of your company's selection process and is worth looking into, but, in my experience, laboratories of similar quality generally price studies similarly. It can be difficult to compare prices because a standard study at one laboratory may have a very different design than a study at a second laboratory, neither of which might match your own idea of a standard study. If you decide to run studies at a laboratory, then I strongly suggest you consider adopting their standard study design and procedures for efficiency reasons and to minimize the chance of errors later.

2.16 Responsibilities of the Study Monitor

If you contract studies routinely at a laboratory, you should expect to be in continual contact with staff there and consider visiting every 2 or 3 years. If that is not practical, then a scheduled video conference call or a meeting with their personnel at scientific meetings can also be productive.

Other ongoing responsibilities of the sponsor are outlined in the OECD Series on Principles of Good Laboratory Practice and Compliance Monitoring, No. 11, January 22, 1998, The Role and Responsibility of the Sponsor in the Application of the Principles of GLP. Although the study director is responsible for verification and identification of the test substance, characterization is often supplied by the sponsor, in which case it should be mentioned in the report. If characterization was not conducted under GLP, then the fact should be mentioned in the study director's signature page as an exception to GLP together with any mitigation (e.g., "Although the test substance was not characterized under GLP, chemical analysis indicating purity, and identity were performed under GMP conditions and a full report is retained by . . .").

References

[1] Diehl KH, Hull R, Morton D, Pfister R, Rabemampianina Y, Smith D, et al. A good practice guide to the administration of substances and removal of blood, including routes and volumes. J Appl Toxicol 2001; 21(1):15−23.

[2] Turner PV, Brabb T, Pekow C, Vasbinder MA. Administration of substances to laboratory animals: routes of administration and factors to consider. J Am Assoc Lab Anim Sci 2011;50(5):600−13.

[3] Hayashi M, Dearfield K, Kasper P, Lovell D, Martus HJ, Thybaud V. Compilation and use of genetic toxicity historical control data. Mutat Res 2011;723(2):87−90.

[4] OECD Guideline for Testing of Chemicals, Genetic Toxicology No. 471, Bacterial Reverse Mutation Test. Organisation for Economic Co-Operation and Development, Paris, 21 July 1997. Available from: < http://www.oecd-ilibrary.org >.

[5] FDA. Guidance for Industry Part 11, Electronic Records; Electronic Signatures—Scope and Application. Available from: http://www.fda.gov/RegulatoryInformation/Guidances/ucm125067.htm; 2003.

[6] FDA. eCFR (Electronic Code of Federal Regulations). Title 21, part 11—electronic records; electronic signatures. Available from: < http://www.ecfr.gov/cgi-bin/text-idx?SID = 1cce2b1d801e978a6c7edd7017a88 10a&mc = true&tpl = /ecfrbrowse/Title21/21cfr11_main_02.tpl; 2015 >.

[7] OECD. The application of the principles of GLP to computerised systems http://www.oecd-ilibrary.org Paris: Organisation for Economic Co-Operation And Development; 1995.

[8] OECD Draft advisory document 161, the application of GLP principles to computerised systems 16 September 2014. Available from: < http://www.oecd.org/chemicalsafety/testing/Draft-OECD-GLP-Guidance-Document-computerised-systems.pdf >.

[9] ICH. International Conference on Harmonisation of Technical Requirements for Registration of Pharmaceuticals for Human Use (ICH) S2(R1) Guidance on Genotoxicity Testing and Data Interpretation for Pharmaceuticals Intended for Human Use. Available from: < http://www.ich.org/products/guidelines/safety/ safety-single/article/guidance-on-genotoxicity-testing-and-data-interpretation-for-pharmaceuticalsintended-for-human-use.html >.

[10] OECD Series on Testing and Assessment No. 198 Report on statistical issues related to OECD test guidelines (TGs) on genotoxicity. OECD Paris 11 July 2014. Available from: < http://www.oecd-ilibrary.org >.

[11] Festing MF, Lovell DP. The need for statistical analysis of rodent micronucleus test data. Comment on the paper by Ashby and Tinwell. Mutat Res 1995;329(2):221−4.

[12] OECD Series on principles of Good Laboratory Practice and compliance monitoring. Number 1 OECD Principles on Good Laboratory Practice (as revised in 1997). <http://www.oecd-library.org>.

[13] Festing MF. Guidelines for the design and statistical analysis of experiments in papers submitted to ATLA. Altern Lab Anim 2001;29(4):427−46.

[14] Festing MF, Altman DG. Guidelines for the design and statistical analysis of experiments using laboratory animals. ILAR J 2002;43(4):244−58.

[15] ICH harmonised tripartite guideline. The common technical document for the registration of pharmaceuticals for human use: safety—M4S(R2). Nonclinical overview and nonclinical summaries of module 2, organisation of module 4. Step 4. January 13, 2004. Available from: < http://www.ich.org/products/ctd.html >.

[16] FDA. Comparison Chart of FDA and EPA Good Laboratory Practice (GLP) Regulations and the OECD Principles of GLP. Available from: http://www.fda.gov/downloads/ICECI/EnforcementActions/ BioresearchMonitoring/UCM133724.pdf; 2004.

CHAPTER 3

Formulation of Test Articles

Annie Hamel[1] and Ray Proudlock[2]

[1]Department of Genetic Toxicology, Charles River Laboratories, Montreal, ULC, Canada
[2]Boone, North Carolina, USA

Chapter Outline

3.1 **Introduction** 52
   3.1.1 Safety 52
   3.1.2 Selecting an Appropriate Formulation 52
3.2 **Formulation Laboratories** 53
   3.2.1 Designing and Equipping a Genetic Toxicology Formulation Area 53
      3.2.1.1 Hoods 55
      3.2.1.2 Storage equipment 55
   3.2.2 Personal Protective Clothing 56
      3.2.2.1 Standard 56
      3.2.2.2 Capital equipment 56
      3.2.2.3 Consumables 57
3.3 **Safety Data Sheets** 57
3.4 **Receipt of the Test Article** 59
3.5 **Formulation Types and Planning** 59
3.6 **Solubility and *In Vitro* Compatibility Testing** 60
   3.6.1 Introduction 60
   3.6.2 Choice of Solvent 61
   3.6.3 Solubility Testing 62
   3.6.4 Calculations and Checking: Small-Volume (*In Vitro*) Assays 64
   3.6.5 Compatibility of Formulation with Culture Medium 65
3.7 **Formulation of Dose Solutions** 68
3.8 **Formulation of Bulk Formulations** 71
3.9 **Formulation of Suspensions** 71
   3.9.1 Aqueous Suspending Agents 71
   3.9.2 Large Volume Suspensions 73
   3.9.3 Small Volume Suspensions 74
3.10 **Chemical Analysis and Stability** 74
References 77

3.1 Introduction

3.1.1 Safety

Genetic toxicology testing usually involves the use of compounds with unknown toxicities and highly hazardous positive control agents. It is the legal and moral responsibility of laboratory management to ensure that an appropriately equipped dedicated laboratory area is available to deal with and contain these types of materials, taking into account that they are likely to have various physical characteristics; for example, powders should not be handled in the same way as volatile liquids. In addition, appropriate PPE (clothing, masks, etc.) must be available to staff handling the materials, and procedures and training should be in place to ensure safe handling and containment. It is the responsibility of staff and management alike to ensure that the prescribed procedures are followed.

Health effects potentially resulting from inappropriate handling of chemical mutagens and cytotoxic drugs (e.g., positive controls, spindle poisons, cytochalasin) used in genetic toxicology are similar to those expected from exposure to radiation and chemotherapeutic drugs [1,2]. These may include:

1. Bone marrow disorders and blood dyscrasia
2. Fetal loss in pregnant women and malformations in the offspring
3. Loss of fertility
4. Painful gastrointestinal disorders, hair loss, nasal sores, and vomiting
5. Liver damage
6. Contact dermatitis, local toxic effects, and allergic reaction
7. Cancer initiation and promotion (one in three people develop cancer in their lifetime)

Although there may be no evidence that staff working with these chemicals have higher incidences of these conditions, minimization of exposure by ensuring appropriate control measures is essential [3]. Precautions apply especially during the formulation process because chemicals are handled in bulk and in concentrated form. In some cases, the risk of exposure can be reduced by purchasing agents in preweighed aliquots.

3.1.2 Selecting an Appropriate Formulation

Two of the first questions that need to be answered when developing a new pharmaceutical or planning a new toxicology testing program for any type of test article are:

1. What will be the route of administration?
2. What vehicles are likely to be compatible with my compound and the chosen route of administration?

Genetic toxicology studies are usually initiated at the start of the testing program and, in the case of *in vitro* studies (including the human *Ether-à-go-go*-Related Gene (hERG) screen for induction of cardiac arrhythmia), often involve a different vehicle. It is important that these questions are answered at the outset so that any formulation development work and associated chemical analysis to support vehicle selection covers all the studies being considered in the test program.

The vehicle and route of exposure for *in vivo* genotoxicity studies usually match the main rodent toxicology studies so that information on toxicity and, when available, information on systemic exposure can be cross-referenced. In the case of a Good Laboratory Practice (GLP) toxicology program, chemical analysis to demonstrate homogeneity, physical stability, and chemical stability, together with preliminary toxicokinetic and acute toxicity results, will be available to support vehicle, route, and dose selection for *in vivo* genotoxicity test(s).

3.2 Formulation Laboratories

Formulation laboratories should be designed to protect individual workers, prevent contamination of the environment, and, as required by GLP, the test facility as a whole.

Toxicity testing facilities are expected to have their own formulation laboratory ("pharmacy") with staff trained in preparing materials for administration to animals by common and specialized routes. However, pharmacy staff are not necessarily adept at dealing with formulations for *in vitro* studies, which usually involve small volumes and highly hazardous cytotoxic and mutagenic materials. For reasons of safety, convenience, and training, and to avoid potential contamination issues, genetic toxicology testing laboratories should have their own separate purpose-designed formulation area. In contrast, formulation (often of suspensions) for use in *in vivo* genetic toxicology work may be assigned to the main pharmacy, which will have the facilities to deal with bulk formulations and will normally be more experienced in dealing with special formulations needed for animal studies (e.g., suspensions, admixture with the diet, inhalation, and infusion). In the case of special routes of administration, the scientist should seek the advice of formulation specialists and a scientist experienced in that route to assist in dose preparation and the in-life phase of the study. Special routes will often complicate sampling and chemical analysis.

3.2.1 Designing and Equipping a Genetic Toxicology Formulation Area

The engineers involved in planning a new laboratory or refurbishing an existing area should be specialists in safe laboratory design; they and laboratory management should be aware of critical aspects of design and national requirements. These aspects, particularly with regard to handling potential mutagens, are outlined here; however, full details of laboratory design are beyond the scope of this book; readers should consult specialist reference manuals [4].

Access to the formulation area should be physically restricted to allow entry of only authorized personnel for safety reasons and to ensure the security and integrity of the test articles. Here, as in the other genetic toxicology laboratories, the flooring should be seamless, physically resilient, solvent-resistant, easy to clean, and skid-proof, and should continue for the first few inches up the wall. Poured epoxy flooring over a concrete base is probably the best option to use. The area should have an anteroom with washing facilities, where staff can change into and out of personal protective clothing when entering and leaving the area. In accord with the principles of OSHA [5], measures to ensure safety and containment should be considered in the following order:

1. Engineering controls
2. Administrative controls
3. Training and enforcement of appropriate work practices
4. Personal protective clothing and equipment

For example, protection from inhalation of chemicals primarily involves ensuring adequate air-flow, for example, powder containment and fume hoods should be used to dispense and formulate materials rather than expecting staff to formulate on the open bench while wearing uncomfortable and constrictive breathing apparatus (which might interfere with efficiency, accuracy, observation, and communication). Individual countries have their own legislation concerning transport, storage, handling, and disposal of chemicals, but useful guidance on the principles of safe handling and disposal of chemicals can be found at the following US government website: http://sis.nlm.nih.gov/enviro/labsafety.html#a1.

The air pressure in the formulation laboratory should be maintained at slightly negative pressure with respect to the anteroom using an extraction system. Fume hoods normally required a balanced air input to avoid excessive negative pressure. In general, minimum air change rates in laboratories are not subject to legal requirements, but 10 air changes per hour seems reasonable given that this figure is often used in designing animal rooms. To simplify design and maintain a standard air change rate in the laboratory, this may involve running the fume hood(s) continuously, if rates are of the constant volume type with a bypass. The extracted air should be vented on the roof with appropriate consideration of the direction of the prevailing wind and precautions should be taken to prevent backflow. The fume hood and powder containment cabinet supplier and the specialist laboratory HVAC (heating, ventilating, and air conditioning) engineer should be consulted and directly involved in the siting of equipment and design of the air-handling system. Efficient air-flow system design is extremely important because it will represent more than half the cost of the pharmacy; poor design will also result in significant additional operational costs in the form of wasted conditioned air—refer to the TSI Laboratory Design Handbook for additional information on air-flow and efficient design [6]. The incoming air should be filtered at a comfortable temperature and humidity to not interfere with the efficiency of operational staff [4,7].

3.2.1.1 Hoods

Test article containers should be opened and contents should be dispensed only in suitable containment devices ("hoods") that are regularly monitored for containment efficiency and air-flow rate. Hoods should be solvent-resistant and easy to clean, with seamless stainless-steel work surfaces and rounded corners. As a minimum, the pharmacy should contain one 4-foot radioisotope-type fume hood. Fume hoods are used for dispensing volatile liquids and, very occasionally, gases.

Fume hoods are not suited for handling powders because the high flow, although directed away from the body of the operator, can generate an aerosol of fine particulates, leading to contamination. Most dispensing involves solids (often powders) and should be performed in a 3-foot-wide powder containment cabinet (similar to a biological containment cabinet class 2B or a laminar-flow cytotoxic drug safety cabinets) extracted via a contained high efficiency particulate arresting air (HEPA) filter to the exterior (e.g., the Xpert station supplied by Labconco). This type of hood provides a lower-speed laminar air-flow away from the operator. Any small amount of particulate generated is captured in the HEPA unit, which is changed regularly as it becomes blocked or after a specified period as per the manufacturers' instructions.

Hoods should be fitted, maintained, and cleaned in accordance with the manufacturers' instructions. They should contain only the items necessary for preparing the current formulation and no bulky items, because these would interfere with the air-flow characteristics. Balances should be situated adjacent to the hood to minimize contamination. Materials should be dispensed into suitable preweighed containers that are recapped inside the hood before being reweighed. The target weight of the dispensed material should be specified as a range so that a calculated amount of vehicle can be added to the dispensed material to achieve the required concentration rather than targeting an exact weight, which would require multiple additions and or removal of material from the weighing vial. Open containers should be held in a rack or hand-held to minimize the chance of spillage. Ancillary items needed for formulation such as pipettes can be conveniently stored adjacently on a stainless-steel cart or in racks next to the hood.

3.2.1.2 Storage equipment

Chemicals should be stored in cabinets:

1. General storage cabinet with chemicals stored in alphabetical or appropriate logical order
2. Lockable store for scheduled drugs (i.e., controlled substances such as phenobarbital)
3. Solvent cupboard
4. Refrigerator set at 4°C
5. Upright freezer set at −20°C

Individual cabinets should be extracted or placed in a glass-partitioned unit providing extraction. Positive controls and cytotoxic agents should be stored separately from test articles. Nonhazardous reagents such as buffers, glassware, and other items should be stored in normal laboratory cabinets.

When not in use, chemical containers should be protected to prevent spills or loss if dropped. Glass vials can be stored in a secondary container (e.g., see-through polycarbonate bottle containing silica gel, if appropriate) and transported in a plastic tool box between work areas.

3.2.2 Personal Protective Clothing

3.2.2.1 Standard

1. Safety glasses with protective sides or face shield
2. Nitrile, neoprene, or latex gloves should be available. The selection should be based on the main solvent being used, referring to the manufacturer's website for details of resistance. Individuals can develop skin sensitization to latex and/or the powder used by the manufacturer, so several types of glove need to be available. Gloves should be changed immediately if exposure suspected or if they become sticky or damaged.
3. Jumpsuit (polyethylene-coated paper or Tyvek® coverall/boilersuit)
4. Disposable protective sleeves, nonslip shoe covers, and head cover
5. NIOSH-approved dust mask

3.2.2.2 Capital equipment

1. Analytical balance, minimum readability 0.1 mg, capacity 300 g or more
2. Top pan balance, readability 1 mg
3. Appropriate calibrated weights to check balance calibration
4. Homogenizer: high shear with a range of probes (e.g., Silverson, Ultra-Turrax, Polytron)
5. Ultrapure water (UPW) and/or deionized water supply

Other equipment

1. pH meter and electrodes
2. Range of stainless-steel spoons, spatulas, and trullae (scoops)
3. Heated stir plates and magnetic followers ("fleas")
4. Mortar and pestle
5. Appropriate glassware including a range of graduated cylinders
6. Pipette controllers, hand-held rechargeable
7. Adjustable micropipettes (regular and positive displacement), single action, and repeater
8. Stainless-steel carts
9. A safelight for use when formulating light-sensitive materials

In addition, a range of equipment needs to be available but not necessarily present in the formulation area, including an autoclave and a laboratory glass-washer. Special formulations are beyond the scope of this chapter, but a ball mill and a set of stainless-steel sieves might be available in the main pharmacy for preparing suspensions of insoluble solids that are not received as fine powders, which is often the case with industrial compounds.

3.2.2.3 Consumables

1. A range of buffering materials, organic solvents, suspending agents, volumetric hydrochloric acid, and sodium hydroxide (stored in tightly sealed bottles to prevent loss by evaporation or reaction with carbon dioxide in the air)
2. Medical wipes and paper towel
3. Weighing paper, weigh boat
4. Aluminum foil
5. Parafilm
6. Disposable syringes and needles
7. Sterilizing filters 0.22 μm, aqueous and solvent-proof types
8. Benchkote or Bench Guard protective paper (supplied in rolls), absorbent on upper side only
9. Micropipette tips, sterile
10. Disposable sterile calibrated pipettes, 2, 5, 10, and 25 mL
11. Disposable screw-top glass vials and containers suitable for preparing and storing formulations; amber containers may be useful when using light-sensitive materials

Note that these lists are not exhaustive and other items may be required in particular cases.

3.3 Safety Data Sheets

Prior to receipt and handling of materials, the program manager in conjunction with the study director(s) is responsible for obtaining information on the test material, often from the sponsor in the case of subcontracted studies. This is used to ensure appropriate handling of the test material but can also facilitate the selection of the vehicle and dose levels. It may also help design other aspects of the study; it may even tell you whether the studies you are planning are appropriate depending on the chemical class of the material and its known or suspected biological activities. For example, volatile agents require contained exposure in the case of in vitro tests, whereas the *in vivo* micronucleus test may not be appropriate for chemicals that cause hemolysis or anemia.

Much of this information can be obtained in the form of a safety data sheet (SDS). Many countries including the United States and Europe are adopting the Globally Harmonized System of Classification and Labelling of Chemicals system developed by the

United Nations and referred to as GHS (see http://www.unece.org/trans/danger/publi/ghs/ghs_welcome_e.html). GHS has developed a standardized SDS that provides information on physical properties, chemical reactivity, and toxicity in a consistent and standardized format using the following section headings.

1. *Identification*: product identifier, manufacturer or distributor name, address, and telephone number, emergency telephone number, recommended use, and restrictions on use
2. *Hazard(s) identification*: all hazards regarding the chemical and required label elements
3. *Composition/information on ingredients*: information on chemical ingredients
4. *First aid measures*: important symptoms/effects, both acute and delayed, and required treatment
5. *Fire-fighting measures*: suitable extinguishing techniques, equipment, and chemical hazards from fire
6. *Accidental release measures*: emergency procedures, protective equipment, and proper methods of containment and clean-up
7. *Handling and storage*: precautions for safe handling and storage, including incompatibilities
8. *Exposure controls/personal protection*: OSHA's Permissible Exposure Limits (PELs), Threshold Limit Values (TLVs), appropriate engineering controls, and personal protective equipment (PPE)
9. *Physical and chemical properties*: the chemical's characteristics
10. *Stability and reactivity*: chemical stability and possibility of hazardous reactions
11. *Toxicological information*: routes of exposure, related symptoms, both acute and chronic effects, and numerical measures of toxicity
12. *Ecological information*
13. *Disposal considerations*
14. *Transport information*
15. *Regulatory information*
16. *Other information*: the date of preparation or last revision

Although the SDS may imply that the material is of low toxicological concern, the information may be unreliable or, as is often the case, inadequate. Unless there is a specific hazard, it is therefore appropriate, convenient, and easier for the staff to handle these materials in the same way as they do positive controls. The scientist in charge of the study should review the SDS for content and any missing information in advance of the use of the material and advise staff of any special precautions (e.g., in the case of volatiles). This can be conveniently done using a standard section in the study protocol/plan. The scientist should also ensure the current version of the SDS is available for staff to consult; if special precautions are required, then the scientist should provide reminders prior to the study (e.g., at a prestudy meeting).

When the scientist/program manager is requesting information in the form of a SDS, the scientist/program manager should also ask for information from the sponsor/chemist regarding the compatibility and solubility of the test article with likely vehicles and relevant information from any early phase (e.g., bioavailability, *in vitro* metabolic profiling, toxicity) investigational studies. Be aware that, in the case of drugs, this information may relate to a different salt form of the test article.

3.4 Receipt of the Test Article

On receipt of the test article, the identity, batch number, expiration date, weight supplied, storage conditions, and physical appearance should be confirmed against the certificate of analysis (COA; where provided) and information given by the supplier in case of error or deterioration. The material should be stored as per the SDS and COA taking into account any additional information provided by the supplier. The receipt date of each lot of the test article should be recorded and marked on the container. These details should be presented in the protocol and in the final report. On arrival in a GLP test facility, and to continue the chain of custody history, it is a standard practice to document the receipt, appearance, location, storage conditions, and usage of test article. This test article disposition and use log should include details of the storage container and its gross weight before and after any removal of material for testing: the difference between before and after is used as a check of the weight of material in each formulation.

At the end of the test program, some of the test article may be sent for confirmation of stability under conditions of storage and use. Alternatively, stability of the test article under the stated storage conditions may already have been established or be ongoing. In any case, confirmation of stability should be stated in the final report.

3.5 Formulation Types and Planning

In GLP toxicology test programs, chemical analysis is required to demonstrate chemical stability, physical stability, and homogeneity for the planned vehicle(s) and concentration ranges to be used in the individual studies. The analytical method is usually developed and the method and formulation are validated in advance of the toxicology studies. Therefore, the nature of the formulations and concentration ranges to be covered should be determined prior to completion of this validation to avoid additional cross-validation work later.

The route of administration for standalone *in vivo* genetic toxicology studies usually matches that used for the rest of the rodent toxicology program (to facilitate dose-setting and allow use of toxicokinetic data, where available) and should be one that mimics human exposure. Oral by intragastric gavage, intravenous bolus injection or infusion, and subcutaneous injection are common routes. Other routes or methods may be considered, such as topical (e.g., dermal, ophthalmic, inhalation, and implant) or capsule; however, if they result in low target organ exposure because of low rates of absorption or low achievable dosages, then other routes may be more appropriate. For example, when evaluating a water-soluble pharmaceutical intended for administration by inhalation, higher systemic exposure levels (in terms of concentration over time) might be achievable using subcutaneous injection or intravenous infusion. These routes may also be significantly less expensive.

For materials that are water-soluble, it usually possible to choose the same vehicle for *in vitro* as well as short-term and long-term *in vivo* studies. In this case, the vehicle will often be isotonic and buffered if given by a parenteral (nonoral) route (e.g., phosphate-buffered saline). However, (water) insoluble compounds are usually administered as suspensions for *in vivo* studies and (to enhance exposure and for practical reasons) as solutions in water-miscible organic solvents for the *in vitro* studies. In the latter case, the final maximum concentration of material in solution in the culture medium/agar is increased by the presence of the solvent ("solubilizing agent"). The disadvantage of this approach is that at least two vehicles need consideration in terms of chemical analysis and formulation validation.

Medical devices are an exception in terms of both formulation and chemical analysis. In this case readers should refer to specific guidelines and procedures published by the Food and Drug Administration (FDA) as well as the ISO 10993 series of standards. These documents undergo continual revision, so the reader should check for any updates prior to embarking on any practical work. In particular, ISO 10993-3 deals with the genotoxicity tests required and ISO 10993-12 deals with sample preparation for testing. In the case of water-insoluble medical devices, extracts are produced under exaggerated conditions using one aqueous solvent and one nonpolar solvent; common extractants are saline, culture medium without saline, and isopropyl alcohol or dimethyl sulfoxide (DMSO). Even though DMSO is polar, it is probably the most frequently used "nonpolar" solvent. Although the guidelines do not specify chemical analysis of the extracts, the manufacturer will normally be aware of the likely major components present based on in-house chemical testing of related extractable and leachable material.

3.6 Solubility and In Vitro Compatibility Testing

3.6.1 Introduction

The purpose of solubility testing is to determine an appropriate solvent for use in the subsequent genotoxicity assays. Subsequent compatibility testing of the solution in culture medium will establish whether the solution requires neutralization. For materials with low aqueous solubility and toxicity, it will also establish the highest dose level to be tested in the subsequent mammalian cell test because the highest one or two dose levels used in that test should show precipitation.

In the case of the subsequent *in vitro* cytogenetic (e.g., chromosome aberration and micronucleus) tests, it is most efficient to test a wide range of dose levels up to the limit established by solubility and compatibility testing, prepare slides, perform a preliminary assessment of toxicity, and then perform detailed analysis on slides from the three or four highest dose levels not showing excessive toxicity. When the material is expected to be highly toxic or when this would involve an excessive amount of work (e.g., in the case of cell mutation assays), a preliminary toxicity test will be required prior to the main biological assay.

3.6.2 Choice of Solvent

The formulation needs to take into account OECD and, in the case of pharmaceuticals, ICH [8] requirements in terms of maximum dose levels; see http://www.oecd.org/env/ ehs/testing/section4healtheffects.htm and http://www.ich.org/products/guidelines/safety/ article/safety-guidelines.html for the latest approved and draft guidelines. If the test article is known or found to be water-soluble at 100 mM, 20 mg/mL, or 20 μL/mL (10 mM or 5 mg/mL in the case of pharmaceuticals), whichever is the lowest, then it should be dissolved in the vehicle selected for the rodent toxicology program. If not soluble at these levels, then it may be necessary to use an organic solvent. Alternatively, it may be possible to dissolve the material directly in the culture medium used for the mammalian cell test; if serum-free medium is used, then it may be possible to use the same formulation for the bacterial mutation test. Note that higher concentrations above the guideline limits may be justifiable when testing a complex mixture or qualifying a pharmaceutical containing a potentially genotoxic impurity. In addition, a correction may be needed for salt form, water, or purity. Organic solvents, where used, should generally be anhydrous to minimize potential development of solvent or test article degradation products.

Generally, aqueous suspending agents such as 1% methyl cellulose are of low toxicity and are compatible with culture medium and S9, so they can be used at the same levels as aqueous solvents. Dilute acids and dilute alkalis can also be used provided that the final formulation does not cause a substantial shift in the pH of the culture medium, because excessive departures from normal physiological conditions can cause irrelevant toxic and genotoxic effects, particularly in cultured mammalian cells. Water-miscible organic solvents are generally less compatible than aqueous vehicles (i.e., they are toxic and inhibit S9 activity), so their dose volume is normally restricted to 100 μL per plate and 1% v/v in bacterial and mammalian cell systems, respectively. Very occasionally, a nonmiscible solvent may be used before further dilution (e.g., solubilization in toluene followed by dilution in DMSO or aqueous surfactant solution)—these solvents are generally more toxic and the final maximum level in the test system should be adjusted accordingly. Because they are not miscible and may degrade plastic culture vessels, nonmiscible solvents should not be used without dilution in a miscible solvent. Similarly, dichloromethane can be used to extract material, but the extract should not be used without evaporation because dichloromethane itself is mutagenic.

An important step in establishment of a new assay involves assessment of maximum compatible dose volumes of commonly used solvents. Otherwise, the compatibility of novel solvents will need to be evaluated in advance of their use. Note that primary cells and the preincubation version of the bacterial mutation test may be less tolerant of solvent levels. Additional solvents that have been evaluated in the bacterial mutation test are listed by Maron and associates [9].

3.6.3 Solubility Testing

Evaluation or confirmation of solubility should be performed in advance of genotoxicity testing based on information supplied by your chemist or, in the case of CROs, your sponsor—do not expect that information to be reliable because it may, for example, be based on a different salt form of a drug undergoing development. Solubility and compatibility testing are not necessarily study-specific and do not follow a formal protocol, so it may be convenient to perform them under an internal non-GLP study number. Copies of the testing procedure and results can be retained with the subsequent genetic toxicology studies, if considered appropriate.

The compatibility of solubilized material should be evaluated with the culture medium to be used in the mammalian cell test as described in the next section. In this way, a maximum practical dose can be established based on solubility and dose volume constraints. Solubility in bacterial mutation test plates does not need to be evaluated unless your facility's standard practice is to only use one nonprecipitating concentration.

When the test shows low solubility in aqueous media, the solubility in nonaqueous solvents compatible with the test system should be assessed. The preferred nonaqueous solvent is usually DMSO, but other water-miscible solvents, including methanol, ethanol, dimethyl formamide, acetone, and acetonitrile, should be tried if the material does not show adequate solubility in DMSO. For volatile solvents, including acetone or viscous solvents like polyethylene glycol, positive displacement pipettes should be used to ensure accuracy when dispensing or measuring. When the test compound exhibits inadequate solubility in aqueous or suitable nonaqueous solvents, then aqueous suspending agents (e.g., 1% methyl cellulose) may be used.

Table 3.1: A selection of vehicles that have been used in regulatory studies at Charles River Laboratories

Vehicle	Bacterial μL/Plate	Mammalian Cell Assays μL/mL
10% CD		200
22% HPCD	200	200
Acetone	100	10
Acetone:THF (3:1)	75	
Acetonitrile	50	10
DMF	100	10
DMSO	100	30
Ethanol	50	20
Ethyl acetate		5
Methanol	50	30
NMP	100	
Toluene	50	
vitE/PG	200	

Notes: [a] vitE/PG 25% vitamin E TPGS/75% propylene glycol.
[b] 22% HPCD aqueous 22% w/v ß-hydroxypropylcyclodextrin in purified water.
[c] 10% CD aqueous 10% w/v sulfobutyl ether ß-cyclodextrin.
[d] NMP N-methyl-2-pyrrolidinone.

For *in vitro* studies, the test article is usually dispensed directly into a preweighed container and then a calculated volume of solvent is added to achieve the target concentration. Glass vials with a screw-top are generally the most practical because they avoid problems with static (which otherwise might causes inaccuracies in weighing), they can be resealed in the hood prior to reweighing, and they are compatible with all solvents. The solvent is added in measured and recorded increments until the test article is dissolved.

This method of formulation avoids wasting material because only the minimum amount used for dosing is needed and the material is formulated directly in the storage container. However, because the formulation is not brought to volume (e.g., in a volumetric flask or measuring cylinder), it introduces a small error because the final volume of the solution will be slightly more than the volume of solvent added. With concentrations more than 60 mg/mL (as is usually the case for mammalian cell tests using nonaqueous solvents), this error can be substantial; slightly less volume of solvent should be added to dissolve the material, and then the final volume should be measured using a variable micropipette before the solution is brought to volume. The theoretical density ("SG") of the dissolved material (typically approximately 3000 mg/mL) can then be calculated to facilitate future formulation.

If the test article is stored at low temperature, then it should be allowed to come to room temperature before dispensing to avoid condensation. Dissolution of the test article can be assisted by warming the mixture with the solvent in a water bath, vortex-mixing, or placing in a sonic bath, provided that this does not result in degradation.

The appearance of the formulation and the method of preparation should be recorded for future reference. To confirm that the material is truly in the solution, the mixture can be transferred to a flat-bottom multiwell plate and examined under an inverted phase-contrast microscope for the presence of insoluble material or centrifuged in a conical tube before examination for sedimentation.

3.6.4 Calculations and Checking: Small-Volume (In Vitro) Assays

The gross weight of the bulk test article should be recorded before and after removal of material for formulation. The difference in weight is expected to be very slightly more than the weight of material dispensed (e.g., there will be a slight loss on the spatula), but the apparent discrepancy should not exceed 5% of the total weight of material dispensed. The container to be used for formulation should be labeled and the gross weight recorded prior to and after addition of the test article (difference = net weight of test article) and then again after addition of the vehicle and dissolution. The net weight of the solvent divided by the specific gravity (SG; per the manufacturer's specification or the Merck index) should equal the stated volume of addition; for dilute aqueous vehicles, the SG can normally be assumed to be 1000 mg/mL. The final total volume of the formulation should be checked with a micropipette. The achieved values for these checks are expected to be within 5% of stated values under normal circumstances.

The volume of vehicle to be added to the test article is calculated as:

Weight of test article × purity ÷ correction for content ÷ target concentration
If there is no correction for purity or content, then those values are equal to 1 (and thus effectively ignored in the calculation). In the case when the final formulation concentration exceeds 60 mg/mL, we recommend you take into account the theoretical volume occupied by the dissolved test article so:
volume of vehicle = weight of test article × purity ÷ correction for content ÷ target concentration − weight of test article ÷ SG
(where SG is the notional/theoretical specific gravity of the test article determined in the solubility test, as described in the previous section.)

Examples

1. I need at least 6 mL of a 50 mg/mL stock solution of compound X in DMSO for use in a standard bacterial mutation test (top dose is 5 mg/plate using a dose volume of 100 μL/plate). If there were no correction for content or purity, then I weigh out just over 300 mg (I do not need to dispense an exact amount); in this case, I find I have added 305.0 mg of compound X, and then the required volume = 305.0 ÷ 300 = 6.1 mL DMSO. After this addition, I expect the weight of the container to increase by 6.1 × 1.100 (SG of DMSO in g/mL) = 6.71 g (±5%).

2. In the same example, the material is supplied as the hydrochloride, which has a molecular weight 1.05-times higher than the free base and contains 4% water. Because the protocol indicates that dosages should be expressed in terms of anhydrous free base, I need to prepare a stock solution at least 1.05×50 mg$\div 0.96 = 54.7$ mg/mL expressed in terms of material as supplied. So, I need to dispense at least 328 mg of material. After weighing, I find that I have added 340.1 mg of material to the formulation container, so I calculate that I need to add:

   340.1 mg $\times 0.96 \div 1.05 \div 50$ mg/mL $= 6.2$ mL (note that amounts are usually only expressed to an appropriate number of decimal places, dependant on the measuring device, although they do not need rounding in your calculation or spreadsheet).

   In this case, I expect the net weight of the solvent to be 6.8409 g ($\pm 5\%$).

3. I need 10.5 mL of a 200 mg/mL solution of the same hydrochloride solution for use in the mammalian cell mutation test $= 10.5$ mL of a 218.8 mg/mL (1.05×200 mg/mL$\div 0.96$) solution expressed in terms of material as supplied (i.e., I need at least 2297 mg of test article). Because the concentration (in terms of material as supplied) is more than 60 mg/mL, I expect the volume of the solute to make a significant contribution to the volume of the solution. I therefore need to make a correction for the notional SG of the compound, which in this example was determined to be 3.1 g/mL (3100 mg/mL) in the solubility test. In this case, I have dispensed 2330.1 mg of material so that:

   Calculated volume of DMSO $= 2330.1$ mg $\times 0.96 \div 1.05 \div 200$ mg/mL

   $- 2330.1$ mg/mL $\div 3100$ mg/mL $= 9.9$ mL.

   After adding 9.9 mL and dissolving the material, I check that the net weight of the solvent is within 5% of the target weight before measuring the total volume to confirm that it is close to 10.5 mL.

   Note that, for the purpose of calculation, you should ensure that the units (dimensions) are consistent throughout. These calculations can be quite complicated so it is best to enter the formulae into a spreadsheet that can be locked as part of an SOP for routine use. The calculations for preparation of stock solutions and dilution should be checked by a second person (ideally the scientist responsible for the study) prior to dosing.

3.6.5 Compatibility of Formulation with Culture Medium

Once an appropriate formulation has been achieved at the desired concentration in the solubility test, the formulation should be assessed for compatibility with the culture medium to be used in the mammalian cell test, if appropriate. The solubilized material is added to culture medium (complete with serum, if appropriate) in a volume calculated to reach the maximum recommended by the relevant ICH or OECD guideline(s) (e.g., 20 μL of a 200 mg/mL solution or 222 μL of a 20 mg/mL aqueous solution added to 2.0 mL medium in the well of a 24-well plate). An inverted microscope should be used to confirm the absence of precipitate and is especially useful at low concentrations, where precipitation might otherwise not be evident. Precipitation can take many forms, including cloudiness, crystallization, and formation of a film on the surface of the medium. Note that excessive precipitation should be avoided in mammalian cell tests because precipitate is often carried over after the exposure period and can result in toxicity or interfere with the quality of slide preparations.

If a significant change in the color of culture medium occurs indicating a significant shift in pH, then the stock formulation should be neutralized by addition of an equivalent amount of alkaline or acid and the dose volume should be adjusted as necessary to avoid irrelevant toxicity that might mask genotoxicity or genotoxic effects as a result of stress [10,11]. Although older guidelines and articles refer to the potential effect of dose solutions on osmolality, osmolarity, or tonicity [12,13], the current specified limits described by ICH and OECD do not have any significant impact on the osmolality of the culture medium. Culture medium is approximately 300 mOs/kg, which is approximately equivalent to 300 mM glucose or 150 mM sodium chloride. Osmolality is proportionate to the same number of particles in solution (i.e., molecules or ions in the case of covalent or ionic compounds, respectively).

Example

The solubility of compound X was evaluated in a range of solvents; it showed low solubility in water (much less than 0.1 mg/mL), was just soluble at 100 mg/mL in DMSO, and showed lower solubility in other water-miscible solvents evaluated, including methanol, acetone, and dimethyl formamide. Therefore, DMSO was chosen as an appropriate solvent for use in the bacterial mutation test, where the standard limit dose of 5 mg/plate could be achieved using a dose volume of 100 µL of a 50 mg/mL solution.

Because Compound X was also to be tested in the *in vitro* chromosome aberration test, the compatibility of DMSO solutions of X was assessed in RPMI culture medium complete with serum (i.e., the culture medium that would be used in the test) as recorded in the table below. Culture medium was added in 2 mL aliquots to each of the 10 wells (numbered 1−10) of a 24-well microplate. A substantial amount of precipitation was seen after addition of 20 µL of the 100 mg/mL stock solution to 2.0 mL culture medium, so 10-fold and 100-fold dilutions of the stock solution were evaluated in the same way. Because precipitation was seen with the 10 mg/mL solution but not the 1 mg/mL solution, an intermediate concentration was also evaluated. The pH of wells showing any apparent change in medium indicator color was measured. The plate was then incubated under the same conditions to be used for the subsequent chromosome aberration test to confirm that there was no change in solubility. Based on these observations, a top dose level of 2560 µg X per mL in culture medium was selected because this would show some precipitation in the culture medium (saturated solution to maximize exposure to the test article). Lower concentrations separated by an interval of two were also evaluated to ensure the dose range included at least one or two doses showing little or no toxicity.

Test Item: X   **Phase: Compatibility with culture medium**   **Vehicle: DMSO**   **Reference no.: 12345**

											Init.	Date			

Medium type (complete) RPMI   **Special instructions:** None

Micropipette ID TI-234

pH meter ID TI-456   0 | Pre-incubation   Post-incubation

Well no.	Culture vol Q mL	Dose vol. R mL	Dilution factor S = Q / R	Volume for dilutions mL — Formulation	vehicle	Formulation conc. T µg/mL	Final conc. T/S µg/mL	Medium color (Pre)	pH† (Pre)	observations (Pre)	Medium color (Post)	pH† (Post)	observations (Post)
1	2.0	0.020	100	–	–	100000	1000	orange	6.8	ppt	N	ND	ppt
2	2.0	0.020	100	0.100	0.900	10000	100	red/orange	6.9	ppt	N	ND	ppt
3	2.0	0.020	100	0.010	0.990	1000	10.0	N	ND	N	N	ND	–
4	2.0	0.020	100	0.025	0.975	2500	25	N	ND	sl. ppt	N	ND	sl. ppt
5													
6													
7													
8													
9													
10													

Init./Date: Init./Date

Key:
† measured if change in indicator color
N normal, ND not determined
ppt precipitate, sl. ppt slight precipitate

Reviewed by/date:

3.7 Formulation of Dose Solutions

Test article is usually dispensed in a powder containment cabinet (or, in the case of volatiles, in a fume hood). Clean or aseptic technique is used throughout. Formulations are prepared and diluted in the powder containment cabinet or a class 2B biological containment cabinet. The stock formulation is prepared by combining the test article with the vehicle, often at the concentration required by the high dose level (e.g., typically 50,000 µg/mL in the case of a bacterial mutation test using a dose volume of 100 µL per plate).

Suggested steps in preparation of solutions and all formulations for use in genotoxicity tests are outlined here. Although the procedural checks may seem lengthy at first glance, they minimize the chance of errors in the formulation and standardize routine calculations.

1. All formulation containers and any vials used for sampling them should be sterile (in the case of *in vitro* tests and for nonoral dosing in the case of *in vivo* studies) and uniquely identified with details of their contents (study number, date, compound name, and concentration). It is often convenient to assign code names or abbreviations to compounds and numbered dose levels (rather than absolute concentrations) for documentation and labeling—these codes should be explained in the formulation records. The stock (usually the high dose level) formulation and dilutions are usually prepared in a suitable glass bottle/vial of adequate volume to accommodate the subsequent formulation.

2. Prior to formulation, two appropriate aliquots of the vehicle should be removed. One of these is the vehicle control and should be set aside (after sampling, if required) to avoid potential contamination. The second aliquot is dispensed in appropriate volumes into the vials for subsequent preparation of lower dose levels by direct dilution from the stock test article formulation.

3. The test article container should be allowed to come to room temperature and then the gross weight should be recorded in the utilization log.

4. The gross weight of the stock formulation vial is measured and recorded.

5. A stainless-steel spatula of a suitable size is wiped with a medical wipe that has been made wet with 70% alcohol (ethanol or isopropanol, 2-propanol). The spatula is used to transfer approximately the minimum required amount of test article to the stock formulation vial. The vial is recapped and weighed to determine the net weight of test article.

6. If less than the required amount of material has been dispensed, then an additional amount is added as noted and the vial is reweighed.

7. The test article container is reweighed and the weight is recorded in the utilization log as a double-check of the amount of material dispensed. The weight of material used should be similar or slightly more than the net weight of material dispensed; any departure from this due to spillage should be recorded in the formulation record.

8. The required calculated volume of vehicle is added and the vial is reweighed to determine the net weight of vehicle added. A gravimetric check of this addition is performed using the formula:

   $(FN - N + W) + (TV \times SGV) + 1000$

   Where:

   FN = Final gross weight of formulation vial

   N + W = Weight of container + test article

   TV = Total volume of vehicle added

   SGV = Specific gravity of vehicle

9. The stock formulation should be mixed until dissolved or (in the case of suspensions) apparently homogenous. Vortex mixing, warming in a water bath, or placing in a sonic bath may be used to enhance dissolution, in which case the details should be recorded. If a stock solution is not expected to be sterile (e.g., in the case of a biological material obtained by fermentation), then it should be filtered/sterilized at this point.

10. All lower-dose formulations are prepared by direct dilution from this stock followed by mixing. When the range of concentrations is very wide, it may be appropriate to prepare the lowest dose levels by dilution from an intermediate dose level. Note that serial dilution is best avoided because this results in compound error, which is especially marked in the case of suspensions.

11. If chemical analysis of formulations is required, then any analytical and retention samples are aliquoted into labeled sterile containers at this point. Because these samples will be transferred to another laboratory or facility, labeling should be comprehensive and include (as a minimum) the study number, test material name, concentration, preparation and sampling dates, volume, site of sample (top, middle, or bottom) in the case of suspensions, and storage conditions. The samples should be accompanied by a form that is used to record the chain of custody. We recommend taking analytical samples in duplicate with back-up (retention) samples taken in triplicate, especially for suspension formulations. The analytical samples will be sent to the analytical laboratory and the back-up samples should be retained by the formulating laboratory for potential analysis (e.g., in case of loss or degradation during transfer or for confirmatory testing in the event of unexpected analytical results for the main samples).

12. The retention samples may be discarded following confirmation of acceptable results of the main samples.

In the Formulation Instruction/Record Sheet, appropriate details have been entered in advance by the responsible scientist. Additional entries made at the time of formulation are entered in the grey cells:

Example Formulation Sheet

Phase: Main Test   **Study No.: ABC 123**
Special instructions: Samples req., take vehicle samples before weighing out compound.

Test Item:	**TI X**	**Vehicle:**	**Dimethyl sulfoxide**
Lot:	**A345**	Abbreviation:	DMSO
Appearance:	**White powder**	Supplier:	
Purity/corr. factor:	**1.0**	Lot no.:	
Theoretical SG:	**Not applicable**	Expiry date:	

Balance ID	Micropipette IDs

Storage:
Appearance:
Specific gravity **SGV**:   **1.10**

Preparation Stock 50 mg/mL DN8

Net weight vial **N mg**

Minimum weight of TI required (in mg) =   **600**   Weight TI **W mg**:

Vol. DMSO to add in mL = mg of TI ÷   **50.0**   Vol vehicle **V mL**

Target final volume (mL):   = W ÷ 50

Measured volume (mL):   must be between 95% and 105% of target

Final wt of vial with TI + vehicle, **FN mg**:

Check, **(FN-N-W) / (TV × SGV) /1000**   must be between 0.95 and 1.05

Appearance of DN8

Dose No.	Formulation conc µg/mL	Vol vehicle mL	Vol DN8 mL	Total mL	*Appearance**
7	15800	6.5	3.00	9.5	
6	5000	8.6	0.950	9.5	
5	1580	9.2	0.300	9.5	
4	500	9.4	0.095	9.5	
3	158	9.5	0.030	9.5	
2	50	9.5	0.0095	9.5	
1	15.8	25.0	0.0079	9.5	

Performed by/date:

* Color and description for stock, description only for dilutions:
CL (clear liquid), SUS (suspension) or if other then describe

All formulations & vehicle prepared in glass vials
& stored RT/Dark for 1 day init./date

Storage ID:

Residual formulations discarded, init./date:

Comments:

3.8 Formulation of Bulk Formulations

In the case of *in vivo* studies where formulations are usually prepared in relatively large volume, it may be easier to bring the formulation to volume in a calibrated vessel (e.g., a measuring cylinder or a calibrated beaker). However, in the case of suspensions especially, there may be some loss of material due to adherence to the measuring vessel, in which case additional precautions may be needed to ensure quantitative transfer of the test article to the final formulation container. For animal studies using suspensions, each dose level is generally prepared independently because of potential error due to adherence of the test article to formulating vessels if prepared by dilution.

If the positive control formulations for *in vivo* studies are prepared by the central pharmacy, then they should follow a protocol (SOP) appropriate for cytotoxic drugs that has been reviewed by the responsible genetic toxicology scientist for safety and accuracy reasons. Some agents (e.g., mitomycin C) are supplied in prealiquoted injectable vials that should be reconstituted by addition of an appropriate volume of solvent and do not require weighing out, thus reducing the chance of error and chemical contamination.

3.9 Formulation of Suspensions

The vehicle for formulation of emulsions (liquid in liquid preparations) may involve a combination of an aqueous suspending agent with a surfactant (emulsifying agent). Emulsions can usually be prepared and diluted, if necessary, in the same way as solutions provided that appropriate procedures are in place to ensure homogeneity (e.g., by mixing using a high-shear homogenizer at the time of preparation). Some emulsions may be unstable and separate ("crack") prior to dosing unless stirred continually. If a cracked emulsion cannot be resuspended by simple methods (e.g., multiple in version of the container) at the time of dosing, then it would normally be considered an inappropriate formulation.

In the case of solid test articles, the material must be a finely ground powder with no large particulate present. If this is not the case, then the test article will need to be ground prior to formulation. This can be done using a ball mill or a mortar and pestle.

3.9.1 Aqueous Suspending Agents

The most common suspending agents are aqueous biological polymers, including methylcellulose (MC), sodium carboxymethylcellulose (CMC), and hydroxypropylmethylcellulose (HPMC). A range of viscosities of suspending agents is available with different molecular weights. In particular, aqueous 1% w/v MC 400 cP has many of the characteristics of an ideal vehicle:

1. Clear, colorless
2. Ideal viscosity; the most commonly used MC has a dynamic viscosity of 400 cP (centipoise) at 2% w/v in water; in comparison, water has a viscosity of approximately 1 cP at room temperature
3. Biologically inert
4. Easily sterilized
5. Not ionic
6. Can be used in combination with surfactants such as Tween 80 to improve wetting and enhance physical stability
7. Is suitable for use in long-term studies
8. Is chemically defined
9. Does not interfere with chemical analysis

Aq. 1% w/v MC can be prepared as follows:

1. Add the required amount of UPW into an appropriate glass Erlenmeyer flask with a stir bar
2. Heat the water until boiling
3. Remove from the heat and allow to cool for 5 min
4. While stirring rapidly, add the appropriate amount of methyl cellulose 400 cPs *gradually* to avoid boil out
5. Transfer the solution and stir bar to a glass bottle with a capacity of twice the volume of the MC and loosely tighten the cap
6. Autoclave the solution at 121°C, 15 psi for 20 min
7. After sterilization, remove the bottle(s) from the autoclave and stir until cold
8. Label the bottle appropriately and store refrigerated
9. Assign an expiration date of 3 months, but note that aq. MC is subject to fungal growth, so any residual amount should be discarded after use

As an alternative to these types of suspending agents, aqueous solutions of ambiphilic cyclodextrins can be used to solubilize hyrophobic compounds. These are occasionally used in toxicology studies and will probably become more widely used in the future.

3.9.2 Large Volume Suspensions

Suggested steps in formulation of large-volume suspensions of a powder in an aqueous suspending agent, as commonly needed for *in vivo* studies, are outlined here.

1. The appropriate amount of test article is dispensed onto a weighing boat (or paper) and then transferred to a mortar. Enough vehicle is added to the weighing boat to wash out any residual test article and is combined with the test article in the mortar. The test article and vehicle are mixed by grinding using a pestle. Additional vehicle is added to form a paste and grinding is continued until a smooth paste is formed. This process is referred to as "trituration" and not only mixes the materials without caking but also helps to reduce the size of aggregates and larger crystals to improve homogeneity.

2. The final required volume of the formulation (weight of test article ÷ required concentration) is calculated and then this volume of purified water is added to a clean glass beaker. The beaker is placed on a level surface and the level of the bottom of the meniscus is marked on the side of the beaker using a marker pen. The water is discarded and the beaker is dried.

3. The paste is transferred to the calibrated beaker and then additional aliquots of the vehicle are added to the mortar and pestle to wash any residual test article into the beaker.

4. Once a sufficient volume of vehicle has been added to reach the calibration mark on the side of the beaker, following gravimetric check if appropriate, the formulation is mixed thoroughly using a high-shear homogenizer (e.g., Polytron, Silverson, or Ultra-Turrax) fitted with a probe of an appropriate size.

5. The mixture is transferred to a labeled clean glass container with a sealable lid. The formulation will usually contain a large number of small bubbles that disappear over time or can be removed by placing the formulation briefly under vacuum.

6. The formulation should be checked for dosability by passing a part through the system that will be used for dosing (e.g., usually a cannula or injection needle in the case of animals studies). If the suspension is not fine enough, then it will either block the cannula or lead to formation of aggregates.

7. Typically, suspensions are stored (often refrigerated) prior to and between use, which helps maintain chemical stability and minimize any microbial growth. During this time, most suspensions will settle and solid material will aggregate ("cake") on the bottom of the storage container. Therefore, any such caked material should be thoroughly dispersed by multiple inversion and gentle shaking. Once dispersed, homogeneity should be maintained by continual shaking, multiple inversion, or stirring on a stir plate.

8. Care should be taken to avoid introduction of bubbles into the formulation just prior to use. If maintained on a stir plate, then it may still be necessary to invert the container several times prior to stirring if solid material is seen to accumulate around the lower inside edge of the formulation container.

3.9.3 Small Volume Suspensions

Very occasionally, for *in vitro* studies where a compatible solvent cannot be found, it may be necessary to formulate the material as a suspension. If the material is in the form of a homogenous fine powder with lumps or large crystals, then it can usually be formulated in a manner similar to that of small-volume solutions. To ensure homogeneity prior to use, the formulation should be thoroughly dispersed by multiple passage into a syringe fitted with an 18-G needle and then, ideally, into a syringe fitted with a 19-G or 20-G needle. If the formulation does not readily pass through the needle, then additional actions will be needed to reduce the particulate size and avoid formation of aggregates, including grinding and use of a high-shear homogenizer.

Small-volume suspensions should be thoroughly dispersed by vortex mixing and multiple inversion prior to and during sampling and/or dosing to ensure homogeneity.

3.10 Chemical Analysis and Stability

As per GLP guidelines, each test article mixed with a vehicle must be tested by appropriate validated analytical methods to determine the stability of the test article in the mixture under the conditions of storage and use in the study. This can be done either before study initiation or concomitantly. Formulations should be tested to confirm achieved concentration; additionally, suspensions should be tested for homogeneity and physical stability. Sample volumes should be representative and should not exceed those used for dosing on the study. The volumes of material involved can be substantial and must be taken into account when calculating test article and formulation requirements. If the decision is made to not include formulation analysis in the study, then this should be mentioned in the final report as a deviation to GLP. In that case, it is particularly important to describe any other factors that support achieving appropriate levels in the test system, including precipitate and signs of toxicity. A typical approach to chemical analysis is described here.

1. Development of the analytical method is necessarily non-GLP and is usually performed at the very start of the toxicology program. Ideally, the method should be specific, sensitive, robust, and reliable and should show a dose-proportionate response (linearity) over a reasonable concentration range.
2. The analytical method validation is used to confirm the suitability of the analytical method over the required concentration range for each of the formulations needed. Reliability and procedural recovery should be established at this point. The analytical method will then be used to confirm chemical stability of formulations over the period of storage and use and, in the case of suspensions, their homogeneity and physical stability. The validation should support the full range of concentrations being used in all of the studies. In the case of suspension formulations, the method will then be used

to confirm that the formulation method produces appropriately homogenous and physically stable formulations. It is therefore vital for the study scientist to communicate directly with the analytical chemist to ensure all required aspects are covered; otherwise, additional validation work (involving additional costs) will be required later. The validation should cover expected storage and use conditions (e.g., refrigerated and room temperature). The results of analysis at time zero are compared with analyses at periodic intervals after preparation (e.g., 48 h, 7, 14, and 28 days). In the case of suspensions, appropriate procedures are used to resuspend the material (e.g., multiple inversion followed by continuous stirring prior to and during sampling).

3. Duplicate samples are normally required for chemical analysis of solutions. One of these is subjected to analysis while the second acts as a backup in case of technical problems.

4. In the case of suspensions, samples are collected from the top, middle, and bottom of the formulation. Ideally, the sample size should be representative of the volume being dosed, and five samples should be collected at each level. Two of these are subjected to analysis while the remaining triplicate samples act as backup in case of problems with the initial analysis (e.g., loss or degradation of original samples, suspected technical error during original analysis, etc.).

5. The number, volume, net weight, and location of all samples should be recorded. The net weight of suspension samples should be used to confirm that the sample volume was accurate. Main samples should be sent to the analytical laboratory (which can often be at a different facility/site) with a copy of the formulation and sample details, whereas the backup samples should be retained in the formulation laboratory to minimize the potential impact of loss or deterioration of samples during transport. Again, it is important for the Study Director to communicate directly with the analytical chemist (designated as Principal Investigator in the case when the analysis is performed off-site) whose contact details should be included in the protocol. The analytical chemist should be sent copies of the protocol and any amendments.

6. If chemical analysis of formulations has demonstrated adequate stability of formulations, then *it is highly recommended* that formulations should be prepared in advance of use and chemical analysis should be used to confirm their suitability confirmed prior to dosing. This will minimize the chance of rejection of part of the study and, in the case of *in vivo* studies, waste of animals.

7. Suspension samples should be diluted in their entirety rather than subsampled to avoid procedural loss.

8. In the case that an Out of Specification (OOS) result is obtained following dose samples analysis, an investigation should be initiated and recorded. Following the completion of the investigation, the Study Director should decide and document an appropriate course of action.

Compatibility of the formulation with storage containers and administration devices (e.g., infusion lines) should be established prior to the study. For infusion studies in particular, especially at low concentrations, it may be necessary to flush the system with the formulation or increase the concentration of the formulation above nominal to ensure the final required concentration is achieved.

Example of a sampling form

Test Item:		Phase: Main	Vehicle: DMSO	Study/Reference no.:	Init./date
Mix formulations by multiple inversion then using a stir bar prior to sampling.					
Analytical samples					—
Vehicle:	2 × 1.00 mL	Remove into glass vials.			
Doses	1 to 10:	Remove 1 × 500 µL sample(s) into glass vials.			
Leave the samples alongside the formulations until the end of dosing.					
Store samples in the formulation laboratory at RT/Dark until shipment. Storage ID:_____					
Ship analysis samples at ambient/Dark to the attention of PI (see protocol).					
Retention samples					—
Vehicle:	2 × 1.00 mL	Remove into glass vials.			
Doses	1 to 10:	Remove 1 × 0.5 mL sample(s) into glass vials			
Leave the samples alongside the formulations until the end of dosing.					
Store retention samples in formulation laboratory at RT/Dark until authorization to discard is obtained from SD. Storage ID:_____					
Sample(s) IDs:_____ transferred for analysis as indicated for analysis samples. Indicate N/R if not required:					
Comments:					
Form prepared					
Form verified					
Form reviewed & approved					
SD approval to discard backup samples					
Backup samples discarded					

References

[1] Power LA, Polovich M. Safe handling of hazardous drugs: reviewing standards for worker protection. Pharmacy Practice News (special edition) 2014;41:51–62. Available from URL: <http://pharmacypracticenews.com/ViewArticle.aspx?d = Special%2bEdition%2b%2f%2b Educational%2bReviews&d_id=63&i=November + 2014&i_id=1118&a_id=28619>.

[2] Health Canada. Carcinogens, mutagens, teratogens and reproductive toxins. Available from URL: <http://www.hc-sc.gc.ca/ewh-semt/occup-travail/whmis-simdut/carcino-eng.php>; 2006.

[3] UK Health and Safety Executive. Safe handling of cytotoxic drugs in the workplace. Available from URL: <http://www.hse.gov.uk/healthservices/safe-use-cytotoxic-drugs.htm>.

[4] DiBerardinis LJ, Baum JS, First MW, Gatwood GT, Seth AK. Guidelines for laboratory design: health, safety, and environmental considerations. 4th ed. New Jersey: Wiley; 2013.

[5] United States Department of Labor. Hazard prevention and control. Available from URL: <https://www.osha.gov/SLTC/etools/safetyhealth/comp3.html>.

[6] TSI. Laboratory design handbook, TSI incorporated. Available from URL: <http://www.tsi.com/ SiteSearch.aspx?searchText = Laboratory%20Design%20Handbook>; 2013.

[7] Furr AK. CRC handbook of laboratory safety. 5th ed. Boca Raton: CRC Press LLC; 2000.

[8] International Conference on Harmonisation of Technical Requirements for Registration of Pharmaceuticals for Human Use (ICH) S2(R1) Guidance on Genotoxicity Testing and Data Interpretation for Pharmaceuticals Intended for Human Use. Available from URL: <http://www.ich.org/products/guidelines/ safety/safety-single/article/guidance-on-genotoxicity-testing-and-data-interpretation-for-pharmaceuticals- intended-for-human-use.html>.

[9] Maron D, Katzenellenbogen J, Ames BN. Compatibility of organic solvents with the Salmonella/microsome test. Mutat Res 1981;88(4):343–50.

[10] Brusick D. Genotoxic effects in cultured mammalian cells produced by low pH treatment conditions and increased ion concentrations. Environ Mutagen 1986;8(6):879–86.

[11] Morita T, Nagaki T, Fukuda I, Okumura K. Clastogenicity of low pH to various cultured mammalian cells. Mutat Res 1992;268(2):297–305.

[12] Brusick DJ. Implications of treatment-condition-induced genotoxicity for chemical screening and data interpretation. Mutat Res 1987;189(1):1–6.

[13] Scott D, Galloway SM, Marshall RR, Ishidate Jr M, Brusick D, Ashby J, et al. Genotoxicity under extreme culture conditions. A report from ICPEMC Task Group 9. Mutat Res 1999;257(2):147–204.

The Bacterial Reverse Mutation Test

Annie Hamel[1], Marise Roy[1] and Ray Proudlock[2]

[1]Department of Genetic Toxicology, Charles River Laboratories, Montreal, ULC, Canada
[2]Boone, North Carolina, USA

Chapter Outline

4.1 Introduction 80
4.2 History 80
4.3 Fundamentals 83
4.4 Equipment 84
4.5 Consumables 85
4.6 Reagents and Recipes 86
   4.6.1 Ampicillin 2 µg/disc 87
   4.6.2 Biotin 0.37 mg/mL 87
   4.6.3 Crystal Violet 5 µg/disc 87
   4.6.4 Glucose 0.4 g/mL 87
   4.6.5 G6P 1M: Glucose-6-Phosphate 88
   4.6.6 HBT: 500 µM Histidine, 500 µM Biotin, 500 µM Tryptophan Solution 88
   4.6.7 Histidine HCl.H₂O 5 mg/mL 88
   4.6.8 KMg 88
   4.6.9 MGA Plates 88
   4.6.10 Minimal Glucose Master (MGM, MGMA and MGMAT) Plates 89
   4.6.11 NADP 0.1 M 90
   4.6.12 Nutrient Agar Plates 90
   4.6.13 Nutrient Broth 90
   4.6.14 Phosphate Buffer 0.2 M pH 7.4 90
   4.6.15 Positive Control and Diagnostic Mutagen Solutions 90
   4.6.16 S9 Fraction 91
   4.6.17 S9 Mix 91
   4.6.18 Tetracycline 1 µg/disc 92
   4.6.19 Top Agar Incomplete: TAI 92
   4.6.20 Top Agar Complete: TAC 92
   4.6.21 Tryptophan 5 mg/mL 93
   4.6.22 VB Salts 50×: Vogel-Bonner Salts 93
4.7 Suggested Phases in Development of the Test 93
4.8 The Bacterial Strains 94
   4.8.1 Genotypes of Routinely Used Strains 95
   4.8.2 Obtaining the Tester Strains 95

Genetic Toxicology Testing.
DOI: http://dx.doi.org/10.1016/B978-0-12-800764-8.00004-5

4.8.3 Receipt of Bacterial Strains   96

4.8.4 Phenotyping of New Isolates   98

4.8.5 Freezing of Selected Isolates   100

4.8.6 Diagnostic Mutagen Test   101

4.9 Routine Testing   105

4.9.1 Designing a Study   105

    4.9.1.1 Metabolic activation system   106

4.9.2 Test Article Considerations   106

    4.9.2.1 Solvent selection   109

    4.9.2.2 Dose volumes   109

    4.9.2.3 Dose levels   109

4.9.3 Positive Controls   113

4.10 Standard Test Procedures   114

4.10.1 Plate Incorporation Method   114

4.10.2 Preincubation Method   115

4.10.3 Standard Study Design   116

4.10.4 Examination of the Plates   118

4.10.5 Interpretation of Results   119

    4.10.5.1 Evaluation of toxicity   119

    4.10.5.2 Validity of the study   119

    4.10.5.3 Criteria for negative/positive/equivocal outcome   120

    4.10.5.4 Unexpected and borderline results   121

4.10.6 Presentation of Results   121

4.10.7 Testing of Volatile and Gaseous Compounds   125

4.11 Screening Tests   126

4.11.1 Simplified Test Systems   126

4.11.2 Screening Tests Using Standard Tester Strains   127

4.11.3 Reduced Format Tests Using Standard Tester Strains   129

4.12 Appendix 1: Growing and Monitoring Suspension Cultures   130

References   134

4.1 Introduction

Bacterial genetic toxicity tests fall into three main categories: back/reverse mutation singular, forward mutation, and DNA repair deficiency systems. Those that detect back mutations (reversion of a point mutation) are the only ones in widespread use and that are generally acceptable for regulatory submissions.

4.2 History

Originally, studies used mutagenic compounds to study the biochemical basis of mutation and to elucidate the structure and organization of the gene. The first demonstration of chemical induction of mutation was described by Auerbach and Robson in 1944 [1] and involved production of mutations and chromosomal aberrations in *Drosophila* using mustard gas and related compounds. Demerec [2] showed that various carcinogenic polyaromatic hydrocarbons also induced mutations in *Drosophila*. Perhaps realizing the simplicity, enhanced sensitivity, and rapidity (based on population size and shorter generation time) of microbial systems, Witkin began work on chemically induced mutation to phage resistance in *Escherichia coli* [3]. Soon afterward, Demerec et al. developed a more practical system quantifying back-mutation from streptomycin dependence to independence in *E. coli* [4,5]. Dependent cells could divide a few times in the absence of streptomycin, allowing a chance for back-mutation (reversion) to streptomycin independence, consequently allowing their growth into visible colonies. Szybalski [6] screened more than 400 chemicals using a variation of Demerec's plate-test method in which the chemical was applied on a filter-paper disk (i.e. a spot test). Ironically, Szybalski was screening for potential antitumor agents as opposed to chemicals that might cause cancer; the test was not particularly successful, probably because it relied on a very specific base-pair reversion at a particular location of the gene, required diffusion of the test substance through the agar, and did not allow for mammalian metabolism.

The *E. coli* mutation system commonly in use today, requiring an auxotrophic trpA mutation to L-tryptophan independence, was originally conceived by Yanofsky et al. [7], and use of the WP2 strain to quantify mutagenesis was described by Hill [8]. The trpA gene is a part of the trp operon and codes for the tryptophan synthetase α chain. The strains used in routine mutation tests generally detect base-pair but not frameshift mutations. These can occur at the site of the original mutation or at a more distant site, which suppresses the original defect. The strains currently used are derived from *E. coli* B and have an incomplete lipopolysaccharide cell wall making them permeable to larger molecules [9]. To some extent, the *E. coli* strains may be considered complementary to the *Salmonella* tester strains described here and are generally used in conjunction with them [10].

The strains constructed by Ames and his colleagues at the University of California in Berkeley were derived from *Salmonella typhimurium* (the causative agent in mouse typhoid fever and a variant of the species *Salmonella enterica*) strain LT2 and were originally used to study genetic aspects of L-histidine synthesis. Mutants were selected based on sensitivity to chemically induced mutation and their relatively low spontaneous mutation frequencies. The mutations in the histidine operon are situated at hotspots that are particularly sensitive to reversion by certain classes of genotoxins, allowing detection of a wide range of chemically induced base-pair substitution and frameshift mutations. The first use of *Salmonella* histidine−requiring mutants to test for mutagenicity involved the carcinogenic methylating agent, cycasin (methylazoxymethanol glucoside), a carcinogen found in some cycad species [11]. The sensitivity of the strains subsequently selected for routine testing was enhanced by deletion of the enzyme responsible for the first step in error-free excision repair (uvrB) and, in the case of the R-factor (pKM101 plasmid) strains, incorporation of the SOS mutagenesis gene umuD (coding for a subunit of DNA polymerase V), which promotes error-prone translesion synthesis. The uptake of large and hydrophobic molecules was enhanced by selection of strains with a deep rough (rfa) mutation that leads to incomplete formation of the smooth outer membrane and associated capsule coating the surface of the bacterium [9]. These strains may be supplemented by a strain with intact excision repair systems (most commonly TA102) so that cross-linking agents such as mitomycin C (which is lethal to excision repair–deficient strains) can be detected.

Xenobiotic metabolic systems that are present in mammals, but not bacteria, are often required for conversion of mammalian mutagens to their ultimate active form. These indirect mutagens could be detected in host-mediated assays in which the test organism was injected into the animal (often intraperitoneally in mouse), recovered, and plated a few hours after treatment of the animal with the chemical [12]. However, recovery was variable and the system was laborious and not very sensitive. Malling [13] used a mouse liver microsomal fraction to convert dimethylnitrosamine to a bacterial mutagen. Bruce Ames successfully adapted Malling's metabolic system using human and phenobarbital or methylcholanthrene-induced rat liver S9 (named after the supernatant postmitochondrial fraction after centrifugation at 9000 g) microsomal preparation with cofactors [14]. In this case, the chemical was mixed with the top agar and bacteria prior to plating to establish the standard plate incorporation bacterial reverse mutation test still in general use today. An important variation of this system for detection of short-lived reactive metabolites involves preincubation of the growing test organisms in the liquid phase with the test material and S9 while shaking before plating. Bartsch et al. [15] used the preincubation system to demonstrate mutagenicity of the dialkylnitrosamines. *Salmonella* strain TA1530 was plated in parallel in selective and survival media, so that mutation frequency could be estimated as in the treat and plate method described later; subsequently, mutagenicity was demonstrated in the same system with strain TA1535. Yahagi et al. [16] used TA98 and TA100 to demonstrate mutagenicity of a range of N-nitrosamines using a preincubation method; interestingly, DMSO (dimethyl sulfoxide, the most widely used organic solvent in mutagenicity testing) inhibited the activity of dimethylnitrosamine and diethylnitrosamine. The preincubation method described by Yahagi et al. and the plate incorporation method versions of the pour plate method are generally the only systems considered acceptable for general regulatory submission. A variation of the preincubation method referred to as "treat and plate" involves removal of the test agent after the preincubation period, and is used where the test agent shows very strong antibacterial activity in preliminary testing. Most regulatory bodies require adherence of testing to OECD guideline 471 [17], which implies that confirmation of "negative results" (i.e., apparent absence of mutagenicity of the test material) is expected. Therefore, the plate incorporation and preincubation methods are often used in tandem or in sequence to provide a complete study. In contrast, a recent revision of ICH guidance that covers testing of pharmaceuticals in the United States, Europe, Japan, and

Canada indicates that a single method and occasion of testing is acceptable when a clear result is obtained [18]. Other bacterial mutation and related methods are available (e.g., liquid fluctuation, spot and spiral plate, differential killing/repair tests), but these do not necessarily meet ICH or OECD criteria and are not recommended for regulatory submission or routine use except when required by specific regulations.

4.3 Fundamentals

The bacterial reverse mutation test detects point mutations, which are the cause of many human genetic diseases and play an important role in tumor initiation and development. The strains have various mutations that inactivate a gene involved in the synthesis of an essential amino acid, either histidine (*Salmonella*) or tryptophan (*E. coli*), so they can only grow in culture medium that is supplemented with that amino acid. When the bacteria are exposed to a mutagen, mutation(s) occur that may restore/reverse the ability of the bacteria to synthesize the amino acid and to continue growth once the limited amount of the amino acid in the top agar is depleted. Relevant mutations involve substitution of individual base pairs or frameshift mutations caused by addition or deletion of a stretch of DNA.

In the plate incorporation method, top agar, the test article formulation, the metabolic activation system or equivalent buffer, and the bacteria are mixed together before pouring onto semi-solid minimal medium containing glucose in a Petri dish/plate. The metabolic activation system usually consists of liver fraction (obtained from rats pretreated/induced by treatment with a chemical) supplemented with appropriate cofactors and is referred to as S9 mix or, more often, simply as S9. The top agar is allowed to set, then the plates are inverted and incubated at 37°C for approximately 65 h before examination. The top agar contains enough of the required amino acid to allow a few bacterial divisions before the amino acid is exhausted, giving rise to millions of microscopic bacterial colonies that give a hazy appearance to the medium referred to as a background lawn. Any preexisting revertants and those bacteria that mutate back (revert) to histidine or tryptophan independence continue to grow, forming macroscopic revertant colonies. A test material formulation that causes a substantial increase in the revertant colony count is regarded as a bacterial mutagen. Usually, increases are dose-proportionate (dose-related; Figure 4.1), but precipitation, toxicity, and limitations on metabolic conversion can have profound effects on the shape of the dose-response curve. The response can be generally linear at low doses, but some compounds such as the interchelating agent 9-aminoacridine show a very steep dose-response curve leading a narrow mutagenic window.

A common variation of the plate incorporation method, the preincubation method, involves incubation of a mixture of the liquid bacterial culture with test article and buffer or S9 mix with shaking for a period of usually 20 or 30 min prior to plating. Because the bacteria are beginning

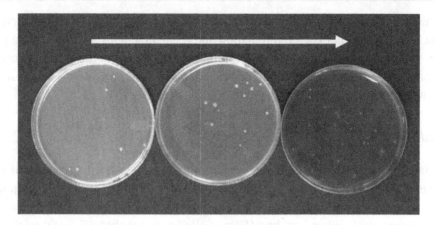

Figure 4.1
Dose-related increase in revertants.

to grow during this relatively high exposure period, and because the test chemical is present at a relatively high concentration, this method can be more sensitive to some classes of mutagen, such as those with short-lived metabolites and volatile agents. In particular, it is usually more appropriate to test short-chain aliphatic nitrosamines, divalent metals, aldehydes, azo-dyes and diazo-compounds, pyrollizidine alkaloids, allyl compounds, and nitro compounds using the preincubation method. However, the preincubation method can be more prone to toxic effects because of the higher test chemical concentration and therefore less sensitive to some chemicals [19]. Both methods use standard 90–100 mm diameter Petri dishes; either and sometimes both methods are generally used in regulatory submissions.

4.4 Equipment

The following is a list of specialized equipment expected to be found in a laboratory performing tests on a routine basis:

- Agar dispensing pump + foot switch + sterile silicon tubing
- Autoclave
- Automatic colony counter with direct data capture system
- Bacterial counting chamber
- Biological containment cabinet class II (externally vented)
- Boiling water bath or microwave
- General laboratory equipment: balances, refrigerator, purified water
- Heating block 45°C
- Incubator 37°C
- Liquid nitrogen cell store or ultralow ($\leq$70°C) freezer

- Microscope(s), ideally a phase contrast for counting bacteria and an inverted for examination of bacterial growth on plates (background lawn)
- Micropipettes (adjustable, repeating, and positive displacement types; range, 2–1000 μL)
- Pipette aids
- Shaker (platform type) or shaking incubator
- Spectrometer or nephelometer
- UV lamp
- Water bath 45°C

4.5 Consumables

Consumables typically used in a testing laboratory (sterile where appropriate) include:

- Bacterial tester strains
- Bacteriological plastic loops
- Crystal violet, ampicillin, and tetracycline in discs or as stock solutions
- Culture flasks
- Disposable bacteriological swabs
- Membrane filters, a range of 0.2 μm filters for aqueous solutions and organic solvents
- Minimal glucose agar (MGA) (plates) Minimal glucose master plates with appropriate antibiotics
- Nutrient agar (plates)
- Nutrient broth
- Phenotype test plates
- Phosphate buffer 0.2 M, pH 7.4
- Pipette tips
- Positive control and diagnostic mutagens
- S9 fraction and cofactors
- Solvents including appropriate anhydrous organic solvents; DMSO in particular is hygroscopic and can develop mutagenic impurities in the presence of small amounts of water. Pure organic solvents should be maintained in an anhydrous condition by addition of a small quantity of a compatible predried molecular sieve (type 4A in the case of DMSO) and stored well-sealed over anhydrous silica gel.
- Spectrometer cuvettes, 1 mL disposable
- Top agar (with and without histidine, biotin, and tryptophan)
- Tubes (disposable glass sample tubes, 13 mm diameter).

Radiation-sterilized standard polystyrene Petri dishes (nominal diameter of 90–100 mm) should be used because ethylene oxide sterilization can leave mutagenic residues. These are used to prepare the bottom agar (MGA) plates. These or six-well MGA plates can also be used to prepare plates for phenotypic testing.

4.6 Reagents and Recipes

The following reagents can be purchased from commercial suppliers such as Moltox or manufactured in-house, in which case we suggest that each recipe should be prepared using a form (an appendix to the Standard Operating Procedure) so that appropriate details including supplier, batch number, and amounts of components can be maintained. It is convenient to create a template for each class of reagent (e.g., solution, plated medium).

In the following recipes, water refers to deionized reverse-osmosis purified water; other forms of purified water including distilled water may be used. Autoclaving is generally for 15 min at 121°C, but large volumes of liquid require a longer time to ensure sterility. Filter-sterilization normally involves the use of a 0.22 μm filter. Reagents should be labeled with identity, preparation date (or batch number), and expiration date.

A calibrated peristaltic pump can be used to dispense media including bottom and top agar into dishes. Laboratories using large numbers of plates should consider purchasing an automatic plate pourer (e.g., Eppendorf, Integra Biosciences AG, Microbiology International), which can be directly linked to sterilizing and plate-labeling systems for sequentially numbering plates. Pre-poured plates can also be purchased from commercial suppliers. Plates should be labeled on the side (e.g., using an indelible marker pen) using a code that corresponds to the study design document to avoid mix-ups or interference with automatic colony counters when labeled elsewhere. Petri dishes/plates have numerous variations, including venting (present or absent), size (internal diameter), ridging around the edge of the plate (stackable vs. slippable), and tabs on the base that can interfere with automatic colony counters; it is a good idea to qualify a specific source and type of plate and then consistently use that to avoid problems. After cooling and a drying period to minimize condensation, plated media can be stored in the plastic bags and boxes in which the original empty plates arrived; care should be taken when using other plastic bags because of potential transfer of toxic impurities into the agar. Pourite (Aurical Company, San Mateo, CA) can be added to semi-solid (agar) media at 100 μL/L to disperse bubbles, which can be a problem with an automatic dispenser. If the poured plates are obtained from a commercial supplier, they can become contaminated during shipment, especially when condensation is present; within 1 or 2 days of arrival, check for and discard any showing microbial growth.

To make the required volume of the reagents listed here, multiply each component by an appropriate constant proportion (e.g., 5 if the recipe describes how to make 1 liter and you need 5 liters). Expiration dates are based on the date of preparation and should take into account the expiration dates of individual components. Expiration dates can be extended provided that results are available in the laboratory to prove the reagent is still fit for its purpose.

Filter paper discs used to test sensitivity/resistance to antibiotics can be purchased or cut from Whatman filter paper No. 1 using a 7-mm hole punch. The absolute amount added to the disc should be optimized so that an appropriate ring of inhibition is formed around the disc in the sensitive strains under the conditions used in the laboratory—amounts indicated herein are for guidance.

Note that some laboratories routinely place antibiotic-resistant strains (e.g., TA98, TA100, TA102) in medium containing appropriate antibiotics, but this does not seem to serve any practical purpose because the bacteria are checked for resistance when they are isolated or subcultured.

4.6.1 Ampicillin 2 µg/disc

Ampicillin sodium salt is dissolved in water at 5 mg/mL and then filter-sterilized. The solution can be stored in a refrigerator for up to 1 year. This solution is diluted to 200 µg/mL with sterile water and then spotted at 10 µL per filter disc to check the strains for the R-factor plasmid pKM101 that confers resistance. The ampicillin discs can be stored in the refrigerator or freezer under desiccating conditions for up to 1 year.

4.6.2 Biotin 0.37 mg/mL

Add 1 liter of water to an appropriate container and heat to boiling point with stirring. Add 370 mg of D-biotin and stir until it is dissolved. The solution should be sterilized by autoclaving or filtration (0.22 µm) and stored at room temperature in ambient light for up to 1 year.

4.6.3 Crystal Violet 5 µg/disc

Crystal violet is dissolved in water at 5 mg/mL and then filter-sterilized. The solution can be stored in darkness in a refrigerator for up to 1 year. The solution is diluted to 500 µg/mL with sterile water and then spotted at 10 µL per filter disc to check strains for the rfa deep rough mutation conferring sensitivity in all *Salmonella* strains. The discs can be stored in the refrigerator for at least 1 year [20].

4.6.4 Glucose 0.4 g/mL

Add approximately 700 mL of water to an appropriate container. Add a magnetic stir bar and 400 g D-glucose in increments while continuously stirring, allowing the sugar to dissolve between additions. Once all the glucose is in the solution, make up to the final volume with water and then filter-sterilize into sterile containers. The solution can also be sterilized by autoclaving, but this tends to cause carmelization, which leads to a slight increase in spontaneous revertant counts. The solution can be stored in a refrigerator for up to 6 months.

4.6.5 G6P 1M: *Glucose-6-Phosphate*

The solution is prepared by dissolving G6P at 260 mg/mL of water; if the sodium salt is used, then it should be dissolved at the rate of 282 mg/mL. Filter-sterilize and then store in a freezer. This expires after 1 year.

4.6.6 HBT: *500 μM Histidine, 500 μM Biotin, 500 μM Tryptophan Solution*

Combine the following volumes of solutions in a measuring cylinder:

- Histidine HCl.H$_2$O 5 mg/mL, 21 mL
- Biotin 0.37 mg/mL, 333 mL
- Tryptophan 5 mg/mL, 20 mL
- Make up to 1 liter with water

Autoclave or filter-sterilize. The solution is stored at room temperature in ambient light and expires after 1 year.

4.6.7 *Histidine HCl.H$_2$O 5 mg/mL*

Add 1 liter of water in an appropriate container; then, add 5 g of L-Histidine.HCl.H$_2$O and stir until dissolved. The solution should be sterilized by autoclaving or filtration and stored in a refrigerator for up to 1 year.

4.6.8 *KMg*

- Potassium chloride (KCl, formula weight 75), 124 mg
- Magnesium chloride (MgCl$_2$.6H$_2$O, formula weight 203), 81 mg

Each mL of solution contains KCl and MgCl$_2$.6H$_2$O in the proportions shown here. Dissolve the salts in water (80% of the final volume) and then make up to full volume with water. Autoclave or filter-sterilize the solution and then store at room temperature in ambient light for up to 1 year.

4.6.9 *MGA Plates*

This agar contains glucose at a final level of 0.4% and is suitable for all tester strains; higher glucose levels may inhibit the growth of TA97a [21]. Other types of agar may be suitable but, because the type of agar can affect the negative/vehicle control count, it is best to use only one type.

Add 15 g Bacto™ agar (BD) and a magnet stir bar to 920 mL water in a 2 L glass Erlenmeyer flask, cover with aluminum foil, and then autoclave. The remaining procedures should be performed using aseptic technique in a laminar flow cabinet. When the solution has cooled to approximately 65°C, gradually add 20 mL VB salts 50 × in increments while stirring, allowing the salts to dissolve completely between additions, and then add 10 mL glucose 0.4 g/mL and stir for at least 1 min. Maintain molten at a temperature of approximately 45°C on a hotplate and dispense 25 mL aliquots into 90–100 mm diameter plastic Petri dishes. Leave the plates on a level surface at room temperature while the agar gels. Allow the plates to cool overnight and then store them inverted (agar side uppermost) in the plastic bags in which the plates were supplied in a refrigerator for up to 6 months (or until they show signs of drying if earlier). Allow the plates to dry at room temperature for 3 days prior to bagging them if excessive condensation is found after overnight cooling/drying.

4.6.10 Minimal Glucose Master (MGM, MGMA and MGMAT) Plates

This agar is similar to MGA but is supplemented with excess histidine, tryptophan and biotin at 333, 333 and 3 μM respectively to allow growth of all the standard (auxotrophic) tester strains. To select for bacteria with appropriate plasmids, ampicillin should be added for the pKM101 strains (including WP2 uvrA pKM101, TA97, TA98, TA100 and TA102); in addition, tetracycline should be added for the pAQ1 plasmid containing strain TA102 — refer to Figure 4.8.1 for plasmid details.

Add 15 g Bacto™ agar (BD), 920 mL purified water, 1.4 mL histidine 5 mg/mL, 2 mL biotin 0.37 mg/mL, 13.6 mL tryptophan 5 mg/mL, 920 mL purified water and a stir bar to a 2 L glass Erlenmeyer flask, cover with aluminum foil, and then autoclave. The remaining procedures should be performed using aseptic technique in a laminar flow cabinet. When the solution has cooled to approximately 65°C, gradually add 20 mL VB salts 50× in increments while stirring, allowing the salts to dissolve completely between additions, and then add 10 mL glucose 0.4 g/mL and stir until homogenous. While the medium is still warm and before the agar starts gelling, dispense 100 mL aliquots into sterile labelled glass bottles. This medium expires after 6 months.

To use for non-plasmid strains, melt the MGM medium in a boiling water bath or microwave then, once cool enough to handle, dispense 25 mL aliquots into standard sterile petri dishes. For the pKM101 strains, melt the medium then, once it has cool enough to handle, add 5 mL ampicillin 5 mg/mL and (for TA102) 333 μL tetracycline 6 mg/mL before dispensing as above. Allow the plates to gel on the level surface of the laminar flow cabinet until cool then replace the lids. Label the plates then store them inverted (agar side up) in the plastic bags in which the dishes came with a small perforation to avoid sweating then store them refrigerated for up to 3 months (MGM) or 1 month (MGMA and MGMAT).

4.6.11 NADP 0.1 M

Dissolve β-nicotinamide adenine dinucleotide phosphate and sodium salt (formula weight 765) at 76.5 mg/mL of water. Filter-sterilize and then store refrigerated in the dark and use on the day of preparation.

4.6.12 Nutrient Agar Plates

The manufacturer of the agar and nutrient broth is not critical; therefore, other equivalent types may be substituted.

Add 15 g Bacto™ Agar (BD), 25 g Oxoid nutrient broth no. 2 powder, and a magnet stir bar to 1000 mL water in a 2-L glass Erlenmeyer flask. Cover with aluminum foil. Stir for a few minutes and then autoclave. Stir to ensure homogeneity and then dispense 25 mL of the mixture into each Petri dish. Leave the plates on a level surface at room temperature while the agar gels. Allow the plates to cool overnight and then store them inverted (agar side uppermost) in the plastic bags in which the plates were supplied in a refrigerator for up to 6 months (or until they show signs of drying if earlier).

4.6.13 Nutrient Broth

Put 1000 mL of purified water into a 2-L Erlenmeyer flask. Add 25 grams of Oxoid nutrient broth no. 2 powder while stirring. Once dissolved, dispense aliquots of the solution into appropriate glass bottle(s) and autoclave at 121°C for 15 min. The solution can be kept at room temperature for 1 month.

4.6.14 Phosphate Buffer 0.2 M pH 7.4

This solution is used to make the S9 mix. It is diluted with an equal volume of sterile water for use as the 0S9 buffer for those plates treated in the absence of S9 mix.

Mix the following two solutions in the proportions shown:

- Sodium dihydrogen phosphate (NaH_2PO_4) 0.2 M, 146 mL
- Disodium hydrogen phosphate (Na_2HPO_4) 0.2 M, 854 mL

Confirm that the pH is in the range of 7.3−7.5 and then autoclave or filter-sterilize it. Store at room temperature in ambient light. This expires after 1 year.

4.6.15 Positive Control and Diagnostic Mutagen Solutions

Stock solutions of 2AA, 2AF, 2NF, 9AC, BaP, DAN, DMBA, MC, MMC, NaAz, and NQO can all be prepared in DMSO in advance of use and then aliquoted in convenient amounts before storing in the freezer for up to 18 months [22] – see section 4.8.6 *Diagnostic Mutagen Test* for a list of chemical names and suggested concentrations. Alternatively, stocks of MMC and NaAz can also be prepared in water. Other positive controls may be substituted when convenient. Volatile positive controls should be avoided because of potential contamination of the incubator.

4.6.16 S9 Fraction

Rats (usually Sprague-Dawley outbred) are pretreated with Aroclor 1254 or phenobarbital plus β-naphthoflavone to promote the levels of xenobiotic metabolizing enzymes [23–25]. S9 fraction is conventionally prepared by homogenization of liver in isotonic 0.15 M potassium chloride at a rate of 1 g wet tissue per 3 mL; after separation by centrifugation, the S9 fraction may be standardized based on protein content by further dilution in potassium chloride solution. Rarely, S9 preparations from other species (e.g., pooled human liver when testing compounds with known human-specific metabolism) or even other tissues may be included when appropriate and justified [26,27]. For benzidine/azo-dyes and diazo-compounds, a reductive metabolic activation system using hamster liver S9 should be included [28–30]. When preparing S9, it is critical for all solutions and labware to be sterile for the liver to be removed under clean conditions by a trained technician.

Most laboratories purchase precertified S9 fraction from a commercial source to avoid issues with handling animals, Aroclor (polychlorinated biphenyls are banned by some countries and some individual companies) and additional biochemical assays. Commercial S9 fraction can be obtained in frozen or lyophilized form; in addition, lyophilized preformulated S9 mix is available from Moltox. Frozen S9 should be thawed entirely immediately before use and mixed well. Thawed S9 degrades fairly rapidly so any excess should be discarded and should not be refrozen for later use.

4.6.17 S9 Mix

The final concentration of S9 fraction in the S9 mix is usually 10% v/v (termed 10% S9); other percentages of S9 may occasionally be appropriate, in which case the volumes of S9 fraction and water should be adjusted. S9 mix also contains the following "cofactors": 8 mM $MgCl_2$, 33 mM KCl, 100 mM sodium phosphate buffer pH 7.4, 5 mM glucose-6-phosphate, and 4 mM NADP [23]; therefore, each mL of 10% S9 mix contains:

- Water, 0.335 mL
- Phosphate buffer 0.2 M pH 7.4, 0.500 mL
- NADP 0.1 M, 0.040 mL
- G6P, 0.005 mL
- KMg, 0.020 mL
- S9 fraction, 0.100 mL

All components should be sterile and added aseptically in the proportions and order listed to a sterile container on ice, kept on ice or refrigerated, and used on the day of preparation.

Unused S9 mix should be discarded and not frozen for future use.

4.6.18 Tetracycline 1 µg/disc

Tetracycline hydrochloride is dissolved in water at 6 mg/mL and then filter-sterilized. The solution is stable when stored in darkness in a refrigerator for up to 1 year. The solution is diluted to 0.1 mg/mL with sterile water and then spotted at 10 µL per filter disc to check for the presence of the pAQ1 plasmid, which confers resistance in *Salmonella* strain TA102.

4.6.19 Top Agar Incomplete: TAI

This is used to make the TAI and, with appropriate supplementation, may be used for phenotype testing.

Add 6 g agar directly to a glass bottle (the bottle size should be $\sim 2\times$ the solution volume), followed by 1 liter of 0.5% w/v sodium chloride solution. Autoclave and, before the agar sets, mix the contents well by swirling.

Store at room temperature in ambient light. Solution expires after 6 months. Before use, the top agar should be melted in a boiling water bath or microwave and then mixed well by swirling.

4.6.20 Top Agar Complete: TAC

This is the top agar used in a routine bacterial mutation system; it contains histidine, biotin, and tryptophan all at levels of 4.5 µM. Although *Salmonella* strains do not require exogenous tryptophan and *E. coli* strains do not require exogenous histidine or biotin, there is less chance of an error if this type of top agar is used for all routine tests.

If necessary, melt the TAI in a boiling water bath or microwave. Add 100 mL HBT per liter of TAI. Normally, the agar is kept molten and used on the same day, but it can be stored at room temperature in ambient light for up to 3 months. Before use, you should ensure that the medium is uniform and completely molten (with no waves/Schlieren pattern) by swirling the bottle. If necessary, continue heating and re-mix until homogenous. Equilibrate in a 45°C water bath before dispensing.

4.6.21 Tryptophan 5 mg/mL

Add 1 liter of water to an appropriate container. Add 5 g of L-tryptophan and mix until it dissolves. The solution should be sterilized by autoclaving or filtration (0.22 μm) and stored in a refrigerator for up to 1 year.

4.6.22 VB Salts 50 ×: Vogel-Bonner Salts

For each liter add approximately 700 mL of water in an appropriate glass container. Heat the water to 45°C using a heated stirring plate and then add salts to the water in the following order while stirring, allowing each salt to dissolve completely before adding the next:

- 10 g magnesium sulfate ($MgSO_4.7H_2O$)
- 100 g citric acid monohydrate ($C_6H_8O_7.H_2O$)
- 500 g potassium phosphate dibasic (K_2HPO_4)
- 175 g sodium ammonium phosphate ($NaNH_4HPO_4.4H_2O$).

Bring the solution to volume with water, mix thoroughly, and then aliquot into appropriate glass bottles. Sterilize the solution by autoclaving and store at room temperature for up to 1 year.

4.7 Suggested Phases in Development of the Test

For laboratories that have not worked on a particular version of the bacterial mutation test before, development may be conveniently divided into four phases:

1. Research: reading literature associated with the assay, particularly the originators of the method, regulatory guidelines, and the associated formative guidance/papers.
2. Setup: optimizing experimental conditions so that high-quality and reproducible results can be obtained. This phase is necessarily non-GLP because the methodology is in the process of being standardized and involves building up stocks of purified and characterized strains, optimizing conditions of bacterial growth, organizing dosing and plating procedures, establishing dose response to routine positive controls, and preparing documentation including instructions used to perform various parts of the test and to record important details so that (in the event of any unexpected results) the effect of potential variables can be assessed. The results of any set-up work should be recorded directly in the raw data, together with any conclusions and recommendations. It is useful to archive the files of this and the subsequent internal validation electronically for potential reference.

3. Internal validation: providing adequate proof that reliable and reproducible results can be produced in the laboratory using the procedures refined during the set-up stage. In a laboratory where subsequent studies will be used for regulatory submission, this phase is expected to be fairly extensive and will include several experiments performed under GLP (with formal protocols and reports) to help generate adequate control databases. Negative (as well as vehicle) control treatments should be included in every experiment to confirm the absence of solvent effects and to rapidly develop a meaningful laboratory control database. Dose-response curves for positive controls and diagnostic mutagens should be generated and limits of toxicity (maximum nontoxic dose volume) should be established for common vehicles/solvents in plate incorporation and preincubation versions of the test. Chemicals from representative classes of mutagen with different physical properties (e.g., poorly soluble, volatile) should be examined. Any paperwork generated including reports should be formally reviewed by the responsible scientist. Then, in the case of GLP facilities and after auditing, it should be archived and readily available for potential inspection by sponsors and regulatory agencies.

4. Routine maintenance and testing: all aspects should follow established SOPs. All checked/audited control results generated (except those from invalid experiments) should be added to the laboratory historical control database.

4.8 The Bacterial Strains

Although the bacterial mutation test is often referred to as a rapid method for evaluation of mutagenicity, it is not necessarily as straightforward as it first appears, partly because of the ongoing effort needed to maintain, monitor, and assess multiple strains for routine testing. Strains obtained externally or that have been rederived must be purified, characterized for appropriate phenotypic characteristics, must have sensitivity to selective (diagnostic) mutagens confirmed, and must be maintained appropriately to provide reliable and reproducible results. The growth characteristics of each strain should be established so that appropriate density working cultures can be prepared from frozen stocks for routine testing using convenient standardized conditions. The frozen stocks should be divided into working cultures (i.e., those used to prepare suspensions for routine testing) and master stock cultures (these are sometimes referred to as master permanents). Master stocks are only used to generate fresh working and master stocks once these become depleted. Details of the suggested procedures are given in the subsequent sections and summarized graphically.

The strains listed here are those mentioned by international guidelines and are those most commonly used for routine testing.

4.8.1 Genotypes of Routinely Used Strains

See Table 4.1.

Table 4.1

Strain Designation	Target Mutation	Repair Deficiency	LPS	Plasmids	Main Mechanism, Sensitivity
S. typhimurium					
TA1535	hisG46	uvrB	rfa		Most base pair substitutions
TA100	hisG46	uvrB	rfa	pKM101	
TA1537	hisC3076	uvrB	rfa		Frameshift, intercalation
TA97a	hisD6610	uvrB	rfa	pKM101	
TA1538	hisD3052	uvrB	rfa		Frameshift
TA98	hisD3052	uvrB	rfa	pKM101	
TA102	hisG428		rfa	pKM101 pAQ1	Base substitution, small deletions, cross-linking, and oxidizing agents
E. coli					
WP2 uvrA	trpE	uvrA			Base substitution
WP2 uvrA pKM101	trpE	uvrA		pKM101	

The uvrB deletion extends through the gal, nitrate reductase (chlorate resistance), and biotin (bio) genes and, like the uvrA mutation in *E. coli*, prevents (relatively error-free) nucleotide excision repair. The pKM101 gene enhances mutability by coding for umuD in an error-prone repair pathway that is otherwise absent in *Salmonella* strains. TA102 was constructed by deletion of the hisG gene and introduction of the pAQ1 plasmid carrying the mutant hisG428 gene; each bacterium contains approximately 30 copies of the plasmid, making the strain much more sensitive to mutagens because a back-mutation of just one copy of the gene will restore the his$^+$ phenotype [31,89].

Although multiple modes of reversion occur in all strains, each strain has a particular mutagen-susceptible sequence (hotspot); hotspots involve repeat sequences in hisD3052, hisD6610, and the A/T-containing codon of hisG428 and the G/C-containing codon of hisG46. The two *Salmonella* hisG46 strains in combination with TA102 or a WP2 strain are reverted by all six possible base substitution mutations [11].

4.8.2 Obtaining the Tester Strains

The *Salmonella* strains could originally be obtained directly from Dr. Ames' laboratory at the University of California at Berkeley; however, that laboratory has not maintained them for many years. Tester strains can be obtained from commercial suppliers or repositories such as: Molecular Toxicology Inc. (Moltox); ATCC; the National Collection of Industrial, Food, and Marine Bacteria (www.ncimb.com); Aberdeen, Scotland, UK (*E. coli* strains and WP2 derivatives); BCCM (Belgian Co-Ordinated Collections of Micro-Organisms); or from a reputable laboratory routinely performing tests in a GLP environment. The bacteria may be classified as potentially hazardous etiologic organisms (e.g., UN No. 3373 biological substance category B); therefore, even though they are attenuated, they may need an import license depending on the country.

Whatever the source, the provenance of the organisms is unlikely to be assured. These strains have been maintained and subcultured over an extended period of time during which they may have become mixed with other strains, mutated, lost or gained plasmids, or have undergone genetic drift. Therefore, any newly arrived strain should be purified and then thoroughly checked for appropriate characteristics as described later. If the organisms have been obtained from a reputable source, then they will have already performed these procedures themselves on a regular basis. If available, details of provenance, passage number, historical control counts, and quality control statements should be obtained from the supplier. These records and subsequent details relating to strain purification, maintenance, storage, subculturing, characterization, and utilization should be maintained in a Laboratory Bacterial Strain Maintenance Log.

Five complementary strains of bacteria are used in a routine study:

1. *S. typhimurium* TA1535
2. *S. typhimurium* TA1537 or TA97a (repurified/rederived form of TA97)
3. *S. typhimurium* TA98
4. *S. typhimurium* TA100
5. *E. coli* WP2 uvrA, *E. coli* WP2 uvrA pKM101, or *S. typhimurium* TA102.

When testing suspect cross-linking mutagens, it is preferable to include a DNA repair-proficient strain such as *S. typhimurium* TA102 or *E. coli* (WP2 or WP2 pKM101) if they are not routinely included. Other strains not mentioned here have been developed with increased sensitivity or to test for specific mutations, or have been engineered with mammalian metabolic enzymes [32,89]; these strains are not generally used for routine screening or regulatory studies.

4.8.3 Receipt of Bacterial Strains

Bacterial cultures may be obtained in freeze-dried (lyophilized), frozen, or liquid suspension forms or on semi-solid agar medium. Shortly after receipt bacteria should be grown up on supplemented minimal glucose master plates containing appropriate antibiotics (for the plasmid-containg strains). This and the isolation procedures described below ensure enventual healthy growth of the bacteria on MGA plates, the presence of the appropriate plasmid and the purity of the cultures. Lyophilized cultures should be reconstituted in nutrient broth and then streaked out onto (minimal glucose) master plates, i.e. MGM, MGMA or MGMAT depending on the plasmid content of the strain — see section 4.6. If unopened, frozen and lyophilized cultures can be stored for up to 2 years when stored at $\leq -70°C$ and $4°C$, respectively. When convenient, frozen suspensions should be thawed rapidly (e.g., by shaking gently in a $37°C$ water bath) and then immediately streaked out on appropriate master plates (MGM, MGMA or MGMAT). Liquid cultures should be streaked out upon receipt. Cultures on agar can be stored in a refrigerator for a few weeks or even months if the culture medium does not dry out; however, viability/recovery of organisms stored at $4°C$ is expected to decline relatively quickly and mutations may accumulate. Bacteria obtained as colonies on semi-solid medium (i.e., as streak, stab, or slopes/slants) should be streaked out as soon as practical; the original material can be kept refrigerated until appropriate stocks of the strains have been built up. Streaks to isolate and purify bacteria prior to characterization may be prepared using a printout of the streak template shown in Figure 4.2 as a guide.

Place the master plate on the template and then load a small amount of the bacterial culture/suspension onto a sterile plastic loop; use this to prepare the streaks in section 1 (1A, then 1B, etc.), use a fresh loop to prepare streaks in section 2, and then use the other side of the loop for streaks in section 3; repeat with a fresh loop for sections 4 and 5. Alternately, a wire loop may be used; the loop should be sterilized before use and prior to streaking each of sections 2 to 5. Wire loops can be dry heat–sterilized using a gas or spirit burner or by infrared using a Bacti-Cinerator and then cooled by touching the surface of the agar before each use.

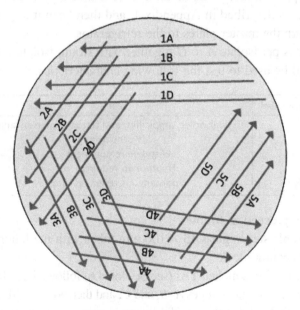

Figure 4.2
Streak template.

The procedure and source of each strain should be recorded in the Maintenance Log; plates should be labeled with strain, date, and study number, which cross-references the paper records. The streaked agar plates should be inverted, incubated for 48–72 h at 37°C, and then stored at 4°C in plastic bags so the medium does not dry out or develop excessive condensation. Discrete isolated colonies will appear in lower number sections of the plate depending on the number of bacteria transferred to section 1 and the type of loop used (wire or plastic).

Take 10 isolated cultures from each strain and streak out each on a master plate labeled with strain, date, study reference, and isolate serial number (1–10). Incubate these master plates at 37°C for 2 to 3 days; then, if not used immediately, store them refrigerated for up to an additional 2 days.

4.8.4 Phenotyping of New Isolates

Routinely, all 10 isolates of each required strain should be characterized. Subsequently, two will be selected for freezing and diagnostic mutagen testing to confirm their suitability.

1. First thing in the morning, pick off a whole isolated colony from the master plate of each of the 10 isolates, use it to inoculate a standard 25 or 30 mL suspension culture, incubate it for approximately 5 hours until there is a density of at least 1×10^9 viable bacteria per mL, as described in Appendix 1, and then keep it at room temperature. Meanwhile, return the master plates to the refrigerator.
2. Label seven plates per isolate A to G together with strain, isolate number, and date. These plates will be used to test the following characteristics:

Plate Label	Test
A	Crystal violet, ampicillin, and tetracycline resistance
B	UV sensitivity
C	Histidine requirement
D	Tryptophan requirement
E, F, G	Spontaneous reversion rate

3. For each culture, proceed as follows:
4. Label six disposable sterile glass 13×100 mm tubes with the letters A to G. Place the tubes in a 45°C heating block.
5. For tubes A to D, add 2 mL molten TAI (see Section 4.6) followed by 100 μL 0.5 mM biotin. Add 100 μL 50 mM histidine to tubes A, B, and C, and then add 100 μL 50 mM tryptophan to tubes A, B, and D. *Note that these additives are in excess of the limiting requirement.*
6. Dispense 2-mL aliquots of TAC into tubes labeled E, F, and G.

7. Ensure that the bacterial culture is uniform by swirling, dispense 100 μL into each tube of top agar, vortex briefly, and then pour the mixture onto the bottom agar in the corresponding MGA plate. Ensure the top agar is evenly distributed by tilting/rotating the plate and then leave the plate on a level surface to set.

8. Once all the plates for all the isolates have been poured, use sterile forceps to add one of each type (crystal violet, ampicillin, and tetracycline) of filter paper discs to plate A. The discs should be approximately equidistant from each other and from the edge of the plate.

9. Mark plate B into five zones of approximately equal width with four vertical lines using a marker pen. Place an opaque barrier over the plate, remove the lid, and place it agar-side up under a low-intensity UV source at a standardized height (15 W at 33 cm); alternatively, the lamp in the biological containment cabinet can be used. Turn the UV lamp on, expose the first sector for 2 s, withdraw the barrier to the next mark, and expose for an additional 2 s, repeating for the third and fourth zones before turning the lamp off. In this way zone 1 will have been exposed for 8 s while zone 5 will remain unexposed. Replace the lid. *UV is particularly damaging to the eyes; therefore, UV-blocking glasses should be worn and exposure of personnel should be minimized. The emission intensity of UV lamps reduces over their working life, so the lamp should be replaced when appropriate. Mitomycin C (0.2 μg/disc) sensitivity can be used as an alternate marker for uvr deficiency.*

10. Once all the isolates have been plated and the agar has set, invert the plates and then incubate them at 37°C for 24 h (plates A−D) or 65 h (plates E−G).

11. After incubation, the plates can be examined immediately or stored at 4°C for a few days.

12. Assess the growth in plates labeled A and record the diameter of any zone of inhibition of growth around the antibiotic discs.

13. For the UV-exposed plates labeled B, record the time taken to inhibit growth (inhibition for repair-proficient strains such as TA102 should take much longer).

14. For the histidine- and tryptophan-deficient plates, labeled C and D, respectively, record the presence or absence of growth.

15. For plates labeled D−F, check the background lawn using a microscope, where necessary, and record the number of revertants for each plate and calculate mean values. These values are referred to as the spontaneous revertant colony counts and reflect the uninduced rate of reversion. The spontaneous count is the phenotypic characteristic most likely to vary from expected.

16. Compare the results with the expected values based on the following chart; isolates that have values outside of expected ranges should be rejected and discarded. We suggest that each laboratory should take into account its own experience with the acceptance criteria and modify them as appropriate in a formal SOP (Table 4.2).

Table 4.2: Expected results for phenotype plates

Strain	Zone of Inhibition mm			UV Kill Time	Count on MGA Plates
	C	A	T	Seconds	Mean[a]
TA1535	>12	>12	>12	2	5−20
TA1537	>12	>12	>12	2	4−15
TA1538	>12	>12	>12	2	6−24
TA97a	>12	<10	>12	2	70−180
TA98	>12	<10	>12	2	20−45
TA100	>12	<10	>12	2	75−140
TA102	>12	<10	<10	>8	190−400
WP2	<10	>12	>12	>8	20−50
WP2 uvrA	<10	>12	>12	2	20−58
WP2 pKM101	<10	<10	>12	>8	50−130
WP2 uvrA pKM101	<10	<10	>12	2	100−200

[a]These values are based on Charles River, Montreal's control range and those summarized in various review articles [32−35] and depend not only on the strain but also on the glucose content of the plate, the volume of the agar, the growth phase and density of the bacterial suspension used and other factors [36−38]. Ranges within an individual laboratory may vary somewhat from these values and may be narrower than those shown here. Isolates with values close to the middle of the acceptable range should be selected for storage and future use to avoid genetic drift.

Note that, in routine testing experiments, values obtained for vehicle control plates with S9 tend to be slightly higher than those without S9.

4.8.5 Freezing of Selected Isolates

Based on the results of the phenotype tests, at least two appropriate isolates of each strain should be grown. Most of each culture will be frozen while the remainder is used to confirm suitability by checking the vehicle or negative control revertant colony count and responses to diagnostic mutagens.

The suggested procedure for growing selected isolates and freezing is listed here.

1. At least 2 days prior to the anticipated diagnostic mutagen test, restreak the selected isolates on nutrient agar plates using the template as a guide.
2. Two days later (first thing in the morning), take one isolated colony from each streak of the restreaked isolates and resuspend in nutrient broth and culture as described in Appendix 1.
3. Once the culture density has achieved $\geq 1.1 \times 10^9$ bacteria/mL, dilute it to 1.1×10^9 bacteria/mL with nutrient broth in a total volume of 30 mL in a sterile container (e.g., a 50 mL centrifuge tube). Discard any surplus culture material.
4. Dispense one 4 mL aliquot of each isolate into a sterile labeled tube and set aside at room temperature for testing as described in the diagnostic mutagen test in Section 4.8.6.

5. To the remaining 26 mL of each bacterial suspension, add 2.3 mL DMSO while agitating by hand. Dispense in 1 mL aliquots into cryovials labeled with strain, isolate, serial number, and date. Transfer the vials to labeled cartons (cryoboxes or similar) and place in the ultralow freezer ($\leq 70°C$) or in labeled canes and then store them in the vapor phase of the liquid nitrogen cell store. When using liquid nitrogen, bacteria are stored separately from cell lines in the vapor phase because the seal of cryovials shrinks at low temperatures, which can allow liquid nitrogen to enter, leading to potential contamination.

6. The cultures should be stored in at least two locations to insure against failure (e.g., running out of liquid nitrogen).

4.8.6 Diagnostic Mutagen Test

Using the 4 mL of liquid culture that was set aside prior to freezing, retest each isolate for phenotypic characteristics as described earlier and plate with selected diagnostic mutagens plus S9 mix or buffer as appropriate in a standard plate incorporation test. Although single or duplicate plates are adequate for testing the mutagenic agents, the DMSO should be tested in triplicate (both with buffer and S9 mix) to give a good idea of the spontaneous rate of reversion in comparison with historical control values and in case of loss of an individual plate (Table 4.3).

Table 4.3: Expected results diagnostic mutagens

Compound	DMSO[a]	Without S9 Mix					With S9 Mix		
		9AC	MMC	2NF	NQO	2AA	2AA	2AF	DMBA
µg/plate	—	50	0.5	1	0.5	1	20	5	20
TA1535	5−25	−	−	−	+	++	++	−	−
TA1537	5−15	++	−	−/+	+/++	+	++	−/+	+/++
TA1538	6−30	−	−	+/++	+/++	++	++	++	+/++
TA97a	70−130	+/++	−	+	−/+	++	++	+/++	+/++
TA98	20−45	−	−	+/++	+/++	++	++	++	+/++
TA100	75−140	−	−	−/+	++	+/++	++	+/++	+/++
TA102	191−400	−	+	−	+	+	+	−	−
WP2 uvrA	25−65	−	−	−	+/++	−	+	−/+	−/+
WP2 uvrA pKM101	100−200	−	−	−	+/++	−	+/++	−/+	+

9AC = 9-aminoacridine; MMC = mitomycin C; 2NF = 2-nitrofluorene; NQO = 4-nitroquinoline-1-oxide;
2AA = 2-aminoanthracene; 2AF = 2-aminofluorene; DMBA = 7,12-dimethylbenzanthracene
− no substantial increase
+ moderate response
++ strong response
[a]Vehicle control tested in the absence and presence of S9.

As with any mutation test, a study design spreadsheet should be generated to specify the contents of each numbered plate and to facilitate calculation and interpretation of results.

The design should include sterility checks of the reagents involved including the top agar, buffer, S9, DMSO, and diagnostic mutagen solutions, i.e., the first 12 plates in the study design. The study design will also indicate the number of MGA plates needed. The rows corresponding to plates 13 to 42 in the example study design are repeated for each isolate tested; the entry in the strain column should indicate the strain and isolate number used. The spreadsheet may also be used to capture the results by direct input or by linking to a data capture system. Depending on the SOPs of the laboratory, the electronic version of the spreadsheet or a printout of the study design should be used to document the procedures and raw data (i.e., the original observations and counts). The bold letters A, B, and C in the spreadsheet example represent the order in which these components are added; the 0 value in the S9 column indicates that buffer is added and the + symbol indicates that S9 mix is used. The abbreviations used in the treatment column are explained later in this section. The spreadsheet should be authorized (signed and dated) by the scientist responsible for the study before use (Table 4.4).

Table 4.4: Study design: diagnostic mutagen test

Plate No.	A Treatment	Dose No.	Dose Vol. μL	Dose μg/Plate	B S9	C Strain	Count	Observations (If Any)
1	–	–	–	–	–	–		
2	Buffer	–	–	–	0	–		
3	S9	–	–	–	+	–		
4	DMSO	0	100	0	–	–		
5	9AC	1	100	50	–	–		
6	MMC	1	100	0.5	–	–		
7	2NF	1	100	1	–	–		
8	NQO	1	100	0.5	–	–		
9	2AA	1	100	1	–	–		
10	2AA	2	100	20	–	–		
11	2AF	1	100	5	–	–		
12	DMBA	1	100	20	–	–		
13	DMSO	0	100	0	0	strain+I		
14	DMSO	0	100	0	0	strain+I		
15	DMSO	0	100	0	0	strain+I		
16	9AC	1	100	50	0	strain+I		
17	9AC	1	100	50	0	strain+I		
18	9AC	1	100	50	0	strain+I		
19	MMC	1	100	0.5	0	strain+I		
20	MMC	1	100	0.5	0	strain+I		
21	MMC	1	100	0.5	0	strain+I		
22	2NF	1	100	0.1	0	strain+I		
23	2NF	1	100	0.1	0	strain+I		
24	2NF	1	100	0.1	0	strain+I		
25	NQO	1	100	1	0	strain+I		

(Continued)

Table 4.4: (Continued)

Plate No.	A Treatment	Dose No.	Dose Vol. μL	Dose μg/Plate	B S9	C Strain	Count	Observations (If Any)
26	NQO	1	100	1	0	strain+I		
27	NQO	1	100	1	0	strain+I		
28	DMSO	0	100	0	+	strain+I		
29	DMSO	0	100	0	+	strain+I		
30	DMSO	0	100	0	+	strain+I		
31	2AA	1	100	1	+	strain+I		
32	2AA	1	100	1	+	strain+I		
33	2AA	1	100	1	+	strain+I		
34	2AA	2	100	20	+	strain+I		
35	2AA	2	100	20	+	strain+I		
36	2AA	2	100	20	+	strain+I		
37	2AF	1	100	5	+	strain+I		
38	2AF	1	100	5	+	strain+I		
39	2AF	1	100	5	+	strain+I		
40	DMBA	1	100	20	+	strain+I		
41	DMBA	1	100	20	+	strain+I		
42	DMBA	1	100	20	+	strain+I		

Where strain + I indicates strain plus isolate number (e.g., TA1535.1).

The suggested procedures for the diagnostic mutagen test are outlined as follows:

1. Label the MGA plates with a unique code for the study number (e.g., a single letter identified in the study design) and with the plate number. The plates should be numbered on the side using an indelible marker pen in case of mix-up of the lids.
2. Calculate the required volumes of each reagent including top agar, buffer, S9, and positive controls based on the study design sheet.
3. Store phosphate buffer 0.1 M pH 7.4 in a refrigerator and keep on ice during use.
4. Prepare an adequate volume of Aroclor 1254 or phenobarbital/benzoflavone-induced 10% rat liver S9 mix. Store refrigerated and keep on ice during use.
5. Melt TAC and then place in a water bath set at 50°C to equilibrate.
6. Set aside an aliquot of DMSO to use as the vehicle control for the test. Prepare formulations of the positive control chemicals (diagnostic mutagens) in DMSO and label them as shown here.

   Note that for laboratories performing tests regularly, it is generally convenient to prepare positive control and diagnostic mutagen solutions in bulk and store in appropriate aliquots deep frozen until use. Alternately, positive controls can be purchased in convenient premeasured aliquots.
7. Label individual test tube racks with treatment: DMSO, 9AC, MMC, 2NF, NQO, 2AA 1, 2AA 2, 2AF, and DMBA. For the DMSO rack, add one sterile

disposable 13 × 100-mm glass tube for the sterility check plus six tubes per isolate; for the remaining racks, add one tube for the sterility check plus three tubes per isolate.

8. Dose each tube with 100 μL of the appropriate control (DMSO or positive as per the rack) using a repeating micropipette (if available). Avoid touching pipette tips against sides of tubes.

9. Arrange the set of 12 sterility-testing tubes in a 45°C heating block as shown here.

9 2AA 1	10 2AA 2	11 2AF	12 DMBA	
4 DMSO	5 9AC	6 MMC	7 2NF	8 NQO
1 Blank	2 Buffer	3 S9		

10. Add 2 mL molten TAC to all tubes in the block, vortex each tube in turn, and pour the contents onto the bottom agar of the appropriate MGA plate. Discard the tube and replace the lid on the plate while ensuring the top agar is evenly distributed by tilting/rotating the plate. Leave the plate on a level surface in a clean area while the top agar gels.

11. Arrange the first set of 30 tubes for testing the first isolate in the 45°C heating block as shown here.

DMSO	2AA 1	2AA 2	2AF	DMBA
DMSO	**2AA 1**	**2AA 2**	**2AF**	**DMBA**
DMSO	**2AA 1**	**2AA 2**	**2AF**	**DMBA**
DMSO	**2AA 1**	**2AA 2**	**2AF**	**DMBA**
DMSO	*9AC*	*MMC*	*2NF*	*NQO*
DMSO	*9AC*	*MMC*	*2NF*	*NQO*
DMSO	*9AC*	*MMC*	*2NF*	*NQO*

12. Add 500 μL buffer to the front three rows of tubes (indicated in italics) and S9 to the back three rows of tubes (indicated in bold).

13. Immediately after, add 2 mL molten TAC to all tubes in the block, then add 100 μL of the appropriate bacterial suspension to all tubes in the block using a repeater pipette, vortex each tube, and pour the contents onto the appropriate plate. Discard the tube and replace the lid on the plate while ensuring the top agar is evenly distributed by tilting/rotating the plate. Leave the plate on a level surface in a clean area while the top agar gels.

   Note that if two technicians are available to perform the assay, it may be more convenient and quicker to add the top agar to the tube using a calibrated dispensing peristaltic pump operated by a foot switch. The operator then immediately adds the bacterial suspension using a multidose pipette before passing the tube to the second technician who mixes the contents of the tube and then pours and distributes it on the surface of the plate. In this case, the bulk TAC is held at 45°C in a water bath and a hot block is not required.

14. Invert and then place the plates in an incubator set at 37°C.

15. Remove the plates from the incubator after 65 h (three overnight incubations). *The OECD guideline indicates that an incubation time of 48−72 h is suitable; however, we recommend that you use a standard incubation time in your laboratory to allow a more direct comparison with historical control counts. The 65 h period is convenient and allows time for growth of most revertant colonies even in the presence of slight toxicity. Note that the colony count for strains with high spontaneous counts particularly tends to drift up with incubation time.*

16. If necessary, store plates refrigerated up to 3 days before examination.

17. Read and record the results of the phenotype confirmation test as before.

18. For MGA plates, where necessary, check the background lawn using a microscope with a total magnification of approximately 100× (10× objective). *Treatment of the excision repair-deficient strains with mitomycin C will usually result in absence of a background lawn.* Record any relevant comments about the plates directly onto a paper or electronic copy of the study design sheet.

19. Count the number of revertants for each plate using the automatic colony counter and record results in the study design sheet electronically or on a printout. Save the file and, if an electronic signature system is not in place, print the results sheet and sign (raw data).

20. Transfer all documents to the Bacterial Strain Maintenance Log file.

21. The responsible scientist should review the results and authorize rejection and disposal of strains that do not meet acceptance criteria.

After confirmation of suitability the frozen cultures are designated as either test batch frozen permanents (set aside to inoculate working cultures for routine experiments) or master permanents (set aside for long-term storage and subsequently used to generate fresh-frozen permanents).

4.9 Routine Testing

4.9.1 Designing a Study

The most widely used study design for routine assessment of chemicals is outlined in OECD guideline 471. Studies for regulatory submission generally follow this guidance and are performed under GLP conditions, in which case any planned deviation from these practices should be described and scientifically justified in the protocol and report.
The potential impact of any unplanned deviation should also be addressed in the report.

The guidelines published by US FDA in the FDA Redbook 2000 [39] and by the US EPA [40] are identical to the international guideline in terms of testing requirements and differ only in terms of layout and, in the case of the FDA, in some aspects of the descriptive information and in the following:

- FDA indicates that no toxicity should be evident at three or more doses in each assay, in each bacterial strain, both with and without metabolic activation. Both FDA and OECD indicate that at least five different analyzable concentrations of the test substance should be used without any indication of what is meant by analyzable. In practice, it is extremely unlikely that a mutagen will be missed if three nontoxic levels are assessed, so it is advisable to include this criterion in any formal protocol.
- FDA indicates that the S9 fraction concentration in the S9 mix should be 10−30% v/v, whereas OECD indicates 5−30%. In practice, most laboratories use 10% S9 by default.
- FDA indicates that detailed information on formulation preparation, storage, and confirmation (where available) should be reported. In practice, this is a GLP requirement and is recommended in any case.

Although the 1997 OECD guideline implies that a confirmatory test is appropriate (in the event of negative results), ICH guidance, which applies to pharmaceuticals to be registered in the United States, Canada, Europe, and Japan and is followed by most other countries, was revised in 2011 and indicates that confirmatory testing is not appropriate in the event of a clear result. Therefore, confirmatory testing is not normally required for submissions involving pharmaceuticals, pharmaceutical impurities, or medical device extracts, except in the case of borderline results. In practice, when an unexpected positive result occurs in a bacterial mutation test, it is usually good practice to investigate the result using appropriate methodology and to preclude the possibility of an error.

4.9.1.1 Metabolic activation system

The S9 mix, used as a model of intact mammalian metabolism, usually contains 10% v/v induced rat liver S9 fraction, although that can be varied between 4 or 5 and 30% depending on the chemical class and guideline being followed.

4.9.2 Test Article Considerations

The bacterial mutation test is used to evaluate a wide range of materials, including organic and inorganic compounds, medical devices, complex mixtures, environmental contamination, pharmaceuticals, household chemicals, impurities, and biological materials. Medical devices are usually extracted and tested as per ISO standards series 10993 (Part 3 Tests for genotoxicity, carcinogenicity and reproductive toxicity and Part 12 Sample preparation and reference materials). The reader should refer to the ISO web page for details of the most recent version of these documents (see https://www.iso.org).

It is important to gather relevant physical and chemical information on the nature of the test article in advance so that appropriate methods of sample preparation and testing are used. At the same time, the chemist involved in the project may be able to give you useful information about potential solvents. This is discussed in part in the Formulation section of this book; therefore, only the test-specific aspects are described here. In addition, despite the efforts of ICH, OECD, ISO, and others, there are national variations and preferences in test requirements, so it is useful to consider the final use of the test article and which regulatory bodies will be involved when designing the study.

For certain chemicals (e.g., pharmaceuticals that have specific effects on mammalian enzymes) it could be argued that the bacterial mutation test is not the most appropriate genotoxicity test; in which case, a mammalian cell mutation study report may be submitted along with appropriate justification for its use. Even so, we suggest that the bacterial test should also be performed because it is generally an expected part of the submission and it is often the most useful test for detection of minor mutagenic components and impurities. Although the test is generally regarded as predictive of long-term adverse effects in humans, the utility and relevance of results obtained with inorganic compounds including metal salts are questionable [41,42].

Regulatory authorities still expect assessment of antibacterial agents even though they may be highly toxic toward the test organisms. In this case it may be appropriate to perform a "Treat and Plate" modification of the preincubation test in addition to the standard test. Using this method, actively growing bacteria are exposed to the test article in suspension for a specified period (often 1 h), centrifuged, washed free of the test material, and plated out in top agar as per the standard method. At the end of the suspension exposure period, the number of viable surviving bacteria is quantified by diluting and plating them in complete medium with excess histidine/tryptophan. In the absence of any effect of the material on bacterial survival, mutagenicity will be evident as an absolute increase in revertant colonies in the normal way. However, at higher dose levels close to the limit of toxicity, the number of induced revertants per billion bacteria (i.e., the induced mutation frequency as opposed to the absolute mutation frequency) must be calculated to determine presence or absence of mutagenicity. The induced mutation frequency is therefore calculated as:

Treated count $-$ vehicle control count $\div$ 10^9 survivors per plate.

Note the importance of using actively growing (log phase) bacteria to ensure fixation of mutations and, therefore, sensitivity, as well as the importance of performing accurate dilutions to quantify survival. Because the treat and plate method involves substantially more work than a standard test and may be less sensitive in some cases, it is generally prudent to run a standard plate incorporation test over an extended dose range (based on available information) to justify following up with this method. For details of the method, refer to Green and Muriel [43] and Mitchell et al. [44].

Biological materials often need special consideration in terms of microbial load: filter-sterilization of formulated material may be appropriate if it is not likely to remove active components. Biological materials that contain amino acids or precursors for histidine or tryptophan can be problematic. In particular, S9 can degrade peptides yielding individual amino acids or oligomers that can be utilized by bacteria in place of histidine and tryptophan. Resulting excessive growth of nonrevertant bacteria leads to a corresponding increase in the number of spontaneous revertant colonies [45]. The increases are typically small, and the problem can usually be readily identified by the increased density of the background lawn. However, particulate material can release high levels of amino acids locally, leading to a densely overgrown area in the immediate area of the particle—such "colonies" can appear identical to normal revertant colonies. When this feeding effect is expected or known to occur, the treat and wash method [46] can be used. This is a minor modification of the treat and plate method mentioned that includes supplementation of bacteria with nutrient broth during the exposure period to enhance growth and sensitivity; it does not require plating for viability because toxic effects are not usually expected with this type of material.

Once bacteria are plated in the top agar, an initial lag occurs before bacteria start multiplying [47]; therefore, the preincubation method is generally preferred for labile/unstable or volatile test agents to ensure exposure of actively dividing organisms. For example, much greater increases in revertant colony counts are obtained with formaldehyde using this method compared with the plate incorporation method.

If the test article belongs to a specific chemical class that gives rise to concern for mutagenicity, it may be appropriate to modify the methodology or the strains tested appropriately; oxidizing or cross-linking agents and hydrazines may justify inclusion of *S. typhimurium* strain TA102, whereas azo-dyes and diazo-compounds, gases, and volatile chemicals and glycosides may require modified methods or metabolic activation preparations. Open source programs (e.g., ToxTree, VEGA, OECD) are available to identify structural alerts in organic chemicals (www.vega-qsar.eu, http://toxtree.sourceforge.net, http://www.oecd.org/chemicalsafety/risk-assessment/theoecdqsartoolbox.htm#Guidance_Documents_and_Training_Materials_for_Using_the_Toolbox). Structural alerts for bacterial mutagenicity are summarized in the Benigni-Bossa rulebase [48]. The VEGA program also identifies specific mutagens with similar alerts that can help determine the appropriate methodology and related positive controls.

A few chemicals are photosensitive (degrade) or are photomutagenic, causing bacterial mutations in the presence of light; laboratories that conduct bacterial mutation tests routinely should consider incorporating ancillary gold/yellow lighting for routine use during formulation and dosing.

4.9.2.1 Solvent selection

As in all toxicity tests, the test article must be prepared in an appropriate form for dosing, taking into account chemical stability and compatibility of the vehicle with the test system (refer to the Formulations chapter for more details). Aqueous solvents such as water and saline are preferred and can be used at levels up to approximately 1 mL per plate before they interfere with gelling of the top agar. If the test article has low aqueous solubility (i.e., less than 5 mg/mL), then organic solvents are often used at a maximal dose of 100 μL per plate. Relatively nontoxic organic solvents include dimethyl sulfoxide, dimethlylformamide, ethanol, methanol, propanone (acetone), and acetonitrile (see also Maron et al. [49] and Vedmaurthy et al. [50]). These solvents should be used in the anhydrous form to maximize solubility and decrease accumulation of potentially mutagenic degradants. Some organic solvents (especially those that are not water-miscible such as toluene and those used in preincubation versions of the test) are more toxic and the dose volume must be reduced below 100 μL/plate. In such cases, it may be more practical to solubilize the test article in the primary solvent and then prepare dilutions in a less toxic organic solvent for dosing. Appropriate solvents are not expected to affect the spontaneous revertant colony rate substantially at nontoxic dose volumes; nevertheless, inclusion of an untreated control group is advisable if a novel solvent is used. When working with novel solvents, it may be appropriate to perform a preliminary compatibility test with one or two of the strains ahead of the study. We suggest you evaluate a range of likely solvents during the validation phase of any assay that is new to the laboratory.

Although OECD recommends three plates per experimental point in a standard assay, it may be desirable to increase this for the vehicle (e.g., a set of triplicate control plates at the start and end of the assay) if the laboratory has limited historical control data or, as mentioned, if it has not used that solvent previously.

4.9.2.2 Dose volumes

For the assays using standard Petri dishes, usually 100 μL of test solution, 100 μL bacterial suspension (containing approximately $1-2 \times 10^8$ viable organisms), and 0.5 mL of sodium phosphate buffer or S9 mix (the metabolic activation system) are mixed with 2.0 mL of overlay/top agar immediately before spreading on the plate. The volume of the test solution can be adjusted when appropriate as described in the previous section.

4.9.2.3 Dose levels

Typically, the test material is assessed at five highest concentrations up to the limit of toxicity or, if nontoxic, at five concentrations up to the standard limit of 5000 μg/plate;

concurrent solvent and strain-specific positive control groups are always required except in the case of a dose-range—finding toxicity test. Usually, the test material is dissolved or extracted or occasionally suspended in the chosen vehicle and a range of dilutions is prepared in the vehicle so that a standard dose volume (typically 100 µL per plate) can be administered throughout. When, for practical reasons, the dose volume is variable and the solvent is not expected to have a significant effect on the spontaneous revertant count, it is justifiable to use only the maximal dose volume for the concurrent vehicle control. It is acceptable to use a different solvent and dose volume for the positive control articles; they are generally dissolved in DMSO or, occasionally, for a few specific positive controls, water, and administered at 100 µL per plate. There is no need to include a separate vehicle control for the positive control; results for this group are compared to the corresponding test material vehicle control because appropriate vehicles are not expected to have any substantial effect on the spontaneous revertant colony count.

Toxic effects of the test material are normally indicated by the partial (Figure 4.3b) or complete absence of a background lawn (in which case colony counts, if any, should not be reported) or a substantial concentration-dependent reduction in revertant colony counts compared with lower concentrations and the concurrent vehicle control. The interval between each concentration should be approximately half log ($\sqrt{10}$). A smaller interval may be used where scientifically justified; this is often appropriate in the case of confirmatory testing and may be justified when the test article is not expected to be toxic. Results should be recorded and reported for at least the five highest nontoxic levels (where available) along with values for the concurrent vehicle and positive controls. Details of toxic effects should be recorded and reported; details for the lowest toxic level can be included in results tables to justify reported levels.

OECD guideline 471 indicates "If precipitation (insoluble material) is observed, at least one or more concentrations can be assessed," which can be interpreted in several ways. In practice, it is extremely unlikely that dosing at levels above the limit of solubility will lead to a false-positive result, and exposure to soluble metabolites and material impurities can be increased at these levels. Therefore, we recommend that all levels including those showing obvious precipitate should be scored. When precipitate interferes with automatic colony counting, revertant colonies should be counted by eye and that detail should be noted in the raw data. Often, precipitation will obscure the background lawn—this detail should be recorded in the raw data. In such cases, it is reasonable to assume that the background lawn is normal and intact if the colony counts are close to expected based on results for adjacent dose levels and the concurrent vehicle control. A phase contrast microscope should be available in the laboratory to facilitate examination for precipitate and to confirm the condition of the background lawn. Sometimes the peak dose for mutagenic and toxic effects can occur at a level slightly higher than the limit of solubility in the agar when an organic

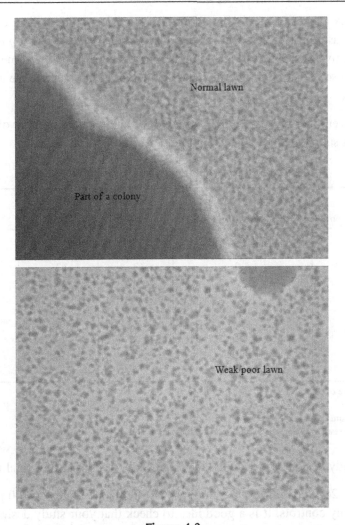

Figure 4.3
Background lawns. The top figure shows a healthy background lawn with part of a normal revertant colony while the bottom figure shows a weak/unhealthy lawn as viwed at low power under a microscope.

solvent is used because the test agent can be present in solution at supersaturated levels during the initial exposure period.

When the test material is in limited supply or when bactericidal effects are suspected, a preliminary toxicity test using one *Salmonella* (often TA100) and one *E. coli* strain (where appropriate) can be used to set dose levels for the subsequent definitive test. In this case, dose levels are usually separated by a factor of 10 and duplicate rather than triplicate plates may be used, although the test material should still be evaluated in the presence and absence of S9 mix because, even in the absence of significant metabolism of the test article, the S9 often acts as a protective agent raising the limit of toxicity. The top dose for the subsequent definitive phase of testing should be one expected to show some toxic effect; six or seven lower dose levels should be included so the target number of five accessible dose levels is achieved.

In the unlikely event that results are not available for an adequate number of dose levels due to toxicity, a supplementary test should be performed (Table 4.5).

Table 4.5: Suggested standard study design: main test

Dose Level/Treatment	Final Conc. (μg/Plate)	Number of Replicates		Number of Strains
		0S9	+S9	
Vehicle	–	3	3	5
1/Test material	1.58	3	3	5
2/Test material	5.0	3	3	5
3/Test material	15.8	3	3	5
4/Test material	50	3	3	5
5/Test material	158	3	3	5
6/Test material	500	3	3	5
7/Test material	1581	3	3	5
8/Test material	5000[a]	3	3	5
Positive control	[b]	3	3	5

0S9 with buffer in place of S9
+S9 with S9
[a]Or 5 μL/plate, maximum dose recommended by OECD.
[b]Dose depends on the test organism, the positive control chemicals, and methodology used.

Based on this study design, you would expect the study to consist of a total of:

10 (treatments) × 2(S9 conditions) × 5 (strains) × 3 (replicate plates) = 300 plates plus appropriate sterility controls. It is a good idea to check that your study design spreadsheet (see later) results in the same number of plates as calculated in the example shown here to minimize the chance of errors. Although the maximum recommended dose for routine testing is 5000 μg per plate, occasionally this may not be achievable for practical reasons (e.g., solubility in the chosen solvent and limitations on dosing volume). Sometimes, a maximum dose above these standard limits may be appropriate (e.g., when testing mixtures or when qualifying a potentially mutagenic impurity in a drug substance). Justification for solvent and dose level selection should be presented in the report.

In the case of non-pharmaceuticals, confirmation of a negative result using a modified methodology is generally required for a regulatory study. The OECD guideline suggests that concentration spacing, the method of treatment (plate incorporation or liquid preincubation), or metabolic activation conditions may be considered appropriate modifications. In practice, it reduces the overall amount of work done if the confirmatory test is performed alongside the original test; the standard plate incorporation method supplies the initial test result while the preincubation method provides confirmatory results. The preincubation method has the added advantage that the concentration of the S9 is effectively increased during the initial exposure and there is direct exposure of bacteria to the test article. In this way, an entire regulatory study can be performed in less than 1 week from the date of test article receipt with only one occasion of formulation.

The work involved in both plate incorporation and preincubation versions of the pour plate test is approximately equivalent. For non-GLP-screening tests, we recommend you use the same pour-plate methodology and S9 conditions that will be used in any eventual regulatory study. The preincubation method can be more sensitive to some chemical classes, which may justify its selection if only one methodology is to be used.

4.9.3 Positive Controls

Positive controls are used to confirm the sensitivity of the test system and the metabolic activity of the S9 mix. Because 2-aminoanthracene is activated by cytostolic enzymes [51], and because its activity can be enhanced using low S9 concentrations, it should not be the only indirect (i.e., metabolically activated) positive control used for routine tests. Example positive controls are listed by OECD and elsewhere; note, however, that mitomycin C is not an appropriate control for *E. coli* WP2 uvrA. For routine testing, each strain is evaluated against a single dose level of an appropriate positive control in both the absence and presence of S9. The dose of positive control should elicit a moderate response as established during the set-up stage of the assay in the laboratory. Intercalating agents such as 9-aminoacridine can have a steep dose-response curve with a narrow mutagenic window between no effect and toxicity, whereas others including the poorly soluble polyaromatic hydrocarbons requiring metabolic activation such as benz[a]pyrene can have a relatively flat dose-response.

Suggested routine positive controls for pour-plate methods and guidance dose levels for the commonly used strains are listed in Table 4.6.

Table 4.6

Strain	Compound	Abbreviation	Conc. µg/Plate	S9
TA1535	Sodium azide	NaAz	0.5	0
TA1537	9-Aminoacridine	9AC	50[a]	0
TA97a	9-Aminoacridine	9AC	50[a]	0
TA98	2-Nitrofluorene or	2NF	1	0
	4-Nitro-*o*-phenylenediamine	NOPD	2.5	0
TA100	Sodium azide	NaAz	0.5	0
TA102	Mitomycin C	MC	0.5	0
WP2 uvrA	4-Nitroquinoline-1-oxide	NQO	0.5	0
WP2 uvrA pKM101	4-Nitroquinoline-1-oxide	NQO	0.2	0

(Continued)

Table 4.6 (Continued)

Strain	Compound	Abbreviation	Conc. μg/Plate	S9
TA1535	2-Aminoanthracene	2AA	2	+
TA1537	Benz[a]pyrene	BaP	5	+
TA97	2-Aminoanthracene	2AA	2	+
TA98	Benz[a]pyrene	BaP	5	+
TA100	Benz[a]pyrene	BaP	5	+
TA102	Danthron	DAN	25	+
WP2 uvrA	2-Aminoanthracene	2AA	20	+
WP2 uvrA pKM101	2-Aminoanthracene	2AA	20	1

[a]A lower dose of 9AC may be appropriate if a preincubation method is used.

4.10 Standard Test Procedures

The procedures used for routine testing largely follow those described in the DIAGNOSTIC MUTAGEN TEST section. Note that we recommend that laboratories new to bacterial mutation testing should use:

Top agar supplemented with biotin plus limited histidine and tryptophan (TAC)
Bottom agar with low 0.4% glucose (MGA)
Nutrient broth without antibiotics

In this way, the media are suitable for use with any of the tester strains and there is much less danger of a mix-up.

The phenotype and diagnostic mutagen checks, spontaneous revertant colony counts (assuming adequate laboratory data are available for the selected vehicle and dose volume), and viability of the bacteria do not need to be confirmed as part of a routine study provided that these characteristics have been established in advance of the experiment. Instead, vehicle and positive control colony counts and the condition of the background lawn are generally considered adequate internal checks.

Fresh bacterial suspension cultures should be inoculated so that they are in the active growth phase with a density of $1-2 \times 10^9$ bacteria/mL at the time of use as described in Appendix 1 using a combination of OD (optical density) measurement and direct counting. Plating for assessing viability is not particularly useful because results are not available to confirm suitability of the culture until later; therefore, it is only considered necessary when the treat and plate modification of the test is used (refer to Modifications of Standard Methods section later).

4.10.1 Plate Incorporation Method

The general procedures are as detailed in the diagnostic mutagen test. A 0.5 mL aliquot of S9 mix (+S9) or phosphate buffer (0S9) is combined with a standard volume (typically 100 μL) of the test solution in sterile tubes in a rack. At least the first and last tubes in the rack should be labeled with a number corresponding to the plate number in the experimental design. The tubes can be stored briefly in the refrigerator, and then 2.0 mL of molten TAC followed by 100 μL bacterial suspension are added to each tube in turn; the tube is vortex-mixed briefly and its contents are immediately poured onto the surface of the corresponding MGA plate. The plates are stacked on a level surface.

Although the order of addition may not be critical, adding the components in this order may help minimize toxicity of the test substance and reduce potential carry-over of bacteria— care should be taken to avoid carry-over of chemicals from one tube to another on the pipette tip. Laboratories with high throughput should purchase a metered peristaltic pump (Wheaton, Cole-Parmer) that is set to dispense 2.0 mL top agar every time a foot switch is depressed. Other components can be conveniently added using air-displacement multidose micropipettes unless a volatile or viscous vehicle is used, in which case a positive displacement pipette system should be used. In this way, all the tubes can be dosed with S9 or buffer and test article in the morning. Subsequently, one operator doses each tube with top agar and bacteria before passing it to a second operative who mixes the contents and pours and stacks the plates. With practice using this type of setup, a team of two technicians can handle an experiment involving formulation and approximately 1200 plates in 1 day. Alternately, when only one technician is available, the tubes with test article and buffer/S9 mix can be placed in a heat block set to 45°C and one block of tubes can be treated and plated at a time.

Once all the plates have been poured and the agar has gelled, they are inverted and incubated at 37°C. Although OECD indicates an incubation period of 48–72 h is acceptable, toxicity of the test solution can reduce the growth rate of the colonies, making them more difficult to detect, especially for strains with higher mutation rates that have more, but smaller, revertant colonies [52]. In addition, even for untreated controls, the colony size tends to increase even at the late stage of incubation. Therefore, we recommend standardizing the incubation period toward the end of this range to facilitate detection of all revertant colonies and to minimize variation in historical control counts. A standard incubation period of 65 h is convenient because it allows the plates to be placed in the incubator at 4:00 PM then removed at 9:00 AM 3 days later.

4.10.2 Preincubation Method

Both versions of the pour-plate (plate incorporation and preincubation) method are generally equally acceptable to regulatory authorities and, when testing non-pharmaceuticals, a combination of the methods is expected to capture nearly all bacterial mutagens. The study design for the two methods is identical and the procedure is very similar.

Using the preincubation method, the test solution is added to each tube, and then S9 mix/ buffer followed by the bacterial suspension are added. The tubes are incubated at 37°C for a standard period of at least 20 (usually 30) min on the platform of an orbital shaker set to a speed just below that causing foaming (typically 180 rpm) in an incubator set to 37°C. It is convenient to incubate the tubes in batches soon after addition of the bacteria. After preincubation, 2.0 mL of molten top agar supplemented with histidine, biotin, and tryptophan is added to each tube in turn, and the contents are mixed briefly by vortexing and then overlaid onto a minimal glucose plate. After the overlay gels, the plates are inverted and then incubated as in the plate incorporation method.

Sometimes it is necessary to modify the method due to the nature of the test article. Studies using these methods may be fully valid and acceptable for regulatory submission provided that appropriate scientific justification for the modification is presented in the report.

4.10.3 Standard Study Design

The Study Design spreadsheet should be generated from a standard template file with plates numbered sequentially prior to the study to specify the contents of each plate and, in the case of GLP studies, who did what and when. The example in Table 4.7 for a single test article covers the sterility control checks, positive controls, and dose levels 0 (vehicle control), 1, and 2 for the first strains. Dose levels 3–8 follow the same layout as doses 1 and 2 at final concentrations of 15.8, 50, 158, 500, 1580, and 5000 µg/plate (typical dose levels for routine testing); this is repeated with each strain in turn. In this case, the final row of the spreadsheet is used to document the staff involved and dates. The preincubation time column is used only in the preincubation version of the test. Blank cells indicate that the additives are the same as in the cell above. The design can be broken down into sections:

1. The first section includes the appropriate sterility controls
2. Positive controls for all strains (typically 30 plates)
3. Vehicle control and the eight dose levels of test material with and without S9 (54 plates) with the first tester strain repeated for each of the other four strains
4. This is repeated for each additional test material tested concurrently—each additional compound tested adds 270 plates plus appropriate sterility controls except when the same solvent/vehicle is used, in which case it would be $48 \times 5 = 240$ plates for each additional compound plus sterility plate(s).

In the example, test article dose number 0 corresponds to the vehicle control and A, B, C indicate the order of additions. Where more than one test article is being assessed, there is no need to duplicate vehicle or positive controls. If this occurs in GLP studies at a Contract Research Organization (CRO), then the test article name should be replaced by a code name to ensure anonymity in case of client review of raw data.

Table 4.7: Study design, example

Plate No.	A Treatment	Dose No.	Dose Vol. μL	Dose μg/Plate	C Strain	B S9	Preinc Time, From to	Count	Observations (If Any)
1	Untreated	−	−	−	−	0			
2	Untreated	−	−	−	−	+			
3	Test article	0	100	0	−	0			
4	Test article	8	100	5000	−	0			
5	NaAz	1	100	0.5	−	0			
6	9AC	1	100	50		0			
7	2NF	1	100	1		0			
8	NQO	1	100	0.5		0			
9	2AA	2	100	20		0			
10	BaP	1	100	5		0			
11	NaAz	1	100	0.5	TA1535	0			
12	NaAz			0.5	TA1535	0			
13	NaAz			0.5	TA1535	0			
14	2AA	1	100	2	TA1535	+			
15	2AA			5	TA1535	+			
16	2AA			5	TA1535	+			
17	9AC	1	100	50	TA1537	0			
18	9AC			50	TA1537	0			
19	9AC			50	TA1537	0			
20	BaP	1	100	5	TA1537	+			
21	BaP			5	TA1537	+			
22	BaP			5	TA1537	+			
23	2NF	1	100	1	TA98	0			
24	2NF			1	TA98	0			
25	2NF			1	TA98	0			
26	BaP	1	100	5	TA98	+			
27	BaP			5	TA98	+			
28	BaP			5	TA98	+			
29	NaAz	1	100	0.5	TA100	0			
30	NaAz			0.5	TA100	0			
31	NaAz			0.5	TA100	0			
32	BaP	1	100	5	TA100	+			
33	BaP			5	TA100	+			
34	BaP			5	TA100	+			
35	NQO	1	100	0.5	WP2uvrA	0			
36	NQO			0.5	WP2uvrA	0			
37	NQO			0.5	WP2uvrA	0			
38	2AA	2	100	20	WP2uvrA	+			
39	2AA			20	WP2uvrA	+			
40	2AA			20	WP2uvrA	+			
41	Test article	0	100	0	TA1535	0			
42					TA1535	0			
43					TA1535	0			
44					TA1535	+			

(Continued)

Table 4.7: (Continued)

Plate No.	A Treatment	Dose No.	Dose Vol. μL	Dose μg/Plate	C Strain	B S9	Preinc Time, From to	Count	Observations (If Any)
45					TA1535	+			
46					TA1535	+			
47	Test article	1	100	1.58	TA1535	0			
48					TA1535	0			
49					TA1535	0			
50					TA1535	+			
51					TA1535	+			
52					TA1535	+			
53	Test article	2	100	5	TA1535	0			
54					TA1535	0			
55					TA1535	0			
56					TA1535	+			
57					TA1535	+			
58					TA1535	+			
Init./date									

4.10.4 Examination of the Plates

After the incubation period, the plates can be examined immediately or stored refrigerated for a few days prior to examination if more convenient. Subsequently, the plates should be stored refrigerated until the results have been compiled and reviewed in case any additional checks are needed. Plates should be evaluated for the quality of the background lawn, the presence of precipitate, and the number of revertant colonies. A microscope should be available to check the quality of the lawn and for the presence of precipitate in case of any doubt following visual examination. Colony counts may be performed "manually" with the aid of a bench-top tally counter and a marker pen. This type of manual counting can be facilitated using a Quebec colony counter illumination system; however, because of the effort involved in manual counting, laboratories performing tests routinely use an automatic colony counter that relies on image analysis to enumerate colonies. Automatic colony counters are generally adjusted to ignore the edge of the plate (which otherwise could be falsely interpreted as bacterial colonies), so a standard mathematical adjustment may be appropriate to provide the equivalent full plate count to allow direct comparison with manual counts. This calculation can be done automatically by systems specifically designed for bacterial mutation testing as follows:

corrected (reported) count = frame count × plate area ÷ frame area

Precipitate, highly colored test article, or minor microbial contamination can interfere with automatic colony counting, in which case a visual count can usually be made.

Depending on the throughput of the laboratory and the GLP status of the test, results may be entered by pen or by direct keyboard entry into the study design, or by direct data capture if an automatic colony counter is used—the latter two methods are preferred because they avoid transcription errors. If precipitation interferes with observation of the background lawn, then this is recorded. Whatever system of data entry is used, it should allow manual input of comments regarding the plates; usually, this is facilitated by the use of standardized abbreviations such as:

cx	microbial contamination obscuring count
c	microbial contamination not obscuring count
il	incomplete lawn (toxicity)
mc	microcolonies (toxicity)
nl	no lawn (toxicity)
poc	precipitate obscuring count
pol	precipitate obscuring assessment of background lawn
ppt	precipitate
vc	visual count
vr	visual recount

4.10.5 Interpretation of Results

4.10.5.1 Evaluation of toxicity

Toxic effects of the test item are normally indicated by the partial or complete absence of a background lawn (colony counts, if any, should not be reported in this case) or a substantial dose-related reduction in revertant colony counts compared with lower dose levels and concurrent vehicle control taking into account the laboratory historical control range; for example, a fold response of less than 0.6-times the concurrent control can be selected empirically to trigger a comment (either considered to be "indicative of toxicity" or, if no supporting information from associated points, "considered to be due to normal variation"). Where precipitation obscures observations on the condition of the background lawn, the lawn can be considered normal and intact if the revertant colony counts are within the expected range based on results for lower dose levels and historical control counts for that strain.

4.10.5.2 Validity of the study

Normally, the bacteria will have been evaluated for appropriate phenotypic markers and response to diagnostic mutagens in advance of use in an individual study. Where these checks are performed concurrently with the study, results for any strain that do not pass the check should be considered invalid.

The spontaneous mean revertant colony counts for each strain should lie close to or within the current historical control range of the laboratory. Note that historical control ranges for the test can drift over time so, providing that the laboratory has sufficient background data, the historical control range should cover only the past 2 years. At a minimum, the historical data should be from at least 10 and preferably 20 independent experiments [53]; the laboratory will have accumulated at least this number of results during their own internal validation of the test. The chosen positive controls (with S9 where required) evaluated concurrently as part of the study should produce substantial increases in revertant colony numbers with the appropriate bacterial strain.

In the case where part of the study is invalid based on criteria described in the protocol (e.g., the positive control does not induce an appropriate response with an individual strain or there is generally poor growth of the background lawn with that strain), detailed results for that part of the study do not need to be reported. The affected part of the study would normally be subjected to an automatic repeat, in which case a protocol amendment with supporting justification may be appropriate for GLP studies if this scenario is not fully covered in the original protocol.

4.10.5.3 Criteria for negative/positive/equivocal outcome

The mean number of revertant colonies for all treatment groups is compared with those obtained for the concurrent vehicle control level. The mutagenic activity of the test item is routinely assessed by applying the following criteria:

The results are considered positive (i.e., indicative of mutagenic potential) if:

- The results for the test item show a substantial increase in revertant colony counts, i.e., response two-times or more the concurrent vehicle control level values, with mean value(s) outside the laboratory historical control range (beyond the 98% tolerance limit). Otherwise, results are considered negative. *Note that this two fold rule is conventional but somewhat arbitrary: depending on a laboratory's experience with the strain it may be more appropriate to require a higher fold increase for strains with a low spontaneous revertant colony count (e.g., TA1537) and a lower threshold for strains with a high spontaneous reversion rate (e.g., 1.5-fold for strains TA97a, TA100, TA102, and WP2 uvrA pKM101). Apparent isolated responses in only a single replicate plate occur only rarely and should be viewed with suspicion; generally, they would be regarded as outliers and reported only in parentheses with appropriate justification for their exclusion from calculation of mean values.*
- The above increase must be dose-related and/or reproducible (i.e., increases must be obtained at more than one experimental point, more than one dose level, more than one occasion, or with different methodologies).

If the second criterion is not met, then the results may be classified as equivocal, and further testing may be appropriate to clarify such results using an appropriately modified study design, (e.g., a narrower dose interval with the appropriate strain) [52]. Parallel testing with appropriate modifications to the test, e.g., using the preincubation method if the original test used the plate incorporation method or also testing TA1537 if the original apparent effect was seen with TA97a. In such cases, if no substantial increase (as defined) is obtained in the confirmatory test, then the results will be considered negative.

It may be that a consistent apparently treatment-related increase in revertant colony counts is obtained on more than one occasion, but the increase does not meet the two fold criterion described. In this case it may be appropriate to consider the outcome as borderline or equivocal, which would put more emphasis on follow-up testing using relevant (often *in vivo*) systems.

4.10.5.4 Unexpected and borderline results

Certain classes of chemicals (i.e., those with structural alerts or with specific modes of biological activity) can be expected to give positive results in the bacterial mutation test. In some cases, bacterial mutagenicity may be due to formation of unique *in vitro* metabolites or degradants; alternatively, the effect may be bacterial-specific and therefore not considered relevant in terms of hazard assessment. In cases where an apparent effect is unexpected for that class of material, it is advisable to check the reproducibility of the results to preclude any experimental error. This is particularly true when an increase in revertant colony counts is seen in only part of the experiment (e.g., in one strain only in the absence but not the presence of S9) and no evidence of genotoxicity has been obtained in other test systems. In this case, only the affected part of the experiment needs repeating over an appropriate dose range using a narrower dose interval, where appropriate. When testing materials in accord with OECD guideline 471, the results of the confirmatory test are normally expected to be very similar to those seen in the initial test even though slightly modified methods may have been used, (e.g., plate incorporation in the initial test and preincubation method in the confirmatory phase).

If the unexpected increase is found to be reproducible, then consideration should be given to the possible presence of a mutagenic impurity in the test article. In this case, different batches of the test material and a highly purified lot of the test material can be compared using the appropriate strain(s). If a substantial difference in response is seen with different batches, then chemical analysis and examination of the synthetic route intermediates can be used to identify the responsible impurity, which, in turn and if stable, could be isolated or synthesized before testing in its pure form.

4.10.6 Presentation of Results

The report should, at a minimum, include all the items listed in the OECD guideline 471 and FDA Redbook 2000 [17,39]. Results should be tabulated to show individual, mean, and standard deviations for revertant colony counts. Any individual counts that are reported but not used for calculation of mean values should be indicated in parentheses and a reason for their exclusion should be footnoted in the tables.

Mean colony counts and their SDs should be rounded and presented to the nearest whole number. Fold values should be reported to a minimum number of significant figures except when clarification is required to define borderline results (e.g., 0.3, 1.8, 11, 1.95). Related values such as concentrations should be decimal-aligned in columns (Tables 4.8 and 4.9).

Results should be presented for all evaluated dose levels for each strain/S9 combination plus at least one toxic level (in cases where toxicity has been observed). At least three of the reported dose levels should not show toxic effects (see next section). Results for all three plates at each reported experimental point should be presented; occasional loss of a plate (e.g., due to microbial contamination) is permissible. Individual plate counts may be considered as potentially erroneous if they are well outside expected levels based on historical control values and results for related plates. In such cases, we suggest reporting the colony count in parentheses and excluding the value from any calculation while presenting justification in a footnote to the table. Although OECD mentions the possibility of using duplicate plates, we advise against it because of the greater potential for invalidating results in the event of loss of an individual plate. Although duplicate plates may be justifiable for the positive controls, the potential very minor savings in workload do not seem to warrant their use.

Negative/spontaneous historical control values for relevant experiments performed within the recent past under similar conditions should be presented in detail to give an idea of how often values at the upper limits occur by chance. If values obtained with different methodologies (e.g., with and without S9, using plate incorporation and preincubation methods) are similar, then historical control values can be presented as combined results for the sake of simplicity. In some laboratories revertant counts for some strains may be somewhat higher in the presence of S9. In that case the laboratory should consider presenting without and with S9 historical control results separately once a sufficiently large database has been accumulated. However, all appropriate details including method, dose volume, and vehicle should be recorded in the historical control database in case there is a reason to consider historical control data for specific conditions separately. The following examples give suggested layouts; footnotes that are not used in a particular report can be deleted. Note that certain authorities also require submission of tabulated summary reports (e.g., eCTD as described by ICH) [54]; these may be supplied separately or in the first (summary) section of the report.

The chart (Figure 4.4) is an example of the historical mean revertant colony counts for triplicate plates obtained in previous QA-audited experiments performed between the first and the last experiment. In this example, the grand mean is 14, SD is 4, and 97.5% of the results fall within the range of 7 to 23 revertants per plate (Table 4.10).

Table 4.8: Compound A: plate incorporation test in the absence of S9 mix.

Strain	Concentration (µg/Plate)	Number of Revertants					Plate Observations[a]			Fold Response[b]
		x_1	x_2	x_3	Mean	SD	x_1	x_2	x_3	
TA1535	0.9% NaCl	27	23	24	25	2				1.0
	15.8	14	18	15	16	2				0.6
	50	12	21	15	16	5				0.6
	158	19	14	$(3)^c$	17	(4)				0.7
	500	31	20	23	25	6				1.0
	1580	19	19	16	18	2				0.7
	5000	7	7	—	7	(0)			il	0.3	T
TA1537	0.9% NaCl	13	16	22	17	5				1.0
	15.8	14	17	16	16	2				0.9
	50	22	13	14	16	5				1.0
	158	14	22	14	17	5				1.0
	500	29	23	27	26	3				1.5
	1580	24	18	14	19	5				1.1
	5000	—	—	—	—	—	il	il	il		T
TA98	0.9% NaCl	31	34	27	31	4				1.0
	15.8	34	26	30	30	4				1.0
	50	41	38	39	39	2				1.3
	158	71	65	83	73	9				2.4	+
	500	143	152	139	145	7				4.7	+
	1580	69	77	103	83	18				2.7	+
	5000	—	—	—	—	—	il	il	nl		T
TA100	0.9% NaCl	143	103	122	123	20				1.0
	15.8	117	135	110	121	13				1.0
	50	103	148	111	121	24				1.0
	158	111	128	113	117	9				1.0
	500	103	143	122	123	20				1.0
	1580	95	106	110	104	8				0.8
	5000	—	—	—	—	—	nl	nl	nl		T
WP2 *uvrA*	0.9% NaCl	43	46	41	43	3				1.0
	50	40	36	44	40	4				0.9
	158	53	43	59	52	8				1.2
	500	46	50	69	55	12				1.3
	1580	41	63	46	50	12				1.2
	5000	21	20	23	21	2				0.5	T

Notes: SD Sample standard deviation;

NA Not applicable

T Toxic as indicated by low revertant colony counts (fold response <0.6) or incomplete/no background lawn (no meaningful count results for plates with il or nl)

L Low count considered due to normal variation rather than toxicity because not clearly dose-related and not outside normal limits based on historical control values

+ Substantial increase in revertant colony counts

[a]Comments on the plate or background lawn: incomplete lawn (il), no lawn (nl), precipitate (ppt), contamination did not obscure count (c), precipitate obscured assessment of background lawn (pol).

[b]Mean revertant count÷concurrent vehicle control value.

[c]Value excluded from the mean because outside expected range based on results for vehicle control and adjacent plates (possible technical error).

Table 4.9: Positive controls for the plate incorporation assay.

Strain	Treatment	Concentration (µg/Plate)	S9	x_1	x_2	x_3	Mean	SD	Fold Response[a]
TA1535	NaAz	0.5	0	327	328	334	**330**	11	12
TA1537	9AC	50	0	356	379	532	**422**	97	22
TA98	2NF	1	0	142	143	96	**127**	27	4.8
TA100	NaAz	0.5	0	537	503	500	**513**	13	5.0
WP2 uvrA	NQO	0.5	0	1180	1201	1170	**1193**	20	27
TA1535	2AA	5	+	247	252	192	**230**	33	15
TA1537	BaP	5	+	104	121	101	**109**	11	6.1
TA98	BaP	5	+	227	263	289	**260**	31	6.2
TA100	BaP	5	+	721	769	749	**746**	24	5.2
WP2 uvrA	2AA	20	+	228	227	206	**220**	12	3.8

Notes: SD Sample standard deviation
0S9 Without S9
+S9 With S9
[a]Fold response in mean revertants compared to concurrent vehicle control.

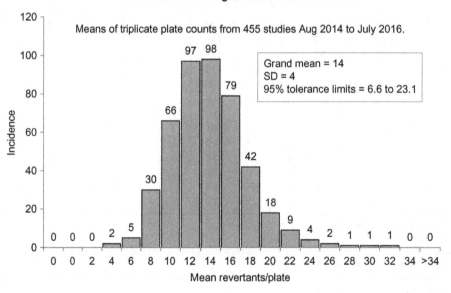

Figure 4.4
Example of historical negative/vehicle control results.

Table 4.10: Historical positive control results

Strain	Treatment	Dose (µg/Plate)	S9	Mean	SD	Range
TA1535	NaAz	0.5	0	320	45	151−655
TA1537	9AC	50	0	337	172	29−2010
TA98	2NF	1	0	166	41	43−330
TA100	NaAz	0.5	0	530	59	250−1003
WP2 *uvrA*	NQO	0.5	0	610	201	82−2220
TA1535	2AA	5	+	380	91	44−699
TA1537	BaP	5	+	110	24	35−189
TA98	BaP	5	+	369	81	179−681
TA100	BaP	5	+	1040	216	408−1669
WP2 *uvrA*	2AA	20	+	300	165	108−2444

Notes: SD Standard deviation
0S9 Without S9
+S9 With S9

Note that in comparison to negative control counts, positive control values can vary widely, so the value of making comparisons of mean values with the values obtained in any specific experiment is limited.

Sometimes it is useful to compare mutagenic potencies of materials tested concurrently (e.g., extracts of soil samples prepared before and after amelioration). In such cases, results are plotted graphically using a spreadsheet program such as Microsoft Excel or OpenOffice. Results obtained at toxic levels should be excluded and then a line of best fit is used to calculate slope expressed as induced revertants (per gram of soil in our example). The dose-response is not necessarily expected to be linear (especially over a wide dose range), so an appropriate transformation may help straighten the curve. Because of this lack of linearity, it is extremely important for equivalent dose levels to be compared; in our example, the doses should be expressed in terms of weight of soil rather than mg of extract.

4.10.7 Testing of Volatile and Gaseous Compounds

The standard plate incorporation and preincubation assays must be specially adapted to allow reliable detection of mutagenic gases and volatiles [55,56]. In both cases bacteria are plated out in the top agar with either buffer or S9 before sealing them in commercially available Tedlar gas sampling bags. Alternatively, they can be exposed in a desiccator jar [57]. As much air as practical is removed before measured amounts of air and the test gas are injected via a septum or valve in the bag using a gas syringe or via a wet gas meter; a flow meter is not suitable for accurate measurement of volume unless it has been calibrated for that particular gas. A range of concentrations of the gas are evaluated; the calculated concentrations should take into account the dead volume of residual air in the plates after the bag has been partially evacuated. Using standard mutagenic gases, the plates can be stacked inverted with lids on as usual. After incubation for the standard period (e.g., 65 h), the bags are vented and removed in a fume cupboard; after the gas has dissipated, plates are evaluated as usual. Note that many types of plastic are porous to gases (Tedlar tends to be less so), and atmospheres of up to 100% gas are possible if the bag is purged with the gas because the bacteria are facultative anaerobes. The laboratory should validate the system using gaseous mutagenic agents. At least one of these can be included in individual studies as proof of competency; otherwise, standard positive controls are sufficient. In the case of volatile materials, a measured amount of test article is added to a glass Petri dish that is immediately sealed in the bag prior to injection of air.

4.11 Screening Tests

Given the importance placed on the outcome of the bacterial mutation test by regulatory authorities, many companies screen their compounds for microbial genotoxicity at a very early stage of the development. At this point, test article availability and resources are often limited, so it is not necessary or feasible to run a full standard test. Individual laboratories may use "cut-down" versions of the Ames test, such as testing only in the presence of S9, using a reduced top dose level, fewer replicate plates, reducing the number of strains examined (often using only TA98 and TA100), or a combination of these [58]. The advantage of this approach is that results can be directly extrapolated to what might be expected in the subsequent GLP test; the disadvantage is that there will be some difficulty in detection of weak mutagens or, in the case of reducing the number of strains, that some mutagens will be missed. However, a positive result in such a test is sufficient to categorize the chemical as a mutagen. Numerous other approaches to preliminary screening have been proposed; some of the modified standard methods and other approaches to screening in current use in the pharmaceutical industry have been summarized and evaluated by Escobar et al. [59].

4.11.1 Simplified Test Systems

Screening tests based on a single or matched pair of test organisms to detect forward mutations or DNA damage generally have very low test material and resource requirements; their main utility seems to be in very early stage screening. However, their predictive ability (in terms of correlation with the eventual Ames test results) seems to be generally weak, so they are only described briefly here. Examples in current use include:

1. Forward mutation systems involve loss of functionality of a non-vital gene leading to drug resistance. Miller et al. [60] described use of strain TA100 to assess induction of forward mutation to 5-fluorouracil resistance in a system with close parallels to the mouse lymphoma mammalian cell mutation assay. An additional mutation was added to the tester strain to prevent cross-feeding (metabolic cooperation). The test uses 30 mg of compound compared with more than 10-times that much for a standard Ames test.

This particular test seemed to perform well during validation with known mutagens but was much less predictive of the Ames test in routine use in one laboratory [59].

2. Bacterial DNA repair tests assess differential killing of matched pairs of tester strains, one of which is repair-deficient. In theory, the repair-deficient strain should be more sensitive to toxins that primarily target DNA [43,61–64]. Toxicity can be assessed using either liquid or semisolid (diffusion-based) systems.

3. Several systems have been developed that detect the biochemical stress response of the organism to DNA damage. These include the "umu test" in which TA1535 incorporates a pSK1002 plasmid containing the umuC gene fused to a lacZ reporter gene. The umuC gene is activated as part of the bacterial SOS response, which, in turn, promotes the β-galactosidase activity associated with lacZ, which is assessed by a colorimetric reaction. Related tests include SOS chromotest in an *E. coli* strain with a deficient cell wall [65]. Vitotox measures induction of a luciferase bioluminescence gene under transcriptional control of a SOS response gene [66,67].

4. Greenscreen and Bluescreen are related licensed reporter gene assays with the same advantages of high-throughput, miniaturization, and low compound requirements. The technology was originally developed in yeast and subsequently transferred to human transformed cell lines. Because the systems use eukaryotic cells, they are not necessarily predictive of the outcome of the Ames test, although they may be capable of detecting a wider range of relevant genotoxic effects [68].

4.11.2 Screening Tests Using Standard Tester Strains

Although some screening tests use non-standard strains or even mixtures of strains, these modifications are not recommended when trying to predict the outcome of the eventual GLP study because of expected lack of correlation, difficulty in interpretation, and reduced sensitivity. Assays using the standard test strains in pure form are discussed briefly.

1. In the Spot Test [69,70] the bacteria are mixed with S9 and top agar and then plated out on MGA using the same components as in a standard bacterial mutation test. A 100-μL volume of test solution is added to a 6-mm filter disc or to a central well created using an alcohol sterilized cork-borer. The test article can also be added directly to the surface of the plate as a solid or as a liquid in a dose volume of 10 μL. During the subsequent incubation at 37°C for 48–72 h, the test article usually diffuses out from center, creating a concentration gradient. Potent mutagens cause a halo around the center, showing an increased density of revertant colonies; often, this halo will have a central zone with no background lawn or with a decreased colony density due to toxicity. The method has obvious deficiencies with respect to sensitivity, its nonquantitative nature, and the requirement for the mutagen (or its active metabolite) to diffuse into the medium.

2. The sloped (gradient) plate method [71] and the Spiral Plate [72–74] both create concentration gradients using physical methods. Although the spiral plates can be analyzed using image analysis equipment, interpretation of results is not as straightforward as in standard testing and both methods use nonstandard equipment; consequently, neither method seems to have gained widespread acceptance.

3. The microsuspension assay was originally developed to detect mutagenic metabolites in urine extract samples [75] to cope with low sample volumes. Bacteria are concentrated to 10-times the normal density by centrifugation and then preincubated with the test sample and S9 (where appropriate) for 90 min prior to plating out in the normal way. Compared with pour-plate methods, a higher density of bacteria are exposed during this preincubation period to high concentrations of the test material, which should mean that a similar response is obtained with reduced compound requirements. However, the bacteria are not dividing during the preincubation period and exposure to the test compound is greatly reduced after plating, both of which are expected to reduce sensitivity of the test as compared with the standard preincubation method. A 96-well version of the microsuspension test has recently been briefly described that simplifies the dosing procedure [59].

4. The BioLum method involves bioluminescent derivatives of the standard test organisms. The bacteria are plated with top agar, S9 (or buffer), and test article in a 24-well plate format that reduces test article usage by at least 95%. Revertant colonies are easy to detect by their phosphorescence and can be scored using a custom-built system [59,76].

5. The fluctuation test originally formulated by Nobel Prize winners Luria and Delbruck was adapted for mutagenicity screening in the 1970s [43,77]. In a more convenient version of the test with very low test article requirements, bacteria are diluted in medium with S9 (where appropriate) before inoculation into microtiter plates [78,79]; both 96- and 384-well versions of the test are used routinely. After overnight incubation, the medium is replaced by medium without histidine/tryptophan before incubation for an additional 3 days; bromocresol purple or bromothymol blue indicator is added at the replenishment point or after completion of incubation and then the proportion of wells showing bacterial growth (as evidenced by pH (color) change and the presence of microscopic colonies) is recorded. Because the bacteria are directly exposed to the test compound during the initial exposure period, and because the spontaneous frequency of mutation can be accurately measured using this method if survival is assessed, it can be more sensitive than pour-plate methods. To optimize sensitivity, the number of viable bacteria dispensed into each well must be controlled to yield approximately 20% positive wells in the vehicle controls. Cultures of TA100 are usually diluted with nine volumes of culture medium immediately before use; a lower histidine concentration may also be appropriate for this strain to optimize the number of spontaneous positive wells [52]. Results can be interpreted using a one-sided chi-square

look-up table [77]; use of the 1% rather than 5% critical significance will help avoid false-positive claims associated with numerous comparisons with the concurrent control. The method may be more problematic and slightly more work than a pour-plate test but, because of its sensitivity, is suited to testing dilute environmental samples, has lower sample requirement, and may be amenable to automation [80–83]. Several commercial kits are available for performing fluctuation tests [84], but they are not necessarily suited to those unfamiliar with genotoxicity testing.

4.11.3 Reduced Format Tests Using Standard Tester Strains

These use the same methods and principles as the standard test except the volume of all components is reduced proportionately. The six-well Miniscreen involves an 80% reduction in volume and consequently utilizes 20% test compound compared with the standard method with a top dose of 1000 μg/well [85]. The 24-well version of Miniscreen is a minor adaptation of a 25-well version originally described by workers in the United Kingdom [86,87] and is now referred to as the micro-Ames [59], or μAmes, with test article usage 95% lower than the conventional Ames test (Figure 4.5). It is advisable to enter results directly into the study design spreadsheet to reduce workload and the chance of transcription error. Where a large increase in revertants is evident, the number of colonies should be estimated (e.g., entering values of >100 and >200 colonies as 101 and 201 in the spreadsheet). An appropriate statistical method can be used to help evaluate the strength of any response because the somewhat arbitrary "two fold rule" to specify positivity is inappropriate, particularly for strains with low background revertant colony counts (i.e., the nonplasmid-containing strains). Results can be extrapolated and compared directly with those obtained using the conventional method. The tests are best suited for use with strains having higher mutation rates because relative increases are easier to identify. The disadvantage of strains with low spontaneous counts can be overcome to some extent by substitution of strains (e.g., using TA97a in place of TA1537) and, in the case of μAmes, by increasing the number of vehicle control replicates from 3 to 12 wells to more accurately define the background rate of reversion. In the 24-well plate version, the compound is added directly on to the bottom agar before addition of a premix of bacteria + S9 (or buffer) + top agar, allowing it to be performed by a single operative in substantially less time than a standard test. Because image analysis systems have not been developed to score plates in these formats, colonies are necessarily scored by eye, which is facilitated using a benchtop tally counter and light box or a Quebec colony counter.

The standard size (positive control) plate illustrates the normal variation in colony size. The smaller colonies probably grow from late-occurring mutants, whereas the larger colonies often show a denser central spot, giving a "poached egg" appearance. These are colonies that have broken out onto the surface of the agar and spread out. Smaller colonies

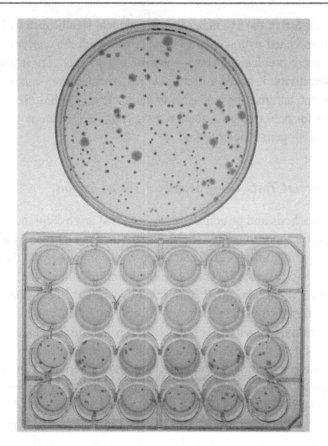

Figure 4.5
Comparison of a standard and a 24-well plate format.

(sometimes torpedo-shaped) are those that remain embedded in the matrix of the medium. The 24-well plate shows a fairly flat dose-response in the presence of S9. The top 12 wells have been treated with the vehicle, whereas the lower wells have been treated with benz[a]pyrene.

4.12 Appendix 1: Growing and Monitoring Suspension Cultures

Technical problems in individual laboratories or experiments such as generally poor background lawns, micro-colonies, and spurious control counts can be due to issues with the top or bottom agar (e.g., top agar too hot or MGA incorrectly formulated). However, problems with individual strains are usually caused by use of unhealthy (often overgrown) suspension cultures or inappropriately maintained stocks. Standardization of culture conditions and appropriate monitoring of growth will help to prevent these issues.

Suspension cultures are usually initiated by addition of freshly thawed bacterial suspension of known density or an isolated colony from a streak into, typically, 25 or 30 mL of nutrient broth in a flask. If a frozen ampoule of bacterial suspension is used, then the suspension should be thawed rapidly in a 37°C water bath while agitating; as soon as the ampoule is thawed, a measured amount of the culture is added to the nutrient broth to dilute the cryoprotectant. The flask is secured on the platform of a gyratory shaker in an incubator and incubated at 37°C at a speed below that causing foaming (typically approximately 100 rpm depending on the shaker and the flask) until, based on growth curve experiments described in the next section, the targeted OD is achieved and the concentration of bacteria has been confirmed by direct count. The density of the culture can also be confirmed by plating, but results will not be available until the next day.

The culture should then be held at room temperature for use on the same day, either for testing or for preparation of frozen aliquots as suggested here. If the suspension is stored chilled for a few hours, then it should be brought to room temperature before addition of top agar to minimize any lag phase and to avoid the possibility of thermal shock [57].

It is important for an optimal and standardized number of actively growing bacteria to be exposed to the test material and its metabolites during the most critical phase of the test (i.e., soon after dosing). Bacteria should have just reached the late log phase of growth at the time of use (target density is $1-2 \times 10^9$ organisms per mL). A common error is to use an apparently very dense overnight culture in late stationary phase that contains a low titer of viable bacteria. Determination of the growth characteristics of bacteria under standardized conditions in the laboratory as described here will ensure that bacterial cultures prepared later for characterization or routine tests achieve an appropriate density at a convenient time in the working day. Accurate assessment of density is complicated by the fact that bacterial size and morphology change during different phases of growth; in addition, bacteria tend to form chains and may clump.

Bacterial density can be estimated by turbidimetric measurement, plate counts, or direct counts using a counting chamber or a Coulter-type particle counter. Whatever method is used, rough pipetting will help disrupt any chains of bacteria prior to measurement. Most laboratories use a spectrometer to measure optical density (OD) of the bacterial suspension at 650 nm as a surrogate for turbidity; a 1/10 dilution in saline may be used because the correlation between OD and density is better at lower concentrations. OD does not correlate directly with turbidity or cell density and can depend on the conditions used; therefore, each laboratory should generate its own standard curve based on the growth curve methods described here. Once the growth characteristics of the strain have been established and the inoculated number of live bacteria and incubation conditions have been standardized, the OD will give a reasonable idea of when the culture has reached an appropriate growth phase.

A Coulter counter suitable for bacterial density measurement may be available in a laboratory that performs cell counts routinely. If not, then a Petroff-Hausser-type bacterial

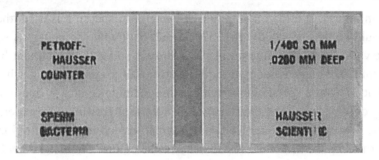

Figure 4.6
A Petroff-Hausser bacterial counting chamber.

counting chamber (Hausser Scientific) (Figure 4.6) or a Helber Thoma chamber (Hawksley) should be purchased. This operates on the same principles as a hemocytometer but has finer divisions and is much shallower (depth 0.01 or 0.02 mm). Bacterial counting chambers are comparatively fragile and expensive ($100–$600) and should be handled and cleaned directly over the bench. Some chambers are supplied with thin and fragile coverslips—obtaining a few (thicker) hemocytometer coverslips to act as replacements is recommended.

A phase-contrast microscope is ideal for performing direct counts but, if not available, a standard microscope can be used with the condenser diaphragm closed down. To focus on the gridlines and locate the appropriate zone near the middle of the mirrored area prior to counting, place the unloaded chamber slide on the stage of the microscope and use a medium power objective (e.g., 10×); then, refocus using a high-power air objective (e.g., 40×). Remove the chamber and clean it and the coverslip thoroughly with a moistened medical wipe (alcohol may help to remove any grease). Place the chamber on a smooth, flat surface and then mount the coverslip on the chamber using a small drop of water (approximately 0.5 µL) in the frosted raised areas on each side of the grid. Position and press down gently on the sides of the coverslip while moving it slightly back and forth to secure it. Prepare a 1 in 10 dilution of the bacterial culture in 0.1 mM copper sulfate in 0.9% saline—copper is toxic and will reduce the motility of the live bacteria to facilitate counting. Use a micropipette to transfer 2.5 µL (for a 0.02 mm deep chamber) of mixture to the silvered central region adjacent to the edge of the coverslip so that the suspension is drawn under the coverslip by capillary action. If the chamber does not fill properly, then clean and reload it. The bacteria should be allowed to settle for a short time before counting.

The central square millimeter of the chamber is ruled into 25 groups of 16 small squares, with each group separated by triple lines, the middle one of which is the boundary. Count the bacteria in a group of 16 small squares (shaded area in Figure 4.7). Bacteria touching the two boundary lines indicated by the arrow are counted while those touching the other

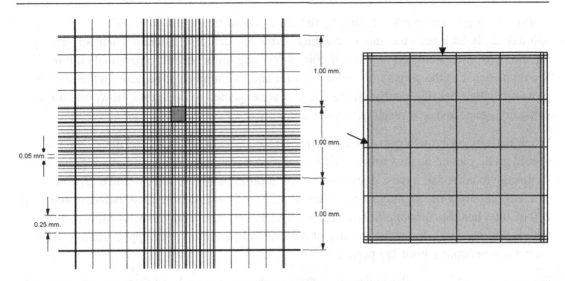

Figure 4.7
Bacterial counting chamber grid.

two lines are ignored. A Denominator-type multichannel bench-top tally counter should be used to facilitate counts.

The volume of a 4×4 square of a 0.02-mm deep chamber is 800×10^{-9} mL; therefore, the bacterial density equal is calculated as:

chamber count $\div$ dilution factor $\div$ 800×10^9 bacteria/mL.

For example, if the culture was diluted with nine volumes of diluent, a count of 120 equates to 1.5×10^9 bacteria/mL ($120 \div 1/10 \div 800 \times 10^9$ bacteria/mL). Although the direct count does not necessarily equal the viable count, virtually all the bacteria counted in a log phase suspension will be viable. The condition of the bacteria in terms of morphology, motility (TA100 in particular is highly motile), and absence of clumping will help confirm their health.

To clean the chamber, carefully slide the coverslip from the chamber. Wipe the coverslip and chamber with a dry paper tissue. Spray the chamber and coverslip with purified water and then wipe dry with a fresh tissue. Clean again with 70% v/v propanol and discard all tissues as appropriate for contaminated material.

The bacteria can also be plated to confirm their density. In this case, the suspension is serially diluted in 0.9% saline to approximately 1000 bacteria/mL (e.g., by two serial 10 µL + 10 mL dilutions using a fresh micropipette tip for each dilution); then, 0.1 mL is either spread directly across the surface of a nutrient agar plate or mixed with 2.5 mL molten top agar at 45°C before spreading across the plate. After a few minutes to allow absorption or gelling on a level surface; the plate should be incubated at 37°C for approximately 24 h before counting colonies. Provided that care is taken when performing the dilutions, the calculated number of colony-forming units per mL of original culture should be equal to the density of viable bacteria and the number of bacteria in the actively growing culture because nearly all the bacteria are expected to be viable. However, some variance is expected as a result of experimental error.

When performing growth curve experiments, OD_{650nm}, viable counts, and direct counts should all be plotted against time. Exponentially growing suspension cultures of *Salmonella* strains are expected to have a doubling time of approximately 30 min, whereas *E. coli* strains generally grow slightly faster. Thus, if a 25 or 30 mL culture flask is inoculated with 200 μL of a healthy *Salmonella* suspension (e.g., as obtained from a frozen culture), then the suspension will achieve the density of the original inoculum after approximately 4.5 h taking into account a brief lag period.

For routine use (i.e., standard testing), if the suspension is inoculated from a freshly thawed frozen suspension of known density, the growth curve experiments can be used to specify inoculation volumes and incubation periods for each of the strains so that suspension cultures can be inoculated and are ready for use at convenient times of the day. Suspensions can be inoculated in the evening at room temperature and then placed in the shaking incubator, which is connected to a timer set to switch the incubator on at a specified time in the early morning so that cultures are ready for use when staff come into the laboratory.

References

[1] Zeiger E. History and rationale of genetic toxicity testing: an impersonal, and sometimes personal, view. Environ Mol Mutagen 2004;44(5):363–71.
[2] Demerec M. Studies of the streptomycin-resistance system of mutations in *E. coli*. Genetics 1951;36(6):585–97.
[3] Witkin EM. Mutations in *Escherichia coli* induced by chemical agents. Nucleic acids and nucleoproteins. Cold Spring Harbor Symp Quant Biol 1947;12:256–69.
[4] Demerec M. Mutations induced by carcinogens. Br J Cancer 1948;2:114–17.
[5] Bertani G. A method for detection of mutations, using streptomycin dependence in *Escherichia coli*. Genetics 1951;36(6):598–611.
[6] Szybalski W. Special microbiological systems: II, observations on chemical mutagenesis in microorganisms. Ann NY Acad Sci 1985;76:475–89.
[7] Berger, et al. Analysis of amino acid replacements resulting from frameshift and missense mutations in the tryptophan synthetase A gene of *Escherichia coli*. J Biochem Mol Biol 1968;34(2):219–38.
[8] Hill RF. Dose-mutation relationships in ultraviolet-induced reversion from auxotrophy in *Escherichia coli*. J Gen Microbiol 1963;30(2):281–7.
[9] MacPhee DG. Development of bacterial mutagenicity tests: a view from afar. Environ Mol Mutagen 1989;14(Suppl. 16):35–8.
[10] Mortelmans K, Riccio ES. The bacterial tryptophan reverse mutation assay with *Escherichia coli* WP2. Mutat Res 2000;455(1–2):61–9.

[11] Hartman PE, Ames BN, Roth JR, Barnes WM, Levin DE. Target sequences for mutagenesis in *Salmonella* histidine-requiring mutants. Environ Mutagen. 1986;8(4):631−41.

[12] Gabridge MG, Legator MS. A host-mediated microbial assay for the detection of mutagenic compounds. Proc Soc Exp Biol Med 1969;130(3):831−4.

[13] Malling HV. Dimethylnitrosamine: formation of mutagenic compounds by interaction with mouse liver microsomes. Mutat Res 1971;13(4):425−9.

[14] Ames BN, Durston WE, Yamasaki E, Lee FD. Carcinogens are mutagens: a simple test system combining liver homogenates for activation and bacteria for detection. Proc Natl Acad Sci USA 1973;70(8):2281−5.

[15] Bartsch H, Malaveille C, Montesano R. *In vitro* metabolism and microsome-mediated mutagenicity of dialkylnitrosamines in rat, hamster, and mouse tissues. Cancer Res 1975;35:644−51.

[16] Yahagi T, Degawa W, Seino Y, Matsushima T, Nagao M, Sugimura T, et al. Mutagenicity of carcinogenic azo dyes and their derivatives. Cancer Lett 1975;1(2):91−6.

[17] OECD Guideline for Testing of Chemicals, Genetic Toxicology No. 471, Organisation for Economic Co-Operation and Development, Paris; 21 July 1997.

[18] ICH Harmonised Tripartite Guideline S2(R1). Guidance on Genotoxicity Testing and Data Interpretation for Pharmaceuticals Intended for Human Use; June 2012.

[19] Gatehouse D, Haworth S, Cebula T, Gocke E, Kier L, Matsushima T, et al. Recommendations for the performance of bacterial mutation assays. Mutat Res 1994;312(3):217−33.

[20] Zeiger E, Pagano DA, Robertson IGC. A rapid and simple scheme for confirmation of *Salmonella* tester strain phenotype. Environ Mutagen 1981;3(3):205−9.

[21] Wilcox P, Wedd DJ, Gatehouse D. Collaborative study to evaluate the inter/intra laboratory reproducibility and phenotypic stability of *Salmonella typhimurium* TA97a and TA102. Mutagenesis 1993;8(2):93−100.

[22] Pagano DA, Zeiger E. The stability of mutagenic chemicals stored in solution. Environ Mutagen 1985;7 (3):293−302.

[23] Maron DM, Ames BN. Revised methods for the *Salmonella* mutagenicity test. Mutat Res 1983;113 (3−4):173−215.

[24] Ong T-M, Mukhtar H, Wolf CR, Zeiger E. Differential effects of cytochrome P450-inducers on promutagen activation capabilities and enzymatic activities of S-9 from rat liver. J Environ Pathol Toxicol 1980;4(1):55−65.

[25] Eliott B, Coombs R, Elcombe C, Gatehouse D, Gibson G, MacKay J, et al. Report of UKEMS working party: alternatives to Aroclor 1254 induced S9 in *in vitro* genotoxicity assays. Mutagenesis 1992;7 (3):175−7.

[26] Hakura A, Suzuki S, Satoh T. Advantage of the use of human liver S9 in the Ames test. Mutat Res 1999;438(1):29−36.

[27] Hakura A, Suzuki S, Satoh T. Improvement of the Ames test using human liver S9 preparation. Methods Pharmacol Toxicol 2004;:325−36.

[28] Prival MJ, King VD, Sheldon Jr. AT. The mutagenicity of dialkyl nitrosamines in the *Salmonella* plate assay. Environ Mutagen 1979;1(2):95−104.

[29] Prival MJ, Mitchell VD. Analysis of a method for testing azo dyes for mutagenic activity in *Salmonella typhimurium* in the presence of flavin mononucleotide and hamster liver S9. Mutat Res 1982;97(2):103−16.

[30] Prival MJ, Bell SJ, Mitchell VD, Peiperl MD, Vaughan VL. Mutagenicity of benzidine and benzidine-congener dyes and selected monoazo dyes in a modified *Salmonella* assay. Mutat Res 1984;136 (1):33−47.

[31] Levin DE, Hollstein M, Christman MF, Schwiers EA, Ames BN. A new *Salmonella* tester strain (TA102) with A.T base pairs at the site of mutation detects oxidative mutagens. Proc Natl Acad Sci USA 1982;79 (23):7445−9.

[32] Watanabe K, Sakamoto K, Sasaki T. Collaborative study of interlaboratory variability in *Salmonella typhimurium* TA102 and TA2638 and *Escherichia coli* WP2/pKM101 and WP2 uvrA/pKM101. Mutagenesis 1995;10(3):235−41.

[33] Gatehouse D. Bacterial mutagenicity assays: test methods. Methods Mol Biol 2012;817:21−34.

[34] Zeiger E. Bacterial mutagenicity assays. Methods Mol Biol NY 2013;1044:3−26.

[35] Wilcox P, Naidoo A, Wedd DJ, Gatehouse DG. Comparison of *Salmonella typhimurium* TA102 with *Escherichia coli* WP2 Tester strains. Mutagenesis 1990;5(3):285−91.

[36] Herbold A, Arni P, Driesel AG, Engelhardt G, Jäger J, Joosten HFP, et al. Criteria for the standardization of *Salmonella* mutagenicity tests: results of a collaborative study II. Studies to investigate the effect of bacterial liquid culture preparation conditions on *Salmonella* mutagenicity test results. Teratog Carcinog Mutagen 1983;3(2):187−93.

[37] Göggelmann W, Grafe A, Vollmar J, Baumeister M, Kramer PJ, Pool BL. Criteria for the standardization of *Salmonella* mutagenicity tests: results of a collaborative study IV. Relationship between the number of his- bacteria plated and number of his+ revertants scored in the *Salmonella* mutagenicity test. Teratog Carcinog Mutagen 1983;3(2):205−13.

[38] de Raat WK, Willems MI, de Meijere FA. Effects of amount and type of agar on the number of spontaneous revertants. Mutat Res. 1984;137(1):33−7.

[39] US FDA Redbook. Short-Term Tests for Genetic Toxicity; 2000.

[40] EPA Health Effects Test Guideline OPPTS 870.5100: Bacterial Reverse Mutation Test.

[41] Hollstein M, McCann J, Angelosanto FA, Nichols WW. Short-term tests for carcinogens and mutagens. Mutat Res 1979;65(3):133−226.

[42] Pagano DA, Zeiger E. Conditions for detecting the mutagenicity of divalent metals in *Salmonella typhimurium*. Environ Mol Mutagen 1992;19(2):139−46.

[43] Green MH, Muriel WJ. Mutagen testing using TRP+ reversion in *Escherichia coli*. Mutat Res 1976;38(1):3−32.

[44] Mitchell I, de G, Dixon PA, Gilbert PJ, White DJ. Mutagenicity of antibiotics in microbial assays: problems of evaluation. Mutat Res 1980;79(2):91−105.

[45] Gatehouse DG, Rowland IR, Wilcox P, Callander RD, Forster R. Bacterial mutation assays. In: Kirkland DJ, editor. UKEMS subcommittee on guidelines for mutagenicity testing, report, part I revised, basic mutagenicity tests: UKEMS recommended procedures. Cambridge: Cambridge University Press; 1990. p. 13−61.

[46] Thompson C, Morley P, Kirkland D, Proudlock R. Modified bacterial mutation test procedures for evaluation of peptides and amino acid-containing material. Mutagenesis 2005;20(5):345−50.

[47] Barber ED, Donish WH, Mueller KR. The relationship between growth and reversion in the Ames *Salmonella* plate incorporation assay. Mutat Res 1983;113(2):89−101.

[48] Benigni R., Bossa C., Jeliazkova N., Netzeva T., Worth A. The Benigni/Bossa rulebase for mutagenicity and carcinogenicity − a module of Toxtree. European Commission report EUR 23241, <http://ihcp.jrc.ec.europa.eu/our_labs/computational_toxicology/doc/EUR_23241_EN.pdf>; 2008.

[49] Maron D, Katzenellenbogen J, Ames BN. Compatibility of organic solvents with the *Salmonella/* microsome test. Mutat Res 1981;88(4):343−50.

[50] Vedmaurthy RB, Padmanabhan S, Vijayan M, Jamal ZA, Kumjumman J, Narayanan ML. Compatibility of different solvents with *Salmonella typhimurium* mutant strains in bacterial reverse mutation assay. Int J Pharm Pharm Sci 2012;4(1):283−4.

[51] Ayrton AD, Neville S, Ioannides C. Cytostolic activation of 2-aminoanthracene; Implications in its use as diagnostic mutagen in the Ames test. Mutat Res 1992;265(1):1−8.

[52] Vennit S, Crofton-Sleigh C, Forster R. Bacterial mutation assays using reverse mutation. Mutagenicity testing: a practical approach. Oxford, UK: IRL Press; 1984.

[53] Hayashi M, Dearfield K, Kasper P, Lovell D, Martis H-J, Thybaud V. Compilation and use of genetic toxicity historical control data. Mutat Res 2011;723(2):87−90.

[54] ICH Harmonized Tripartite Guideline. The Common Technical Document for the Registration of Pharmaceuticals for Human Use: Safety−M4S (R2), Nonclinical Overview and Nonclinical Summaries of Module 2. Organisation of Module 4.

[55] Hughes TJ, Simmons DM, Monteith LG, Claxton LD. Vaporization technique to measure mutagenic activity of volatile organic chemicals in the Ames/*Salmonella* assay. Environ Mutagen 1987;9(4):421−41.

[56] Araki A, Noguchi T, Kato F, Matsushima T. Improved method for mutagenicity testing of gaseous compounds by using a gas sampling bag. Mutat Res 1994;307(1):335—44.

[57] Mortelmans K, Zeiger E. The Ames *Salmonella*/microsome mutagenicity assay. Mutat Res 2000;455 (1—2):29—60.

[58] Zeiger E, Risko KJ, Margolin BH. Strategies to reduce the cost of mutagenicity screening with the *Salmonella* assay. Environ Mutagen 1985;7(6):901—11.

[59] Escobar PA, Kemper RA, Tarca J, Nicolette J, Kenyon M, Glowienke S, et al. Bacterial mutagenicity screening in the pharmaceutical industry. Mutat Res 2013;752(2):99—118.

[60] Miller JE, Vlasakova K, Glaab WE, Skopek TR. A low volume, high-throughput forward mutation assay in *Salmonella typhimurium* based on fluorouracil resistance. Mutat Res 2005;578(1—2):210—24.

[61] Slater EE, Anderson M, Rosenkranz HS. Rapid detection of mutagens and carcinogens. Cancer Res 1971;31:970—3.

[62] Kada T, Tutikawa K, Sadaie Y. *In vitro* and host-mediated "rec-assay" procedures for screening chemical mutagens; and phloxine, a mutagenic red dye detected. Mutat Res 1972;16(2):165—74.

[63] Leifer Z, Kada T, Mandel M, Zeiger E, Stafford R, Rosenkranz HS. An evaluation of tests using DNA repair-deficient bacteria for predicting genotoxicity and carcinogenicity. A report of the U.S. EPA's Gene-TOX Program. Mutat Res 1981;87(3):211—97.

[64] de Flora S, Zanacchi P, Camoirano A, Bennicelli C, Badolati GS. Genotoxic activity and potency of 135 compounds in the Ames reversion test and in a bacterial DNA-repair test. Mutat Res 1984;133(3):161—98.

[65] Quillardet P, de Bellecombe C, Hofnung M. The SOS Chromotest, a colorimetric bacterial assay for genotoxins: validation study with 83 compounds. Mutat Res 1985;147(3):79—95.

[66] Verschaeve L, Van Gompel J, Thilemans L, Regniers L, Vanparys P, Van der Lelie D. VITOTOX bacterial genotoxicity and toxicity test for the rapid screening of chemicals. Environ Mol Mutagen 1999;33(3):240—8.

[67] Westerink WM, Stevenson JC, Lauwers A, Griffioen G, Horbach GJ, Schoonen WG. Evaluation of the Vitotox and RadarScreen assays for the rapid assessment of genotoxicity in the early research phase of drug development. Mutat Res 2009;676(1—2):113—30.

[68] Simpson K, Bevan N, Hastwell P, Eidam P, Shah P, Gogo E, et al. The bluescreen-384 assay as an indicator of genotoxic hazard potential in early-stage drug discovery. J Biomol Screen 2013;18 (4):441—52.

[69] Iyer VN, Szybalski W. Two simple methods for the detection of chemical mutagens. Appl Microbiol 1958;6(1):23—9.

[70] Ames BN, McCann J, Yamasaki E. Methods for detecting carcinogens and mutagens with the *Salmonella*/ mammalian-microsome mutagenicity test. Mutat Res 1975;31(6):347—64.

[71] McMahon RE, Cline JC, Thompson CZ. Assay of 855 test chemicals in ten tester strains using a new modification of the Ames test for bacterial mutagens. Cancer Res 1979;39(3):682—93.

[72] de Flora SA. "Spiral test" applied to bacterial mutagenesis assays. Mutat Res 1981;82(2):213—27.

[73] Diehl M, Fort F. Spiral *Salmonella* assay: validation against the standard pour-plate assay. Environ Mol Mutagen 1996;27(3):227—36.

[74] Claxton LD, Houk VS, Warren S. Methods for the spiral *Salmonella* mutagenicity assay including specialized applications. Mutat Res 2001;488(3):241—57.

[75] Kado NY, Langley D, Eisenstadt E. A simple modification of the *Salmonella* liquid-incubation assay. Increased sensitivity for detecting mutagens in human urine. Mutat Res 1983;121(1):25—32.

[76] Aubrecht J, Osowski JJ, Persaud P, Cheung Ackerman JR, Lopes SH, Ku WW. Bioluminescent *Salmonella* reverse mutation assay: a screen for detecting mutagenicity with high throughput attributes. Mutagenesis 2007;22(5):335—42.

[77] Green MH, Muriel WJ, Bridges BA. Use of a simplified fluctuation test to detect low levels of mutagens. Mutat Res 1976;38(1):33—42.

[78] Gatehouse D. Detection of mutagenic derivatives of cyclophosphamide and a variety of other mutagens in a "microtitre"® fluctuation test, without microsomal activation. Mutat Res 1978;53(3):289—96.

[79] Gatehouse DG, Delow GF. The development of a "microtitre®" fluctuation test for the detection of indirect mutagens, and its use in the evaluation of mixed enzyme induction of the liver. Mutat Res 1979;60(3):239−52.

[80] Bridges BA. The fluctuation test. Arch Toxicol 1980;46(1−2):41−4.

[81] Näslund M, Kolman A. On the sensitivity of the fluctuation test. Mutat Res. 1980;73(2):409−13.

[82] Reifferscheid G, Maes HM, Allner B, Badurova J, Belkin S, Bluhm K, et al. International round-robin study on the ames fluctuation test. Environ Mol Mutagen 2012;53(3):185−97.

[83] Hubbard SA, Green MHL, Gatehouse D, Bridges JW. The fluctuation test in bacteria. In: Kilbey BJ, Legator M, Nichols W, Ramel C, editors. Handbook of mutagenicity test procedures. 2nd ed. Elsevier; 1984. p. 141−60.

[84] Pant K. In: Steinberg P, editor. Ames II™ and Ames liquid format mutagenicity screening assays, in high-throughput screening methods in toxicity testing. Hoboken (NJ, USA): John Wiley & Sons, Inc.; 2013.

[85] Diehl MS, Willaby SL, Snyder RD. Comparison of the results of a modified miniscreen and the standard bacterial reverse mutation assays. Environ Mol Mutagen 2000;35:72−7.

[86] Brooks TM. The use of a streamlined bacterial mutagenicity assay, the MINISCREEN. Mutagenesis 1995;10(5):447−8.

[87] Burke DA, Wedd DJ, Burlinson B. Use of the Miniscreen assay to screen novel compounds for bacterial mutagenicity in the pharmaceutical industry. Mutagenesis 1996;11(2):201−5.

[88] Josephy PD, Gruz P, Nohmi T. Recent advances in the construction of bacterial genotoxicity assays. Mutat Res 1997;386(1):1−23.

CHAPTER 5

The Mouse Lymphoma TK Assay

Mick Fellows[1] and Melvyn Lloyd[2]

[1]AstraZeneca Innovative Medicines and Early Development, Cambridge, UK
[2]Covance Laboratories Ltd, North Yorkshire, UK

Chapter Outline

5.1 Introduction   139
5.2 History   141
5.3 Provenance of the Cells   143
5.4 Spontaneous Mutation Frequency   144
5.5 Materials   145
   5.5.1 Safety   145
   5.5.2 Growth Medium   145
   5.5.3 Cell Culture   146
   5.5.4 Metabolic Activation   147
   5.5.5 Test Item   148
   5.5.6 Vehicle   148
   5.5.7 Positive Controls   148
5.6 Study Design   148
   5.6.1 General Test Conditions   148
   5.6.2 Preliminary Toxicity Test   150
   5.6.3 Main Mutation Test   151
      5.6.3.1 Posttreatment procedures   151
      5.6.3.2 Expression period   151
      5.6.3.3 Viability assessment and mutant selection (microtiter version)   152
      5.6.3.4 Viability assessment and mutant selection (agar version)   152
      5.6.3.5 Analysis of results   153
      5.6.3.6 Acceptance criteria   155
5.7 Evaluation Criteria   155
5.8 Predictivity of the MLA   156
References   158

5.1 Introduction

The mouse lymphoma L5178Y $tk^{+/-}$ assay (MLA) is a standard *in vitro* mammalian cell gene mutation test. Partly because it is also sensitive to chromosome-breaking agents, it is the most

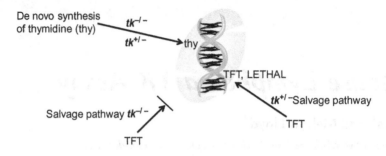

Figure 5.1
Cells with and without functional thymidine kinase can use the nucleotide de novo synthesis pathway. $tk^{-/-}$ cells cannot phosphorylate thymidine in the salvage pathway or the toxic base analogue trifluorothymidine (TFT).

widely used and accepted gene mutation test for screening and regulatory testing of chemicals, particularly drug candidates and medical devices. The assay investigates forward mutation at the thymidine kinase (tk) gene locus, such as the change from $tk^{+/-}$ to $tk^{-/-}$ with consequent loss of thymidine kinase (TK) enzyme activity. TK catalyzes the initial phosphorylation of thymidine deoxyriboside (dThd) to form deoxythymidylate (dTMP). TK allows cells to salvage thymidine for use in DNA synthesis; deficiency in this enzyme is not lethal because cells are able to survive using the de novo DNA synthetic pathway. Because mouse lymphoma L5178Y 3.7.2C cells are heterozygous at the tk locus ($tk^{+/-}$), a single mutagenic event in the tk^+ gene on chromosome 11b can lead to forward mutation to the $tk^{-/-}$ genotype with a phenotype having little or no TK activity. Loss of functional tk^+ expression renders cells resistant to toxic thymidine analogues that can be phosphorylated by TK (e.g., trifluorothymidine [TFT]). Accordingly, TFT is used to select $tk^{-/-}$ mutant clones in a background of $tk^{+/-}$ cells [1] (Figure 5.1). Mutation frequency is estimated by comparing the cloning efficiency (CE) of cells in medium with and without the selective agent; mutagenic activity is determined by treating cultures with different concentrations of test compound and examining the potential for dose-related increases in mutant frequency (MF).

Theoretically, a wide variety of mutagenic events can lead to TFT resistance, including small mutations within the tk^+ gene (genetic mutations), larger clastogenic chromosomal events within and beyond the tk^+ gene altering chromosome 11b structure (including deletions, translocations, and mitotic recombinations), and, as has been proposed, loss of whole chromosome 11b via chromosomal nondisjunction or aneuploidy [2]. However, there is still much debate regarding whether the MLA can reliably detect *in vitro* aneugenicity; recently, it has been demonstrated that the MLA cannot consistently detect seven well-characterized anuegens [3]. In view of this, the MLA should not be considered a reliable primary screen for aneugenicity.

Mutant ($tk^{-/-}$) clones can have slow or wild-type growth rates. The difference in mutant clone growth has been attributed to different mechanisms of DNA damage; for example,

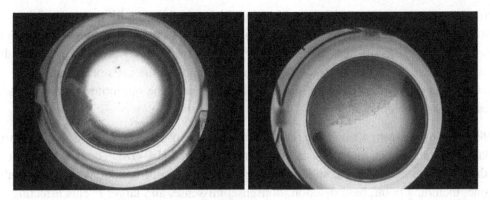

Figure 5.2
Small (left) and large (right) TFT-resistant colonies in wells of a 96-well plate.

chromosomal mutations extending beyond the *tk* gene produce small slow-growing mutant clones, and intragenic mutations produce large wild-type–growing clones [4] (Figure 5.2). However, because it has also been shown that small mutants can result from other mechanisms [5,6], mutant colony size should be used only as an indicator and not as a definitive measure of a chemical's mode of mutagenic action.

Although the TK version of the MLA is the most widely used of the *in vitro* mammalian cell gene mutation assays, a variant of the assay measures mutation at the HPRT (hypoxanthine-guanine phosphoribosyl transferase) locus of the same cell line or Chinese hamster ovary cells. This assay measures gene mutation only; the *hprt* gene is X-linked and mainly point mutations are detected, but *hprt* is a large gene and changes of 30 to 40 kilobases have also been reported. The assay has a low spontaneous mutation rate (typically 5–15 mutants per 10^6 viable cells) and a long expression period (7 days) by comparison with the TK assay. It can be a useful assay, for example, to complement preexisting *in vitro* chromosome aberration data, but it lacks the versatility of the TK assay and is not commonly used.

5.2 History

L-5178 cells were derived in the 1950s from a DBA/2 mouse with transplanted leukemia from a thymic tumor that had been induced by 3MC [7]. This tumor line was later used to create the established cell line L5178Y [8]. The cells were treated with ethyl methanesulfonate to create a thymidine kinase–deficient ($tk^{-/-}$) cell line [9]. From these, heterozygous ($tk^{+/-}$) cells were isolated using treatment with the folate reductase inhibitor amethopterin (amethopterin blocks TK de novo synthesis and, hence, preferentially kills $tk^{-/-}$ cells). The resultant L5178Y $tk^{+/-}$ mouse lymphoma clone 3.7.2C was used to develop the MLA [10] in the 1970s by Don Clive and associates [10,11]. Jane Cole modified the original soft agar plate method by cloning at limiting dilution in liquid medium in 96 microwell plates to assess viability and MF using a "microtiter" fluctuation test technique [12,13]. The agar and microtiter versions of the assay are equally acceptable; however, because the agar can affect the plating efficiency of the cells or contain particulate that might interfere with image analysis systems, the microtiter version of the test can be less problematic.

In 1988, the results from a small interlaboratory trial testing 63 chemicals in the MLA to validate its potential as a mutagenesis assay were published [14–18]. The trial concluded that the assay was effective and suitable for detecting a range of mutations in a mammalian cell line, including point, base deletion, nonsense, missense, and larger events affecting chromosomes such as deletions and possibly aneuploidy (now of doubt, see previous text and Fellows et al. [3]). As the understanding of the types of genetic damage that could be detected by the MLA increased, its potential to be used as an alternative to the chromosome aberration assay was proposed. It was suggested that this was possible due to the nature of induced small mutant clones being indicative of chromosomal mutation [19]. In the early 1990s, the International Conference on Harmonisation (ICH) was formed to harmonize procedures for testing pharmaceuticals. ICH initially published documents in 1995 [20] and 1997 [21] detailing genotoxicity testing strategy and aspects of test procedures. These included guidance on performance of the MLA and the proposition that, at least for pharmaceutical testing, the MLA was an acceptable screen for gene mutation and clastogenicity. The OECD Test Guideline 476 on performance of mammalian cell gene mutation assays was published in 1997 [22] and included more detailed testing guidance, including specific advice on acceptable levels of insolubility, pH, and osmolality, with the aim of avoiding some of the concerns over sensitivity of the MLA. OECD guidance on *in vitro* mammalian cell mutation testing is currently being updated—the TK forward mutation tests will be the subject of a new and separate guideline that the reader should consult for specific guidance on dose level limits when testing nonpharmaceuticals. The utility of the MLA to detect chromosome-damaging agents (as well as mutagens) was clarified in ICH guideline S2B [21], where continuous treatment in the MLA for 24 h in the presence of the test chemical was considered appropriate for detection of certain groups of chemicals (e.g., nucleosides) that were not detected after 3 to 4 h of exposure, allowing detection of division-dependent clastogens. In 2011, the ICH guidance was updated into a single document, S2(R1) [23], reducing the highest test concentration for mammalian cell *in vitro* screens from 5000 µg/mL or 10 mM to 500 µg/mL or 1 mM. Thus, the advice for testing pharmaceuticals became significantly different from the testing regimes in other industries.

Testing requirements for the MLA have been extensively debated at the International Workgroup on Genotoxicity Tests for the MLA (IWGT-ML), which have steered the assay's development since the late 1990s [24–28]. Recommendations on acceptability and interpretation of results from this group have been incorporated into the regulatory guidelines and are described in more detail later. These include acceptable limits on MF for negative control cultures, a standard method for assessing toxicity based on relative total growth (RTG), a standardized Global Evaluation Factor (GEF) used to resolve the significance of borderline increases in mutation frequency, and the requirement for positive control chemicals to induce increases in the number of small colonies to confirm the assay sensitivity to clastogenic activity [27,28].

5.3 Provenance of the Cells

Before any laboratory considers setting up the MLA, they should ensure they are using cells of appropriate provenance. It is not unusual for researchers to inadvertently use inappropriate cell lines. For example, work at the German Collection of microorganisms and Cell Cultures showed that out of 598 leukemia or lymphoma cell lines analyzed, 31% were either contaminated with mycoplasma, with another cell line, with both, or were not the cell line described by the supplier [29–31]. Furthermore, continual subculturing can lead to genetic drift and instability of the karyotype [32]. Fortunately for modern researchers, as part of an International Life Sciences Institute/Health and Environmental Sciences Institute (ILSI/HESI) and Genetic Toxicology Testing Committee (GTTC) project to provide well-characterized cells as close to the original isolate as possible, cells that can be traced back to Don Clive's laboratory with minimal subculturing have now been expanded and deposited at the European Collection of Animal Cell Cultures (ECACC) and Japanese Collection of Research Bioresources Cell Bank (JCRB) and are internationally available for any group wishing to establish or reestablish the MLA. The spectral karyotyping of these cells has been confirmed and shows a composite karyotype with a modal chromosome number of 40 and the aberrations detailed in Figure 5.3. This result is essentially the same as the previously published karyotype by SKY®-FISH [33]. The three observed differences were considered to be due to improved resolution in karyology. Specifically:

1. The previous spectral karyotype indicated as T(18;6) is now identified as T(6;18)
2. Previously identified as chromosome 6 in origin 6 (T6;14) is now identified as 14 (T14;6)
3. Previously identified as chromosome 15 (T15;18;14) is now identified as chromosome derivative 18 (t15;18;14).

It is considered that this karyotype is currently the most up-to-date for the L5178Y $tk^{+/-}$ 3.7.2C subline and should be used for comparative purposes if any researcher wishes to spectral karyotype their cells [34].

Accordingly, it is recommended that investigators should consider setting up the MLA purchase cells from GTTC characterized source. Researchers using cells with other

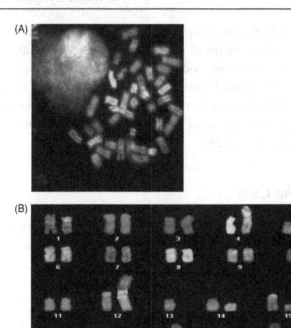

Figure 5.3
L5178Y mouse lymphoma $tk^{+/-}$ clone 3.7.2C spectral karyotype. (A) Fluorescently stained metaphase. (B) Arranged karyotype demonstrating pseudo-color resolution of spectrally labeled chromosomes. Arranged karyotype demonstrating cytogenetic aberrations at chromosome 4, Dp(4); chromosome 5, T(15;5); chromosome 6, T(18;6); chromosome 9, T(9;6); chromosome 14, del T(14;6); chromosome 15, T(5;15); a derivative chromosome demonstrating a portion of chromosome 15 at the proximal end, chromosome 18 at the intermediate section, and chromosome 14 at the distal end; T(15;18;14); and Rb(Dp12;13).

provenance should consider performing a similar karyotype analysis as described or, as a minimum, confirm that the cells have an appropriate modal chromosome number (i.e., 40) and the presence of two copies of chromosome 11.

All researchers should also establish that their cells are free from mycoplasma before use.

5.4 Spontaneous Mutation Frequency

Even when using L5178Y cells of appropriate provenance, it is still important to ensure the spontaneous MF of the cells used is both stable and within IWGT acceptable limits. Several factors that may affect the MLA spontaneous MF were considered in Fellows et al. [34]. These include the requirement for using appropriately heat-inactivated (56°C for 30 min) donor horse serum in culture medium, titration of methotrexate (amethopterin) concentration used to cleanse stocks of $tk^{-/-}$ mutants (0.3 μg/mL was optimal in Fellows' laboratory but other laboratories should confirm this), and avoiding excessive cell culturing. Methotrexate resistance is important because it indicates that formation of dTMP is not possible. Amethopterin is an analogue of dihydrofolate, the precursor of tetrahydrofolate. Tetrahydrofolate is the precursor of N5,N10-methylenetetrahydrofolate which is the one-carbon donor and electron donor in the methylation reaction causing reduction of tetrahydrofolate to dihydrofolate and subsequently conversion of dUMP (deoxyuridylate) to dTMP. Because this pathway for production of dTMP is nonfunctional in the $tk^{-/-}$ cells, treatment with amethopterin purges these mutants from the general cell population. Growing cells for a few days after amethopterin treatment will allow them to regain a suitable background MF and will provide cells for subsequent use. Once cells of appropriate spontaneous MF are derived, cells should be frozen in large batches and cultured for no more than 2 weeks from frozen before use to maintain an acceptable and consistent spontaneous MF.

5.5 Materials

5.5.1 Safety

When testing compounds where the hazards are unknown, it is always prudent to consider them as potential mutagens. Where available, safety data should be consulted and appropriate precautions should be taken. Class II safety cabinets, where the air flow protects the materials under test and the operator, should be used for all compound and cell manipulations. The use of sterile equipment and reagents is essential and aseptic techniques must be used to prevent contamination. Appropriate laboratory clothing and/or equiptment should be worn.

5.5.2 Growth Medium

Roswell Park Memorial Institute (RPMI) 1640 medium is typically used for cell culture throughout the assay. It contains 2 mmol/L L-glutamine and is supplemented with heat-inactivated donor horse serum, 2 mmol/L sodium pyruvate, 1% (v/v) Pluronic F68, 200 IU/mL penicillin, and 200 μg/mL streptomycin.

1. RPMI 1640 is most commonly used for culturing mouse lymphoma cells as described here, although Fischer's medium may be used. Medium can be buffered with HEPES and/or sodium bicarbonate and usually contains phenol red as a pH indicator.
2. Antimicrobial and antifungal agents (e.g., penicillin/streptomycin or gentamicin and amphotericin B)
3. A surfactant (e.g., Pluronic F68) is included to maintain single-cell suspensions.

4. Donor horse serum is necessary for cell growth. It is advisable to screen serum prior to use for rate of cell growth, CE, and spontaneous and induced MFs. Typically, medium containing 10% v/v horse serum (RPMI 10) should be used for normal subculturing procedures. Medium containing 20% v/v horse serum (RPMI 20) is recommended when plating cells for determination of CE and mutant selection. For short (pulse) treatment exposure, it is advisable to reduce serum concentration to between 2.5% and 5% (v/v) to minimize potential protein binding of the test item. For 24-h exposure, it is advisable to maintain serum at 10% (v/v) to ensure good cell growth during the exposure period.

5. Heat inactivation of the serum at 56°C for 30 min deactivates thymidine phosphorylase, which may be present in batches of horse serum and degrades TFT [34].

5.5.3 Cell Culture

1. All cell cultures should be maintained in a humidified CO_2 incubator at 37 °C. L5178Y mouse lymphoma cells are suspension cultures and, hence, can be maintained in roller cultures. However, this is not essential for normal growth.

2. L5178Y $tk^{+/-}$ (3.7.2C) mouse lymphoma cells should be used for the assay. Cells of appropriate provenance are available from the ECACC and JCRB.

3. Within each laboratory a "Master Stock" of cells should be expanded and, following minimal culturing, frozen in medium with 10% serum without surfactant or in 100% serum, both of which should contain 10% DMSO as a cryo-protectant. Cells will not tolerate immediate immersion into liquid nitrogen and therefore must be slowly frozen, for example, by placing ampoules of the suspension in Nalgene® Mr. Frosty freezer containers containing isopropyl alcohol. When placed in a −80 °C freezer (overnight), these containers provide the critical 1°C/min cooling rate required for successful cryopreservation of cells. Cells should be frozen in ampoules at a standard density (e.g., 2×10^6 cell/vial) and finally stored in a freezer maintaining temperatures of ≤ 150 °C or the gas phase of a liquid nitrogen container. Note that certain makes of ampoule tend to leak, especially if not tightened to the right torsion, so it is not advisable to store them in the liquid nitrogen phase.

4. From the master stock, subsequent "Assay Stocks" should be prepared by taking a vial from frozen, fast-thawing (e.g., in a waterbath at 37 °C), minimal culturing and purging of $tk^{-/-}$ mutants. Prior to counting, cells should be disaggregated by shaking the cultures to maintain single cell suspensions. The following is an example of a purging procedure.

   Purging of $tk^{-/-}$ mutants (cleansing). Once cells are in exponential growth in RPMI 10 at 2×10^5 cells per mL, they are incubated with medium containing

9 μg/mL thymidine, 15 μg/mL hypoxanthine, 22 μg/mL guanine (THG), and 0.3 μg/mL amethopterin for 24 h. Cultures are centrifuged at 200 g to remove amethopterin, washed once in RPMI 10, centrifuged again, then resuspended in RPMI 10 + THG before incubation for another 24 h to allow recovery of thymine monophosphate synthesis. Stock THG and methotrexate solutions may be made up as $100 \times$ concentrations and stored at $-80\,°C$.

Purged Cell Assay Stocks should then be aliquoted into ampoules at 2×10^6 cells per vial and then frozen and stored as described for master stocks. Before use, new Assay Stocks should be screened for mycoplasma and appropriate CE, spontaneous MF, and sensitivity to positive controls. The population doubling time of the cell cultures should be confirmed: typically, L5178Y cells have a doubling time of 8 to 10 h.

5.   For each assay a vial of cells should be taken from freeze, fast-thawed in a 37°C water bath, and used with minimal culturing. When cells are in exponential growth, subcultures are established in an appropriate number of flasks, usually aiming to maintain concentrations between 10^5 and 10^6 cells/mL. If cells are not to be subbed daily, then it is acceptable to culture from lower concentrations, but at least 10^7 cells should be maintained for each subculture.

5.5.4 Metabolic Activation

Many mutagens are pro-mutagens and require metabolic activation. Accordingly, tests should be conducted in the absence and presence of an exogenous metabolizing system. The default metabolic activation system includes rat liver postmitochondrial ("S9") fraction with appropriate cofactors, i.e., S9 mix. S9 fraction is usually prepared from male rats induced with Aroclor 1254 or phenobarbital/5,6-benzoflavone and is stored frozen at $-80°C$ prior to use. If another metabolic activation system is used, then its use should be justified in the study report. S9 is commercially available (e.g., from Molecular Toxicology Inc., Boone, NC, USA). Each batch of S9 fraction should be checked for sterility, protein content, ability to convert known promutagens to bacterial mutagens, and cytochrome P-450-catalyzed enzyme activities (alkoxyresorufin-O-dealkylase activities). If obtained commercially, then this will be done by the supplier who will provide a certificate of analysis that should be maintained with the study raw data.

Typically, S9 mix contains glucose-6-phosphate (G6P, 692 mmol/L), β-nicotinamide adenine dinucleotide phosphate (NADP, 33.6 mmol/L), potassium chloride (KCl, 150 mM), and S9 fraction in the ratio 1:1:1:2 (other cofactor mixtures may also be used). The S9 mix is added to cell cultures at a 1:20 dilution, resulting in a final S9 fraction concentration of 2% v/v. Other S9 concentrations (1%−10% v/v) may be appropriate for specific chemical classes as indicated in OECD Guidelines.

5.5.5 Test Item

1. The test item is formulated in a suitable vehicle prior to administration to the test system. Aqueous vehicles are preferred but, if the test item is not adequately soluble in them, it should be formulated as a solution in a water-miscible organic solvent. It is important to achieve full solubility in the primary vehicle.
2. Stock test solutions prepared in aqueous vehicles should be prepared aseptically or filter-sterilized.

5.5.6 Vehicle

1. Aqueous vehicles (such as water or physiological saline) may be added to the test system at a final concentration up to 10% v/v. Poorly soluble test items may be formulated directly in tissue culture medium.
2. Organic solvents such as dimethyl sulfoxide (DMSO), ethanol, acetone, or dimethylformamide (DMF) may be added at a final concentration of up to 1% v/v.
3. If other vehicles need to be used, then their effect on MFs may need to be checked prior to treatment or by inclusion of untreated controls in the experimental design.

5.5.7 Positive Controls

1. Positive controls are included in each mutation test as a quality control measure to ensure that the test system is capable of responding to known mutagens. Ideally, batches of positive controls are made in advance at $100 \times$ final concentration and aliquots are frozen at $-80°C$. Each laboratory should establish stability of any frozen stocks.
2. In the absence of S9, 4-nitroquinoline-1-oxide (NQO) or methyl methane sulfonate (MMS) are routinely used in a variety of laboratories. However, it should be noted that MMS is a volatile mutagen and a potential human carcinogen, and therefore should be used with caution. It is also not possible to stably freeze MMS aliquots. Accordingly, many laboratories may not consider MMS to be a suitable positive control.
3. In the presence of S9, benzo[a]pyrene (BP), cyclophosphamide (CPA), or 3-methylcholanthrene (3MC) may be used.
4. Appropriate concentrations of positive controls that give adequate responses should be determined by the individual testing laboratory.

5.6 Study Design

5.6.1 General Test Conditions

Figure 5.4 shows a typical study design for the microtiter version of the MLA.

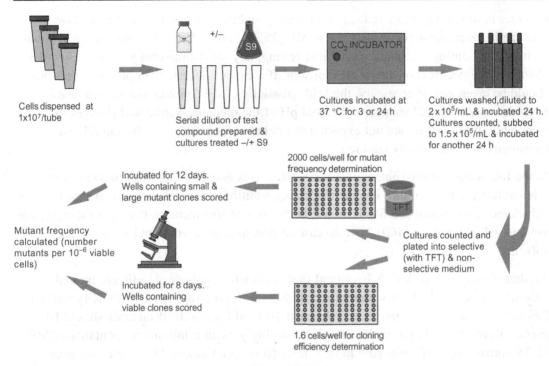

Figure 5.4
The microtiter MLA: typical study design.

Usually, a preliminary toxicity test is needed to establish an appropriate concentration range for the subsequent mutation test and involves short-term (3 to 4 h) exposure in the absence and presence of S9. For pharmaceuticals, a prolonged 24-h exposure test is required (unless a clear mutagenic effect is seen after short-term exposure) and may also be justified for poorly soluble materials and suspected antimetabolites. The 24-h exposure is performed only in the absence of metabolic activation because prolonged exposure to S9 is known to be toxic and the relevant enzymes degrade over time. Both short and long exposures may be performed concurrently to minimize the in-life phase of the test and reduce efforts involved in formulation.

For compounds not freely soluble in culture medium, the lowest precipitating concentration (observed at the end of treatment) should be the highest dose level analyzed. Examination for precipitate should be made on treatment and at the end of the exposure period. Where the test item is freely soluble in the culture medium, the highest concentration tested for pharmaceuticals should be a maximum of 1 mM or 500 µg/mL (whichever is lower); in other cases, the highest concentration should usually be 10 mM or 5000 µg/mL (whichever is lower). Higher concentrations may be justifiable when testing complex mixtures or biological materials. Readers should consult the latest OECD and ICH guidelines to confirm these limits.

Changes in osmolality of more than 50 mOsm/kg and fluctuations in pH of more than one unit can be responsible for an increase in MF [35,36]. The pH of the culture medium should be monitored during preliminary solubility testing; any substantial change will cause color change if the medium contains a pH indicator. If a change is seen, then pH measurements should be taken and, if necessary, the acidity/basicity of the formulations should be adjusted to avoid any substantial change in the final pH of the medium. Substantial changes in osmolality of the culture are not expected at final concentrations of ≤ 10 mmol/L, so measurement is not usually required.

In the following sections, unless otherwise stated, it is assumed that short treatments are for 3 h and that the final culture volume (following addition of the cell suspension, test item, or vehicle/positive control and S9) is 10 mL at the time of treatment. In that case the treatment volume will normally be 100 μL in the case of nonaqueous solvents and 1 mL for aqueous solvents.

To detect increases in MF, it is critical that sufficient numbers of cells are treated, subcultured, and selected for mutation assessment, taking into account toxicity and the laboratory's expected negative MF. At least 10 (and ideally 100) mutants should be carried through all stages of the assay. Accordingly, with a minimum spontaneous MF of 35 mutants per 10^6 cells (the lowest acceptable spontaneous MF in the soft agar version of the MLA), at least 3×10^6 cells per culture should be treated. This assumes that with lowest survival of 10%, 3×10^5 surviving cells would contain approximately 10 mutants. In practice it is advisable to treat at least 5×10^6 to 1×10^7 cells. For the 24-h exposure, it is usual to test 2×10^6 cells in 10 mL culture to allow for growth over the exposure period. Ideally, following both short and long exposure, each subsequent subculture should carry over 5×10^6 cells.

5.6.2 Preliminary Toxicity Test

Usually, single cultures are tested. For short exposure in the absence and presence of S9, 5×10^6 cells per culture are resuspended in RPMI 1640 medium containing 2.5% to 5% v/v horse serum (RPMI 2.5 or 5) and seeded into sterile, disposable 50 mL centrifuge tubes. For the 24-h exposure, at least 2×10^6 cells per culture are resuspended in RPMI 10 and seeded into 75-cm^2 tissue culture flasks. Vehicle or test item solutions are added together with S9 mix. The cultures are then incubated at $37 \pm 1°C$ for the appropriate treatment period in a humidified incubator gassed with 5% (v/v) CO_2 in air. Following treatment exposure, cultures are maintained as indicated in the posttreatment procedures. After the expression period, relative survival growth is calculated (see Section 5.6.3.5.1).

5.6.3 Main Mutation Test

Dose levels are selected based on preliminary test results and should span the range from nontoxic down to approximately 10% RTG. In the case of relatively nontoxic compounds, the upper dose will be limited by solubility or maximum required concentration. Cell numbers, volumes of individual components, and other details of treatment procedures are identical to those of the preliminary tests. However, a minimum of five concentrations should be tested; if only single cultures are used at each experimental point, then at least eight dose levels should be tested. For nontoxic compounds, halving concentrations up to the maximum achievable concentration is acceptable; for toxic compounds, it is useful to test narrower concentration spacing to ensure that a concentration of 10–20% survival is achieved. For the main test only, positive control compounds (in the absence and presence of S9) are included to demonstrate the sensitivity of the test, the effectiveness of the exogenous metabolic activation system, and the ability to induce both small and large colony mutants.

5.6.3.1 Posttreatment procedures

After 3-h exposure of 5×10^6 cells per culture, the cultures are centrifuged ($200 \times g$) for 5 min, washed with medium, recentrifuged, and resuspended in 25 mL RPMI 10 in 75-cm^2 tissue culture flasks or other suitable vessels. This assumes that if all cells had survived treatment, then the cell concentration is 2×10^5 cells/mL. This gives a true indication of cell growth and accounts for cell loss during the treatment incubation period. After 24-h exposure, the cultures are centrifuged ($200 \times g$) for 5 min, washed, recentrifuged, and resuspended in 10 mL of RPMI 10. Cell counts are determined for each culture using an automated cell counter (e.g., Coulter counter) or hemocytometer and adjusted (where sufficient cells survive) to between 1×10^5 and 2×10^5 cells/mL.

5.6.3.2 Expression period

TK has a limited half-life; therefore, in newly mutated $tk^{-/-}$ cells, sufficient residual TK remains to phosphorylate TFT, resulting in toxicity. Therefore, L5178Y cells are allowed a recovery ("expression") period of 2 days in culture following treatment before addition of TFT so that TK is no longer expressed in the $tk^{-/-}$ mutants. L5178Y cells maintain exponential growth if cultured below approximately 1×10^6 cells/mL. Hence, it is important to subculture during the expression period as described here.

5.6.3.2.1 Expression period day 1

One day after the end of the respective treatment periods, cell counts are performed on all cultures and the density is adjusted (where possible) with RPMI 10 to give between 1×10^5

and 2×10^5 cells/mL while ensuring sufficient cells are carried over (e.g., where possible 5×10^6 cells per culture). If substantial toxicity is seen such that cultures are already at or below 2×10^5 cells per mL, then they should not be subcultured.

5.6.3.2.2 Expression period day 2

Two days after the end of the respective exposure periods, all cultures are counted and the cell concentrations are readjusted (where possible) by adding RPMI 20. The higher serum content enables effective growth for plating and incubation to determine TFT resistance when cultures are restricted in microwells or in agar.

5.6.3.3 Viability assessment and mutant selection (microtiter version)

For mutant selection plating, cultures are counted and selected cultures are adjusted to 1×10^4 cells/mL with RPMI 20 (i.e., to give an average of 2000 cells/well when plated at 0.2 mL per well). Sufficient cell preparation for each culture should be made to plate into two 96-well plates (e.g., approximately 45 mL). These plates may be labeled "TFT plates." For viability plating, a further dilution of these cultures in RPMI 20 is performed to achieve 8 cells/mL in 45 mL (i.e., to give an average of 1.6 cells/well when plated at 0.2 mL/well). TFT is prepared at a concentration of 0.3 mg/mL in RPMI media. TFT is light-sensitive, so solutions should be protected from light. TFT solution aliquots may be prepared and stored frozen at $-80°C$ for at least 6 months. To solutions prepared for TFT selection, before plating, TFT is added to each culture to give a final concentration of 3 μg/mL.

5.6.3.3.1 Colony counting (microtiter version)

Mutant plates are typically incubated for 10 to 14 days and viability plates are typically incubated for 7 to 10 days in a humidified incubator at $37 \pm 1°C$ gassed with 5% v/v CO_2 in air. Although automated plate scoring systems are available for 96-well plates, these are usually scored by eye using background illumination with a light box or using an inverted microscope. Colonies should be defined as large (greater in area than one-quarter of the well) or small (less than one-quarter of the area of the well) (see Figure 5.2). Small colonies are distinguishable from the debris of dead (unselected) cells by their refractive properties under an inverted microscope; they appear brighter when back-lit. Contaminated wells should not be scored and heavily contaminated plates should be discarded. If wells or plates are lost, then MF calculations must be adjusted to take this into account.

5.6.3.4 Viability assessment and mutant selection (agar version)

A total of 3×10^6 cells/culture are suspended in RPMI 20 containing 0.22% w/v soft agar (prepared from stock 2% Noble agar melted and held at 70°C) and TFT (3 μg/mL) and distributed into three 100-mm dishes. The absolute CE at the time of selection is determined by seeding a total of 600 cells into three 100-mm dishes in RMPI 20 containing

0.22% w/v soft agar. Dishes are left for agar to set at room temperature prior to incubation in a humidified incubator at $37 \pm 1°C$ gassed with 5% v/v CO_2 in air. It is important to ensure that the batches of agar used maintain appropriate cell CE.

5.6.3.4.1 Colony counting (agar version)

After 10 to 14 days, colonies may be counted by eye or by using an automated colony counter (e.g., Loats Associates, Inc. High Resolution Colony Counter System for the Mouse Lymphoma Assay). Image analysis systems should be validated to ensure accurate quantitation of large and small mutant colonies. If one agar plate is lost due to contamination or other cause, then the average colony count is determined from the average of the two remaining plates.

5.6.3.5 Analysis of results

Calculations may be performed manually, but commercial or internally validated computer software may also be used.

5.6.3.5.1 Relative suspension growth

Suspension growth (SG) is a measure of the growth in suspension over the treatment and the expression periods. In its simplest form it would be the ratio of the number of cells at the start of treatment divided by the number of cells at the end of the expression period. However, calculation of SG needs to take into account the fact that cells are subcultured during this period and only a proportion of the cells are carried over as indicated here:

$$\text{SG short exposure} = \frac{\text{Day 1 cell count}}{\text{Day 0 cell count}} \times \frac{\text{Day 2 cell count}}{\text{Day 1 cell count}^1}$$

$$\text{SG 24-h exposure} = \frac{\text{Day 1 cell count}}{\text{Day 0 cell count}} \times \frac{\text{Day 2 cell count}}{\text{Day 1 cell count}^1} \times \frac{\text{Day 3 cell count}}{\text{Day 2 cell count}^1}$$

where the Day 0 cell count is the density at the start of treatment.

[1]Density after adjustment.

The theoretical optimum SG is approximately five fold per day. Relative suspension growth (RSG) is calculated as percent SG compared to the concurrent vehicle control and is used as a measure of toxicity:

$$\text{RSG} = \frac{\text{Individual culture SG}}{\text{Control SG}} \times 100\%$$

5.6.3.5.2 Toxicity assessment

CE (i.e., the number of viable cells that will form a colony under the relevant selection conditions) in either selective or nonselective medium in the microtiter assay is based on the zero term of the Poisson distribution. P(0) is estimated from the proportion of wells in which a colony has *not* grown, (i.e., the number of empty wells divided by the total number of wells plated):

P(0) = Number empty wells ÷ umber wells plated

CE (microtiter) = $-\ln$ P(0) ÷ Number of cells per well

where ln P(0) is the natural log ($\log_e$) of the proportion P(0).

CE in the agar assay is a function of the number of colonies counted per plate and the seeding density of the plate.

RTG is used as the definitive measure of toxicity and is the product of RSG and viability (CE) in nonselective medium at the time of selection for TFT-resistant mutants.

Relative cloning efficiency (RCE) is:

%RCE = CE ÷ Mean control CE × 100%

Relative total growth (RTG) is:

%RTG = %RSG × %RCE÷100%

5.6.3.5.3 MF assessment (microtiter version)

MF for each culture is calculated as the CE in selective (TFT) medium. It is corrected for viability in nonselective medium from the same culture and expressed as mutants per 10^6 viable cells, i.e.,

MF (per 10^6 cells) = [CE (mutant)/CE (viable)] × 10^6 cells

Small and large colony MFs are calculated in an identical manner using the relevant number of wells empty of small and large colonies, as appropriate. It is common to only score small and large colonies for controls to ensure assay acceptance and for any positive concentrations to give an indication of potential mutagenic mechanism (i.e., large colonies may be associated with gene mutation and small colonies may be associated with damage at the chromosomal level).

5.6.3.5.4 MF assessment (agar version)

MF is calculated as the number of mutant colonies (total of three dishes) divided by the number of cells seeded and adjusted by the absolute CE at the time of selection, and is reported as TFT-resistant mutants per 10^6 viable cells. Absolute CE is calculated as the ratio of the total number of viable colonies to the number of cells seeded. MFs are normally derived from sets of three dishes for both mutant colony count and viable colony count. To allow for losses due to contamination or other reasons, an acceptable MF can be calculated from a minimum of two dishes per set. Small and large colony MFs along with total MF should be calculated separately.

5.6.3.6 Acceptance criteria

The assay is considered valid if the following criteria agreed in consensus documents published by the MLA workgroup [24−28] are met:

1. The mean MFs in the vehicle control cultures should fall within the normal ranges (50−170 mutants per 10^6 viable cells for the microwell assay, 35−140 mutants per 10^6 viable cells for the agar assay).
2. At least one positive control concentration should show either an absolute increase in mean total MF of at least 300×10^{-6} (at least 40% of this should be in the small colony MF) or an increase in small colony MF of at least 150×10^{-6} above the concurrent vehicle control.
3. The mean RTG for the positive controls should be greater than 10%.
4. The mean cloning efficiencies of the negative controls from the Mutation Experiments should be within the range 65−120% on Day 2.
5. The mean SG of the negative controls from the Mutation Experiments should be between the range 8 and 32 following short exposure or between 32 and 180 following 24-h exposure.
6. At least four (duplicate cultures) or eight (single cultures) concentrations are available for analysis, and for toxic test agents the highest concentrations analyzed and reported should ideally show RTG between 10% and 20%. However, if there is absolutely no indication of a concentration relationship, highest concentrations showing 20−25% RTG may be acceptable. Furthermore, negative concentrations showing less than 10% RTG may be included in analysis [25].

5.7 Evaluation Criteria

If the acceptability criteria are fulfilled, then the test item will be considered as mutagenic in this assay if:

1. The MF of any test concentration exceeds the sum of the mean control MF plus the GEF (126×10^{-6} for microtiter and 90×10^{-6} for agar) [27]. Positive concentrations giving less than 10% RTG are usually rejected from analysis and a test item would not be regarded as mutagenic if the only concentration giving a positive result was <10% RTG. Test items that give small increases in MF only at concentrations between 10%

and 20% RTG should be evaluated with caution because these apparent increases may be an artifact of toxicity.

2. The increases are concentration-related, as defined by a statistically significant trend.

The test item will be considered positive in this assay if both of these criteria are met and negative if neither of the criteria are met. Results that only partially satisfy the assessment criteria described are considered on a case-by-case basis. However, evidence of a weak trend in the absence of an increase in MF achieving GEF would normally be considered to be a negative result. In other circumstances, repeat testing is recommended. Positive responses only seen at concentrations of high toxicity are unlikely to be biologically relevant, but testing using other endpoints may be required to confirm this (e.g., where possible a follow-up with an *in vivo* study such as the *in vivo* hematopoietic cell micronucleus assay would help with such interpretation). For positive results, colony sizing will also be taken into consideration: increases in large colony MF are indicative of small genetic events (such as point mutations), whereas increases in small colony MF are indicative of potential clastogenic events. However, this should only be taken as an indication of mutagenic mechanism, not as definitive evidence.

Clearly negative or positive results do not need to be repeated. Other results should be repeated on a case-by-case basis.

5.8 Predictivity of the MLA

Along with other *in vitro* mammalian cell genotoxicity assays, the predictivity of the MLA for identifying carcinogens has often been questioned. Several publications from the past decade have highlighted this [37–41]. For example, the retrospective review by Kirkland et al of genotoxicity data from ICH-recommended tests indicated that out of 105 noncarcinogens, the MLA unequivocally correctly identified only 41 as being negative [37]. This suggested a "false-positive" rate for the MLA as high as 61%. An assay with such a high "false-positive" rate would seem to be of little value in any screening paradigm. The paradox is that the MLA is still routinely used for screening in many industries. Accordingly, either the lack of specificity suggested by Kirkland et al. is not real (which is the perception gained by the authors over the past 25 years) or a surprisingly large number of novel chemicals are positive in *in vitro* mammalian cell genotoxicity tests.

Kirkland et al.'s review on the specificity in the MLA considered the inability of the MLA to correctly identify noncarcinogens as being nongenotoxic. Unfortunately, oncogenicity data are not available for the majority of novel compounds tested in the MLA. However, at least in pharmaceutical research, it is possible to consider a compound's primary pharmacological target and mechanism and relate this to any positive result, with the possibility of deducing beyond reasonable doubt the mechanism of a false-positive finding, therefore changing a false positive into a mechanistically interpretable result. This was done for 355 compounds tested in the MLA at AstraZeneca, Alderley Park, UK, between 2001 and 2010 [42]. Three hundred and three compounds were concluded to be negative (85% of the total number of compounds tested). Only 52 compounds were concluded to be positive (15% of the total compounds tested) (Figure 5.5). All of these 52 compounds were positive at concentrations of less than 1 mM. Furthermore, only 19 compounds were positive by a mechanism that could not be related to the compounds primary pharmacological activity or were positive in other genotoxicity assays. This indicated that, when used in an experienced laboratory using modern protocols, the MLA had an "unexplainable positive" rate of only 5% (Figure 5.6), confirming its value as an appropriate *in vitro* genotoxicity screen.

Although cancer bioassay data were not available for the 355 compounds, because 97% of them were not bacterial mutagens and all were tested as potential drug substances, it must be assumed that the majority are probably not DNA-reactive carcinogens [42]. At least for pharmaceuticals, it appears that the MLA does not generate as many positive results as

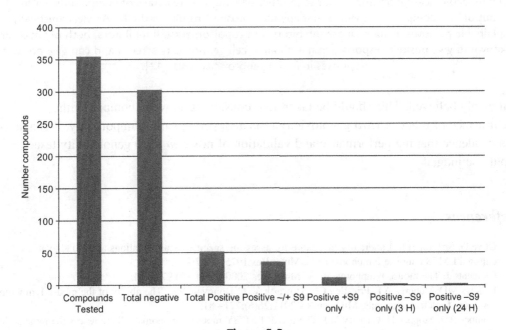

Figure 5.5

Results of 355 compounds tested in the MLA at AstraZeneca, Alderley Park, between 2001 and 2010.

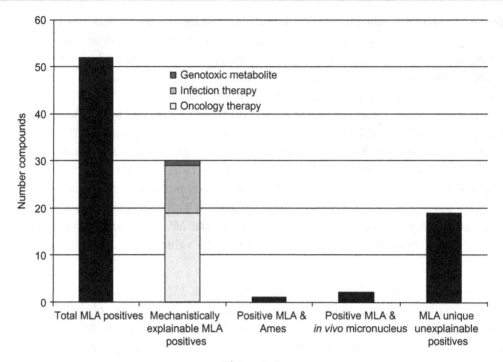

Figure 5.6

Pharmacological target and response in other genetic toxicity assays of compounds, with 52 out of 355 compounds giving S9-independent positive results in the MLA. Mechanistically explainable positives include kinase inhibitors and topoisomerase II inhibitors, both of which are known to give positive responses in mammalian cell genotoxicity screens and can give positive responses in *in vivo* genotoxicity tests [42].

commonly believed. This should be taken into consideration when comparing the performance of other *in vitro* genotoxicity tests and, perhaps more importantly, it is against this incidence that the performance and validation of novel *in vitro* genotoxicity tests should be judged.

References

[1] Clive D, Spector JFS. Laboratory procedure for assessing specific locus mutations at the TK locus in cultured L5178Y mouse lymphoma cells. Mutat Res 1975;31:17−29.
[2] Clements J. The mouse lymphoma assay. Mutat Res 2000;455(1−2):97−110.
[3] Fellows MD, Doherty AT, Priestley CC, Howarth V, O'Donovan MR. The ability of the mouse lymphoma TK assay to detect aneugens. Mutagenesis 2011;26(6):771−81.
[4] Combes RD, Stopper H, Caspary WJ. The use of L5178Y mouse lymphoma cells to assess the mutagenic, clastogenic and aneugenic properties of chemicals. Mutagenesis 1995;10(5):403−8.
[5] Blazak WF, Stewart BE, Galperin I, Allen KL, Rudd CJ, Mitchell AD, et al. Chromosome analysis of trifluorothymidine-resistant L5178Y mouse lymphoma cell colonies. Environ Mutagen 1986;8(2):229−40.

[6] Blazak WF, Los FJ, Rudd CJ, Caspary WJ. Chromosome analysis of small and large L5178Y mouse lymphoma cell colonies: comparison of trifluorothymidine-resistant and unselected cell colonies from mutagen-treated and control cultures. Mutat Res 1989;224(2):197−208.

[7] Law LW. Increase in incidence of leukemia in hybrid mice bearing thymic transplants from a high leukemic strain. J Natl Cancer Inst 1952;12(4):789−805.

[8] Fischer GA. Studies of the culture of leukemic cells *in vitro*. Ann NY Acad Sci 1958;76(3):673−80.

[9] Liechty MC, Hassanpour Z, Hozier JC, Clive D. Use of microsatellite DNA polymorphisms on mouse chromosome 11 for *in vitro* analysis of thymidine kinase gene mutations. Mutagenesis 1994;9:423−7.

[10] Clive D, Flamm WG, Machesko MR, Bernheim NJ. A mutational assay system using the thymidine kinase locus in mouse lymphoma cells. Mutat Res 1972;16:77−87.

[11] Clive D, Johnson KO, Spector JF, Batson AG, Brown MM. Validation and characterization of the L5178Y/TK$^{+/-}$ mouse lymphoma mutagen assay system. Mutat Res 1979;59(1):61−108.

[12] Cole J, Arlett CF, Green MH, Lowe J, Muriel W. A comparison of the agar cloning and microtitration techniques for assaying cell survival and mutation frequency in L5178Y mouse lymphoma cells. Mutat Res 1983;111(3):371−86.

[13] Cole J, Muriel WJ, Bridges BA. The mutagenicity of sodium fluoride to L5178Y [wild-type and TK$^{+/-}$ (3.7.2C)] mouse lymphoma cells. Mutagenesis 1986;1(2):157−67.

[14] Mitchell AD, Myhr BC, Rudd CJ, et al. Evaluation of the L5178Y mouse lymphoma cell mutagenesis assay: methods used and chemicals evaluated. Environ Mutagen 1988;12:1−18.

[15] Mitchell AD, Rudd CJ, Caspary WJ. Evaluation of the L5178Y mouse lymphomacell mutagenesis assay: intralaboratory results for sixty-three coded chemicals tested at SRI international. Environ Mutagen 1988;12:37−101.

[16] Caspary WJ, Daston DS, Myhr BC, et al. Evaluation of the L5178Y mouse lymphoma cell mutagenesis assay: interlaboratory reproducibility and assessment. Environ Mutagen 1988;12:195−229.

[17] Caspary WJ, Lee YJ, Poulton S, et al. Evaluation of the L5178Y mouse lymphoma cell mutagenesis assay: quality-control guidelines and response categories. Environ Mutagen 1988;12:19−36.

[18] Myhr BC, Caspary WJ. Evaluation of the L5178Y mouse lymphoma cell mutagenesis assay: intralaboratory results for sixty-three coded chemicals tested at Litton Bionetics, Inc. Environ Mutagen 1988;12:103−94.

[19] Clive D, Turner NT, Krehl R, Eyre J. The mouse lymphoma assay may be used as a chromosome aberration assay. Environ Mutagen 1985;7(Suppl. 3):33.

[20] International Conference On Harmonisation, 1996-last update, ICH S2A. Genotoxicity: specific aspects of regulatory genotoxicity tests for pharmaceuticals. Available: <http://www.ema.europa.eu/docs/en_GB/document_library/Scientific_guideline/2009/09/WC500003146.pdf>.

[21] International Conference On Harmonisation, 1997-last update, ICH S2B Genotoxicity: a standard battery for genotoxicity testing of pharmaceuticals. Available: <http://www.fda.gov/downloads/Drugs/GuidanceComplianceRegulatoryInformation/Guidances/ucm074929.pdf>.

[22] OECD. *In Vitro* mammalian cell gene mutation test. In: OECD guidelines for the testing of chemicals, test guideline 476. Paris: OECD. Available: <http://titania.sourceoecd.org/vl=1382924/cl=17/nw=1/rpsv/cw/vhosts/oecdjournals/1607310x/v1n4/contp1-1.htm>; 1997.

[23] International Conference On Harmonisation, 2011-last update, ICH Topic S2(R1) guidance on genotoxicity testing and data interpretation for pharmaceuticals intended for human use. Available: <http://www.ich.org/products/guidelines/safety/article/safety-guidelines.html>.

[24] Moore MM, Honma M, Clements J, et al. Mouse lymphoma thymidine kinase locus gene mutation assay: international workshop on genotoxicity test procedures workgroup report. Environ Mol Mutagen 2000;35:185−90.

[25] Moore MM, Honma M, Clements J, et al. Mouse lymphoma thymidine kinase gene mutation assay: follow-up international workshop on genotoxicity test procedures, New Orleans, Louisiana, April 2000. Environ Mol Mutagen 2002;40:292−9.

[26] Moore MM, Honma M, Clements J, et al. Mouse lymphoma thymidine kinase locus gene mutation assay: international workshop on genotoxicity test procedures workgroup report-Plymouth. UK 2002. Mutat Res 2003;540:127−40.

[27] Moore MM, Honma M, Clements J, et al. Mouse lymphoma thymidine kinase gene mutation assay: follow-up meeting of the international workshop on genotoxicity testing-Aberdeen, Scotland, 2003-assay acceptance criteria, positive controls, and data evaluation. Environ Mol Mutagen 2006;47:1−5.

[28] Moore MM, Honma M, Clements J, et al. Mouse lymphoma thymidine kinase gene mutation assay: meeting of the international workshop on genotoxicity testing, San Francisco, 2005, recommendations for 24-h treatment. Mutat Res 2007;627:36−40.

[29] MacLeod RA, Dirks WG, Matsuo Y, Kaufmann M, Milch H, Drexler HG. Widespread intraspecies cross-contamination of human tumor cell lines arising at source. Int J Cancer 1999;83(4):555−63.

[30] Capes-Davis A, Theodosopoulos G, Atkin I, Drexler HG, Kohara A, MacLeod RA, et al. Check your cultures! A list of cross-contaminated or misidentified cell lines. Int J Cancer 2010;127(1):1−8.

[31] Drexler HG, Dirks WG, Matsuo Y, MacLeod RAF. False leukemia-lymphoma cell lines: an update on over 500 cell lines. Leukemia 2003;17:416−26.

[32] Hughes P, Marshall D, Reid Y, Parkes H, Gelber C. The costs of using unauthenticated, over-passaged cell lines: how much more data do we need?. BioTechniques 2007;43(5):575 577−8, 581−2 passim

[33] Sawyer JR, Binz RL, Wang J, Moore MM. Multicolor spectral karyotyping of the L5178Y Tk$^{+/-}$ −3.7.2C mouse lymphoma cell line. Environ Mol Mutagen 2006;47(2):127−31.

[34] Fellows MD, McDermott A, Clare KR, Doherty A, Aardema MJ. The spectral karyotype of L5178Y TK (+/ −) mouse lymphoma cells clone 3.7.2C and factors affecting mutant frequency at the thymidine kinase (tk) locus in the microtiter mouse lymphoma assay. Environ Mol Mutagen 2014;55(1):35−42.

[35] Brusick D. Genotoxic effects in cultured mammalian cells produced by low pH treatment conditions and increased ion concentrations. Environ Mutagen 1986;8:879−86.

[36] Scott D, Galloway SM, Marshall RR, Ishidate Jr. M, Brusick D, Ashby J, et al. Genotoxicity under extreme culture conditions. A report from ICPEMC Task Group 9. Mutat Res 1991;257:147−204.

[37] Kirkland D, Aardema M, Henderson L, Muller L. Evaluation of the ability of a battery of three *in vitro* genotoxicity tests to discriminate rodent carcinogens and non-carcinogens I. Sensitivity, specificity and relative predictivity. Mutat Res 2005;584(1−2):1−256.

[38] Kirkland D, Pfuhler S, Tweats D, et al. How to reduce false positive results when undertaking *in vitro* genotoxicity testing and thus avoid unnecessary follow-up animal tests: report of an ECVAM Workshop. Mutat Res 2007;628(1):31−55.

[39] Kirkland D, Speit G. Evaluation of the ability of a battery of three *in vitro* genotoxicity tests to discriminate rodent carcinogens and non-carcinogens III. Appropriate follow-up testing *in vivo*. Mutat Res 2008;654(2):114−32.

[40] Matthews EJ, Kruhlak NL, Cimino MC, Benz RD, Contrera JF. An analysis of genetic toxicity, reproductive and developmental toxicity, and carcinogenicity data: I. Identification of carcinogens using surrogate endpoints. Regul Toxicol Pharmacol 2006;44(2):83−96.

[41] Matthews EJ, Kruhlak NL, Cimino MC, Benz RD, Contrera JF. An analysis of genetic toxicity, reproductive and developmental toxicity, and carcinogenicity data: II. Identification of genotoxicants, reprotoxicants, and carcinogens using *in silico* methods. Regul Toxicol Pharmacol 2006;44(2):97−110.

[42] Fellows MD, Boyer S, O'Donovan MR. The incidence of positive results in the mouse lymphoma TK assay (MLA) in pharmaceutical screening and their prediction by MultiCase MC4PC. Mutagenesis 2011;26(4):529−32.

CHAPTER 6

The In Vitro *Micronucleus Assay*

Ann Doherty[1], Steven M. Bryce[2] and Jeffrey C. Bemis[2]

[1]*AstraZeneca Innovative Medicines and Early Development, Cambridge, UK*
[2]*Litron Laboratories, Rochester, NY, US*

Chapter Outline

6.1 Introduction 163
6.2 Practical Considerations 165
    6.2.1 Regulatory Guidelines 165
    6.2.2 Good Laboratory Practice (GLP) 165
    6.2.3 Cell Types 166
    6.2.4 Laboratory Proficiency 166
    6.2.5 Controls 166
    6.2.6 Metabolic Activation 167
    6.2.7 S9 Rat Liver Homogenate 167
    6.2.8 Experimental Design 167
    6.2.9 Cytotoxicity Measures 167
        6.2.9.1 *Methods used to determine cytotoxicity in the absence of cytochalasin B 168*
        6.2.9.2 *Method used to determine cytotoxicity in the presence of cytochalasin B 168*
    6.2.10 Historical Controls 169
6.3 Methods 169
    6.3.1 Mononuclear Assay 169
    6.3.2 Binuclear Assay 169
    6.3.3 Centromeric Labeling 169
    6.3.4 Nondisjunction Assay 170
6.4 Materials 171
    6.4.1 Mononuclear Assay 171
    6.4.2 Binuclear Assay 172
    6.4.3 Centromeric Labeling 172
    6.4.4 Nondisjunction Assay 172
6.5 Protocols 172
    6.5.1 S9 Mix 172
    6.5.2 Mononuclear Assay 173
        6.5.2.1 *Treatment schedules 173*
        6.5.2.2 *Cell culture and treatment 174*
        6.5.2.3 *Slide preparation 174*

Genetic Toxicology Testing.
DOI: http://dx.doi.org/10.1016/B978-0-12-800764-8.00006-9

       6.5.2.4 Coding of slides   175

       6.5.2.5 Analysis of slides (microscope)   175

       6.5.2.6 Analysis of slides (semiautomated scoring)   176

    6.5.3 Binuclear Assay   177

       6.5.3.1   Treatment schedules   177

       6.5.3.2   Human peripheral blood lymphocytes   178

       6.5.3.3   Donors   178

       6.5.3.4   Lymphocyte culture   178

       6.5.3.5   Staining and analysis   179

       6.5.3.6   Coding of slides   179

       6.5.3.7   Analysis of slides   179

       6.5.3.8   Evaluation of results (acceptance criteria and statistics)   180

       6.5.3.9   Criteria for a valid assay   180

       6.5.3.10 Evaluation of data   180

    6.5.4 Centromeric Labeling   181

       6.5.4.1 FISH using a programmable hotplate such as HYBrite™ or Thermobrite™   181

       6.5.4.2 Alterative protocol for FISH   182

       6.5.4.3 Slide checking   182

       6.5.4.4 Slide scoring   183

    6.5.5 Nondisjunction Assay   183

       6.5.5.1 FISH method   183

       6.5.5.2 Slide checking   183

       6.5.5.3 Slide scoring   183

6.6 Flow Cytometric Method   184

    6.6.1   Equipment   184

    6.6.2   Consumables   185

    6.6.3   Reagents and recipes   185

    6.6.4   Suspension Cell Protocol   187

       6.6.4.1 Treatment, preliminary assessments   187

       6.6.4.2 Cell harvest   187

       6.6.4.3 Complete nucleic acid dye A staining   187

       6.6.4.4 Simultaneous cell lysis and nucleic acid dye B staining   188

    6.6.5   Attachment Cell Protocol   188

       6.6.5.1 Treatment, preliminary assessments   188

       6.6.5.2 Cell harvest   188

       6.6.5.3 Complete nucleic acid dye A staining   189

       6.6.5.4 Simultaneous cell lysis and nucleic acid dye B staining   189

    6.6.6   Flow Cytometric Data Acquisition   189

    6.6.7   Flow Cytometric Data Analysis   193

       6.6.7.1 Independent cytotoxicity assessment   194

       6.6.7.2 Criteria for a valid assay   194

       6.6.7.3 Criteria for positive/negative outcomes   194

    6.6.8   Creating an Analysis Template   195

    6.6.9   Example Plate Layout   198

    6.6.10 Example Results Table   199

    6.6.11 Advice for Test Article Exposure   200

       6.6.11.1 Suspension cells   200

       6.6.11.2 Attachment cells   201

6.6.11.3 *Metabolic activation   202*
6.6.11.4 *Positive controls   202*
6.6.12 Use of Multichannel Aspirator with Bridge   202
6.6.13 Plate Placement During Nucleic Acid Dye B Photoactivation   203
6.6.14 Updates and Future Work   203
References   203

6.1 Introduction

Micronuclei in erythrocytes have been identified for more than 100 years as the Howell-Jolly bodies seen in hematology. The first suggestion of the use of micronucleus frequency as a quantitative measure of chromosomal damage was provided by Evans et al. [1], although a spindle poison had previously been found to induce micronuclei in ascites tumor cells *in vivo* [2]. In the early 1970s, two independent research groups described the use of micronuclei production in rodent bone marrow erythrocytes as a measure of chromosomal damage in animals exposed to mutagens *in vivo* [3,4]. Countryman and Heddle [5] were the first to develop an *in vitro* method using cultured peripheral lymphocytes. Because the expression of micronuclei is dependent on the cell undergoing division, it is important to be able to identify cells that have divided at least once during or after treatment. A breakthrough in this area came when Fenech and Morley [6] proposed the cytokinesis-block method. This utilizes cytochalasin-B, a mycotoxin isolated from *Helminthosporium dematioideum*, to inhibit cytokinesis without blocking mitosis [7]. This results in the formation of binucleated cells, allowing easy identification and scoring of cells that have undergone nuclear division after treatment.

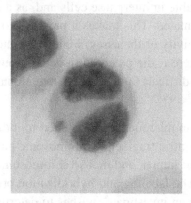

Image 1: Photograph of a micronuclei in a binucleate human lymphocyte cell (the image was captured from an acridine orange preparation in fluorescent colors and then the negative image was used to convert to grayscale).

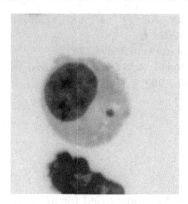

Image 2: Photograph of a micronuclei in a mononucleate L5178Y cell (the image was captured from an acridine orange preparation in fluorescent colors and then the negative image was used to convert to grayscale).

Micronuclei are DNA fragments that are separate from the main nucleus and have originated from acentric chromosome or chromatid fragments or whole chromosomes that fail to be included in the daughter nuclei at the completion of telophase during mitosis because they did not attach to the spindle during the segregation at anaphase. Thus, micronuclei may result from clastogenic or aneugenic mechanisms, for example, chromosome breakage leading to acentric fragments or interference with chromosomal segregation at anaphase. The *in vitro* micronucleus test is an umbrella term for many differing micronucleus tests, such as those with and without cytochalasin B and a variety of treatment and recovery schedules. Rapidly dividing cells can be used for the mononuclear micronucleus protocol and require a robust measurement of toxicity, such as population doubling.

Micronuclei are readily detectable in interphase cells and, as a result, can be scored rapidly by eye or analysis can be automated. This makes it practical to score thousands of cells per treatment, increasing the sensitivity of the assay. Finally, because micronuclei may arise from lagging chromosomes, there is the potential to detect aneuploidy-inducing agents, a class of genotoxin that can be difficult to detect in conventional chromosomal aberration tests [8,9] (Figure 6.1).

The presence of a centromere in micronuclei is assumed to indicate the presence of a whole chromosome rather than an acentric fragment. Chromosome paints are commercially available for the centromeres of human and mouse chromosomes and have fluorescent labels incorporated [10−12]. The labeling and hybridization procedures for detection of centromeres can be used when an investigator wishes to determine whether an increase in micronucleated cells is the result of clastogenic and/or aneugenic events.

Finally, probes can be used to label specific individual chromosomes and evaluate whether they are inappropriately segregated into the two daughter nuclei of binucleate cells at

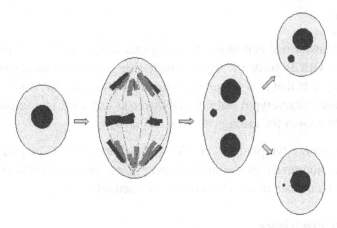

Figure 6.1
Overview of micronucleus formation with micronuclei originating from either a whole
chromosome or a chromosomal fragment in binucleate and mononucleate cells.

interphase. This *nondisjunction assay* can be incorporated into the standard cytochalasin
block micronucleus test to identify aneugenic agents [13].

6.2 Practical Considerations

6.2.1 Regulatory Guidelines

The OECD guideline 487 for the *in vitro* mammalian cell micronucleus test was introduced
in 2010 and, at the time of writing this chapter, most recently revised on September 26,
2014. The latest versions of OECD guidelines can be obtained at http://www.oecd-ilibrary.
org/. Studies for regulatory submission are normally conducted in accordance with OECD
guidelines under GLP.

6.2.2 Good Laboratory Practice (GLP)

The practical methods described in this chapter have all come from a pharmaceutical
laboratory and, as such, the methods have all been conducted according to good laboratory
practice (GLP) requirements.

Generally, GLP refers to a system of management controls for laboratories and research
organizations to ensure the consistency and reliability of results as outlined in the
OECD Principles of GLP and national regulations. GLP applies to nonclinical studies
conducted for the assessment of the safety of chemicals to humans, animals, and the
environment.

6.2.3 Cell Types

Many primary or transformed cell lines are appropriate to use for *in vitro* micronucleus testing. The current OECD guideline has not made firm recommendations of the choice of cell types but it suggests that it is important, when evaluating chemical hazards, to consider the *p53* status, genetic (karyotype) stability, DNA repair capacity, and origin (rodent vs. human) of the cells chosen for testing (refer Guideline 474).

In this chapter, the mouse lymphoma L5178Y cell line clone 3.7.2C is used as an example of the mononuclear micronucleus test method and primary human lymphocytes are used as an example of the binucleate blocked micronucleus method.

6.2.4 Laboratory Proficiency

The OECD guideline for the micronucleus test requires laboratories to show proficiency in the conduct of the micronucleus assay prior to routine testing. This requires performance of a series of experiments with positive reference substances acting via different mechanisms, including at least one with and one without metabolic activation, and one acting via an aneugenic mechanism (Table 6.1).

6.2.5 Controls

Concurrent positive and solvent/vehicle controls both with and without metabolic activation (S9) are required in each experiment. The positive controls should demonstrate the ability of the cells to respond to both clastogens and aneugens and the capability of the metabolic activation system used for the assay, such as S9. The positive controls should allow

Table 6.1: Examples of reference substances recommended for assessing laboratory proficiency and for the selection of positive controls as listed by OECD

Category	Substance	CASRN
1. Clastogens Active Without Metabolic Activation		
	Methyl methanesulfonate	66-27-3
	Mitomycin C	50-07-7
	4-Nitroquinoline N-oxide	56-57-5
	Cytosine arabinoside	147-94-4
2. Clastogens Requiring Metabolic Activation		
	Benzo(a)pyrene	50-32-8
	Cyclophosphamide	50-18-0
3. Aneugens		
	Colchicine	64-86-8
	Vinblastine	143-67-9

micronucleus formation at concentrations expected to provide reproducible increases over background, demonstrating the sensitivity of the test system [9].

6.2.6 Metabolic Activation

In vitro assays generally require the use of an exogenous source of metabolic activation unless the cells are metabolically competent, although, of course, exogenous metabolic activation systems cannot entirely mimic *in vivo* conditions. The most commonly used system is a cofactor-supplemented postmitochondrial fraction (S9) prepared from the livers of rodents treated with enzyme-inducing agents such as Aroclor 1254 [14]. A combination of phenobarbitone and β-naphthoflavone [15] is considered equally effective as Aroclor 1254 for inducing mixed-function oxidases and may be a preferred alternative in certain countries given that Aroclor is considered to be a persistent environmental pollutant and is difficult to obtain commercially.

6.2.7 S9 Rat Liver Homogenate

The postmitochondrial fraction (S9) of a rat liver homogenate can be prepared in-house or, more conveniently, purchased from MolTox Inc. (Boone, North Carolina, USA). Its metabolic capacity is demonstrated by key enzyme assays and the ability to activate reference bacterial mutagens. S9 fraction is stored in liquid nitrogen or at $-80\,^{\circ}\mathrm{C}$ until used. S9 is added to a cofactor solution to form the S9 mix, which is then added to cultures.

6.2.8 Experimental Design

The experimental design can include a dose range–finding phase to assess cytotoxicity. Alternatively, the main test can be conducted with a large number of dose levels (10–20), and then doses can be selected to score based on the cytotoxicity. At least three scorable concentrations must be scored and selected across the dose range to achieve a maximum of 50% toxicity. Dose intervals were one-half log or 80% when the toxicity curve was very steep.

6.2.9 Cytotoxicity Measures

Appropriate toxicity measurements are required for *in vitro* genotoxicity assays to set an appropriate maximum dose level for evaluation, unless the high dose is limited by other factors, such as solubility in the culture medium. In addition, assessment of toxicity must be incorporated in the main experiment itself, even if performed in a preliminary experiment. A comparison of cytotoxicity measures for the *in vitro* micronucleus tests was undertaken previously [16, 17]. Relative cell counts (RCC), relative increase in cell counts (RICC), and relative population doubling (RPD) for treatments without cytokinesis block were compared against the replication index (RI) for treatments with cytokinesis block.

6.2.9.1 Methods used to determine cytotoxicity in the absence of cytochalasin B [16] (reproduced with permission of the author)

1. *Relative cell count*
    RCC was determined as:

$$\text{Final count treated cultures} \div \text{Final count control cultures} \times 100\%$$

2. *Relative increase in cell count*
    RICC was determined as:

$$\frac{\text{Increase in number of cells in treated cultures (final − starting)}}{\text{Increases in number of cells in control cultures (final − starting)}} \times 100$$

3. *Relative population doubling*
    RPD was determined as:

$$\frac{\text{Number of population doublings in treated cultures}}{\text{Number of population doublings in control cultures}} \times 100$$

where

$$\text{Population doubling} = \frac{[\log(\text{Posttreatment cell number}/\text{Initial cell number})]}{\log 2}$$

6.2.9.2 Method used to determine cytotoxicity in the presence of cytochalasin B

Replicative index
    RI was determined as:

$$\frac{\dfrac{(\text{No. binucleated cells} + 2 \times \text{No. multinucleate cells})}{\text{Total number of cells treated cultures}}}{\dfrac{(\text{No. binucleated cells} + 2 \times \text{No. multinucleate cells})}{\text{Total number of cells control cultures}}} \times 100$$

No two cytotoxicity endpoints give the same result. In particular, RCC markedly underestimated the toxicity compared with other measures [16] and, therefore, is no longer recommended for use in the test [9]. Furthermore, using these estimations of cytotoxicity and the limit of 50% survival, all the mutagens and aneugens tested were appropriately identified as positive in the *in vitro* micronucleus assay. Accordingly, it was clear that testing beyond 50% survival was not necessary to identify the potential of these agents to induce micronuclei [16].

6.2.10 Historical Controls

The laboratory should establish historical positive and negative control databases during assay development and validation. Negative controls should be consistent with published negative control data, where they exist, for that cell culture system. The laboratory's historical negative control database should initially be built with a minimum of 10 experiments but would preferably consist of at least 20 experiments conducted under comparable experimental conditions [9]. The negative control values for an individual test should ideally be within the 95% control limits of that distribution based on percentile values. Historical positive and, in particular, negative control results distributions showing ranges, means, standard deviation, 95% limits, and number of replicates/experimental points involved should be presented in every report. Laboratories should use quality control methods, such as control charts to monitor potential drift over time.

6.3 Methods

6.3.1 Mononuclear Assay

The mononuclear micronucleus assay is described in mouse lymphoma L5178Y cells, clone 3.7.2C, which were obtained from Dr J. Cole, (MRC Cell Mutation Unit, University of Sussex, Brighton, UK). This clone was confirmed to have the expected karyotype [18], including two copies of Chromosome 11 as detected by fluorescent *in situ* hybridization (FISH). The average doubling time of the cells is approximately 9–10 h. Cells from our laboratory have been lodged in the European cell culture collection along with full SKYFISH karyotype (for details see Mouse lymphoma chapter Section 4).

6.3.2 Binuclear Assay

The binucleate micronucleus assay is described in separated human lymphocytes and the average cell cycle of 18–20 h in pooled human lymphocytes from at least two donors of the same sex. Human peripheral blood lymphocytes should be obtained from young (approximately 18–35 years of age), nonsmoking individuals with no known illness or recent exposures to genotoxic agents (e.g., chemicals, ionizing radiation) at levels that would increase the background incidence of micronucleate cells [9].

6.3.3 Centromeric Labeling

Centromeric labeling provides a method of identifying whether a micronucleus contains a centromere. In our laboratory all positive results are followed-up by centromeric labeling to

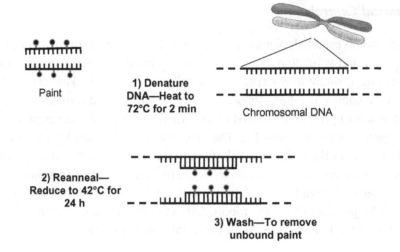

Figure 6.2
Fluorescent *in situ* hybridization (FISH) cartoon of the FISH technique showing denaturation and reannealing steps.

understand mechanisms of micronucleus induction. The presence of a centromere signal in the micronuclei is assumed to indicate the presence of a whole chromosome. The FISH technique is used with commercially available centromeres of mouse and human chromosomes and have fluorescent labels incorporated; CY3 label is red and FITC label is green when viewed through a fluorescent microscope with the appropriate filters (Figure 6.2).

6.3.4 Nondisjunction Assay

Nondisjunction can be examined in binucleate human lymphocytes by using centromere-specific probes to examine distribution of pairs of chromosomes between the two nuclei [13].

Cytochalasin B blocks cells at cytokinesis, leading to an accumulation of binucleate cells. The incorporation of centromere-specific probes allows visualization of chromosome segregation and distribution in the individual nuclei of the binucleate cell. When using two centromere-specific probes, the normal distribution of chromosomes would be two copies in each nucleus written as a 2:2 distribution. Nondisjunction is the malsegregation of chromosomes due to the failure of chromosomes on the metaphase plate to divide to each daughter nuclei and may be determined by a 3:1 or 4:0 distribution of centromere-specific signals (Figure 6.3).

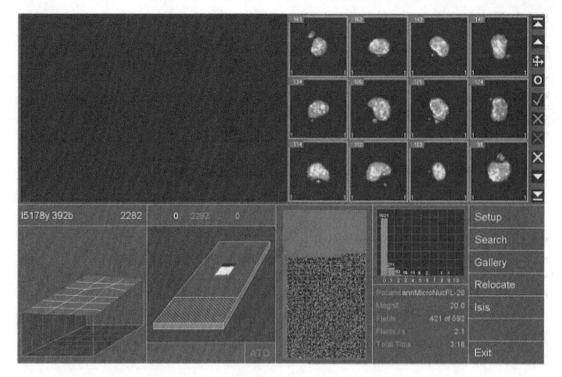

Figure 6.3

Cartoon of cell division with dark and light small circles representing individual centromere-specific probes: (A) 2:2 normal distribution of chromosomes to daughter nuclei; (B) 3:1 nondisjunction of the chromosome represented by a light circle; (C) 4:0 nondisjunction of the chromosome represented by a light circle; (D) both a 3:1 nondisjunction of the chromosome represented by a light circle and 4:0 nondisjunction of the chromosome represented by a dark circle; and (E) both a 3:1 nondisjunction of the chromosome represented by a dark circle and loss of one copy of the chromosome represented by a light circle in a micronuclei.

6.4 Materials

6.4.1 Mononuclear Assay

- Medium for L5178Y cells: RPMI 1640 medium (Invitrogen, Paisley, UK) supplemented with 10% heat-inactivated donor horse serum, 2 mmol/L L-glutamine, 2 mmol/L sodium pyruvate, 1% v/v Pluronic F68, 200 IU/mL penicillin, 200 μg/mL streptomycin
- 4'-6-Diamidino-2-phenylindole (DAPI) in Vectasheild™ mounting medium refractive index 1.45
- Fresh phosphate buffer (0.66% w/v potassium phosphate monobasic plus 0.32% w/v sodium phosphate dibasic, pH 6.4−6.5)
- Acridine orange (AO) hemi (zinc) chloride (12 mg AO/100 mL buffer)

6.4.2 Binuclear Assay

For human lymphocytes:

- Accuspin System Histopaque-1077
- RPMI medium with serum and PHA: PB Max Karyotyping Medium (Gibco Invitrogen) containing HA16, 0.01 mg/mL (Remel, UK)
- Cytochalasin B 6 μg/mL

6.4.3 Centromeric Labeling

- 20X SSC stock solution: 3 M NaCl (17.53 g/100 mL) plus 0.3 M trisodium citrate (8.82 g/100 mL)
- 2X SSC (1 in 10 dilution of stock)
- 2X SSC with 0.1% Tween-20 (100 μL Tween-20 in 100 mL of 2X SSC)
- 0.4X SSC with 0.3% Tween-20 (20 mL 2X SSC + 80 mL water plus 300 μL Tween-20)
- The pan-centromeric paint, either human for binucleate assay or mouse for mononuclear assay, is available from Cambio UK Star FISH paints (light-sensitive)

All solutions are prepared fresh on day of use from stock of 20X SSC, which is stable for 1 year and stored at room temperature

6.4.4 Nondisjunction Assay

Because the nondisjunction assay described is in primary human lymphocytes, it uses the same medium as the binuclear assay (see Section 6.4.2). Nondisjunction is determined by examining the segregation of centromere-specific probes in the binucleate lymphocyte; therefore, the centromere probe materials are same as those in centromeric labeling (see Section 5.4).

- Human centromeric-specific chromosomes (light-sensitive) probes are available from four suppliers: Cambio, Abbot, MP Biomedicals (formerly Qbiogene), and Poseidon DNA Probes (Kreatech Biotechnology NL). Concentrated probes are needed to allow mixing. The program used for centromere-specific probes includes a denaturation step at 72 °C for 2 min followed by 16–40 h at 42 °C.

6.5 Protocols

6.5.1 S9 Mix

- *Buffer solution A:* 3.12 g NaH_2PO_4 in 500 mL distilled water
- *Buffer solution B:* 14.2 g $Na_2HPO_4 \cdot 2H_2O$ in 100 mL distilled water
- *Magnesium chloride solution:* 8.14 g $MgCl_2 \cdot 6H_2O$ and 12.3 g KCl in 100 mL distilled water

- 79 mg nicotinamide adenine dinucleotide phosphate (NADP)
- 38 mg glucose-6-phosphate sodium salt (G6P)

The sterilized cofactor solution may be formulated as a stock batch, aliquoted into sterile 20 mL vials, and stored at $-80\,^\circ$C for 12 months.

To prepare a 0.2 M phosphate buffer (pH 7.4):

> Mix 60 mL of buffer solution A and 440 mL of buffer solution B. If necessary, adjust to pH 7.4 and sterilize using 0.22-micron filter unit.

To prepare cofactor:

> Weigh 79 mg NADP and 38 mg G6P monosodium salt and dissolve in:
> 12 mL Phosphate buffer
> 0.5 mL Magnesium chloride
> 9.5 mL Distilled water

The cofactor solution is filter-sterilized using a 0.22-micron filter.

Immediately prior to use, snap-thaw the S9 fraction and add 5–20 mL cofactor solution and mix well. Then, add 0.5 mL of the S9 mix per 10 mL culture (Table 6.2).

6.5.2 Mononuclear Assay

6.5.2.1 Treatment schedules

To detect an aneugen or clastogen acting at a specific stage in the cell cycle, it is important for cells to be treated with the test substance during all stages of their cell cycle. The cell cycle time should be established using bromodeoxyuridine incorporation and this value should be used to ensure that cells have been treated for at least 1.5-times the cell cycle (Table 6.3).

Table 6.2

Cofactor Constituent		Amount	Final Concentration in Cofactor Solution
Phosphate buffer	NaH_2PO_4	12 mL	0.11 mmol/L
	$Na_2HPO_4 \cdot 2H_2O$		
Magnesium chloride	$MgCl_2 \cdot 6H_2O$	0.5 mL	19 mmol/L
	KCl		37.5 mmol/L
NADP		79 mg	4.7 mmol/L
G6P		38 mg	6.12 mmol/L
Distilled water		9.5 mL	
Rat S9 fraction		5 mL	20%

Table 6.3

Cell lines treated without cytoB	+ S9	Treat for 3−6 h in the presence of S9; remove the S9 and treatment medium; add fresh medium and harvest 1.5−2.0 normal cell cycles later
	− S9 Short exposure	Treat for 3−6 h; remove the treatment medium; add fresh medium and harvest 1.5−2.0 normal cell cycles later
	− S9 Extended exposure	A: Treat for 1.5−2.0 normal cell cycles; harvest at the end of the exposure period B: Treat for 1.5−2.0 normal cell cycles; remove the treatment medium; add fresh medium and harvest 1.5−2.0 normal cell cycles later

This table was present in the 2011 version of the OECD guideline and is still very useful for consideration of extended recovery times needed for expression of some forms of genotoxic damage such as aneugenicity.

6.5.2.2 Cell culture and treatment

L5178Y cells are cultured in supplemented RPMI 1640 and maintained at 37 °C in a humidified atmosphere of 5% CO_2 in air.

Remove cells from liquid nitrogen, wash in medium, resuspend in fresh medium, and grow for 3−4 days to get sufficient cells for a micronucleus test.

To set up test cultures, cells are disaggregated and counted, and the volume is adjusted with fresh medium to an appropriate concentration (usually 1×10^4 to 2×10^5 cells per mL) and 10 mL aliquots dispensed into 25 cm^2 tissue culture flasks, and then incubated until required for assessment of cytotoxicity and micronucleus frequency.

Cells are then exposed to the test compound for 3 h or 24 h (see Table 6.1). The cells for the micronucleus test are removed from the culture for cytospinning and the remaining cells are grown in culture for cell counts to determine population doubling.

6.5.2.3 Slide preparation

1. Individual cultures are vortexed and, when possible, 850 μL is dispensed into a Megafunnel™ and centrifuged at 1000 rpm for 8 min using a Shandon Cytospin 4.
2. Slides are removed from the cytocentrifuge and left to air-dry completely.
3. Slides are fixed with 90% methanol for 10 min.
4. For manual scoring, slides are dipped in fresh phosphate buffer and stained in a solution of AO for 1 min. Slides are then placed in buffer for 10 min, followed by another 15 min in fresh buffer.
5. Alternatively, for automated scoring using the MicroNuc™ module of the Metafer system, slides may be stained immediately with DAPI or stored until ready for analysis

and then stained. Slides are stained by adding antifade containing DAPI counterstain, mounted with large (22 × 40 mm) coverslips, placed in card trays, and stored flat, protected from light prior to scoring on Metafer [15]. Following addition of antifade and prior to scoring, slides are examined under the microscope for the presence of nucleated cells (blue from DAPI counterstain).

6. Alternatively, after staining, slides are air-dried and stored protected from light.
7. Slides are analyzed using an automated scoring system or scored "by eye." Whatever method is used, results are recorded appropriately.

6.5.2.4 Coding of slides

To prevent bias in the micronucleus scoring, slides must be coded prior to scoring.

1. The Study Director generates a code sheet. All cultures are allocated a slide code.
2. The slide codes are written or printed on adhesive labels together with the study number.
3. The code labels are applied to the appropriate slides according to the code sheet. A blank label is also placed on the reverse of the frosted end of the slide to cover all identification marks.
4. Ideally, someone not involved in the micronucleus analysis should perform the coding, but when this is not possible, it will not invalidate the study.

The code sheet must then be sealed and only opened after all analyses are complete for decoding.

6.5.2.5 Analysis of slides (microscope)

1. Slides are "wet"-mounted (carefully avoiding air bubbles) prior to scoring with phosphate buffer and a glass coverslip. Microscopic analysis is performed using a fluorescence microscope with suitable filter sets for AO (i.e., an Olympus BG-12 excitation filter and 0-530 barrier filter).
2. The cells are identified by the following staining properties of AO: nuclei and micronuclei (DNA) are stained yellow/green and the cytoplasm is stained red. Micronuclei are identified according to the criteria of Countryman and Heddle [16]. Less than one-third of the main nuclei size, the stain intensity should be similar to the main nuclei and all membranes must be intact and circular. The size of micronuclei can indicate an aneugenic response is some cases (Hashimoto 2010), but care must be taken not to overinterpret these data because some compounds with large amounts of breakage also provide large micronuclei as damage appears to accumulate.
3. Counting is performed on electronic digital counters and data are recorded on paper.
4. Relative proportions of micronuclei are determined in a total of 1000 mononuclear cells per each of two replicate cultures so that 2000 mononuclear cells are scored for each dose.
5. In the event of an equivocal result, analysis may be extended up to 4000 mononuclear cells.

6. Peer review of slide analysis may be undertaken. In the event of unusual results, the study director or other senior cytogeneticist may reexamine and should comment on findings of any peer review. In our laboratory, we also conduct a yearly comparison of scoring among all trained scorers to check for drift.

6.5.2.6 Analysis of slides (semiautomated scoring)

The automated system used in our laboratory is the MicroNuc program by MetaSystems [19,20]. This program has been written to detect micronuclei in binucleate cells and contains classifiers that are easily modified to determine the size and shape of nuclei and micronuclei and are adaptable to mononuclear screening.

The slides are scanned on Metafer using $\times 20$ magnification objective and an 8-slide automatic stage. The classifier developed by MetaSystems to score binucleate cells has been modified to score mononucleated L5178Y cells and is deliberately oversensitive to detect all aberrant divisions.

Slides are scanned using the Metafer 4 master station comprising a Zeiss Axioplan Imager Z1 equipped with a Maerzhaeuser stepping motor stage that can scan eight slides unattended. The MicroNuc module is run on the Metafer MSearch platform v3.4.102 (MetaSystems GmbH, Altlussheim, Germany). Images are acquired on a Peltier cooled grayscale digital CCD camera Axiocam MRm (Carl Zeiss). The plane of focus is determined at a number of grid positions that are distributed evenly across the scan area. A predetermined scan area for the Shandon Megafunnel is used for all slides. The scan area is set to deliberately avoid the outside margins of the cell preparation area, because this area contains cellular clumps that cannot be scanned accurately.

The nuclei classifier for scanning mononuclear preparations is set to the following criteria: object threshold, 20%; minimum area, 10 μm^2; maximum area, 400 μm^2; maximum relative concavity of depth, 0.9; aspect ratio, 2.5; maximum distance between nuclei, 0 (this feature is designed for binucleate scoring capabilities); maximum area asymmetry, 90%; region of interest radius, 40 μm; and maximum object area in region of interest, 90 μm^2.

The criteria for the micronuclei are set to: object threshold, 10%; minimum area, 1 μm^2; maximum area, 55 μm^2; maximum relative concavity of depth, 1; aspect ratio, 3.5; and maximum distance, 35 μm.

Once the slides are scanned, the images collected in the "gallery" are arranged in order of the number of micronuclei they contain. Images are then visually assessed on screen and the number of cells containing true micronuclei are counted, thus allowing rejection of artifacts or cell debris from cytotoxicity. The automated scoring is set to capture 2500 cells.

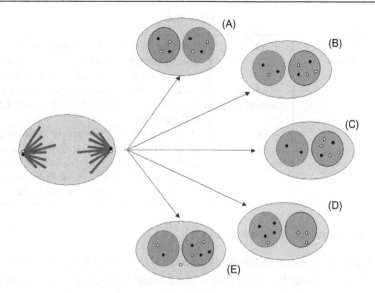

Figure 6.4

Screenshot of the automated micronucleus system, Metafer™, showing the gallery of mononuclear cells with micronuclei.

Criteria for evaluation

Micronuclei evaluated should be less than one-third the diameter of the main nucleus, separate from the main nucleus with intact cytoplasmic membrane, and located within the cytoplasm area; cells containing three or less micronuclei are assessed (Figure 6.4).

6.5.3 Binuclear Assay

6.5.3.1 Treatment schedules

One of the most important considerations in the performance of the *in vitro* binucleate micronucleus test is ensuring that the cells being scored have completed mitosis during the treatment period or, when used, the posttreatment incubation period (Table 6.4).

This table was present in the TG487 version from 2011 and is now removed from the current version; however, it is still a useful guide.

Table 6.4

Lymphocytes, primary cells, and cell lines treated with cytoB	+ S9	Treat for 3–6 h in the presence of S9; remove the S9 and treatment medium; add fresh medium and cytoB; and harvest 1.5–2.0 normal cell cycles later
	− S9 Short exposure	Treat for 3–6 h; remove the treatment medium; add fresh medium and cytoB; and harvest 1.5–2.0 normal cell cycles later
	− S9 Extended exposure	*A:* Treat for 1.5–2 normal cell cycles in the presence of cytoB; harvest at the end of the exposure period *B:* Treat for 1.5–2.0 normal cell cycles; remove the test substance; add fresh medium and cytoB; and harvest 1.5–2.0 normal cell cycles later

6.5.3.2 Human peripheral blood lymphocytes

Human lymphocytes have been extensively used in the *in vitro* binucleate micronucleus assay [21–23]. Cytochalasin B is required when human lymphocytes are used because cell cycle times will be variable within cultures and among donors, and because not all lymphocytes will respond to phytohemogglutinin (PHA). PHA obtained from Remel is HA15 or HA16 and may be used to stimulate T-cell division; however, HA16 in its purified form will provide more consistent stimulation of lymphocytes and should be batch-tested along with the serum used to obtain optimal growth.

6.5.3.3 Donors

Blood donors should be younger than age 45 years, healthy, nonsmoking individuals with no known recent exposures to genotoxic chemicals or radiation. Micronucleus frequency increases with age [24].

6.5.3.4 Lymphocyte culture

Lymphocytes may be separated prior to culture initiation or at the end of treatment; however, it is faster and simpler to separate the lymphocytes at culture initiation.

Lymphocytes are separated by layering fresh whole blood mixed 1:1 with medium onto Accuspin System Histopaque-1077 and centrifuged at $800 \times g$ for 15 min or $1000 \times g$ for 10 min. The mononuclear cell layer is then removed and washed in PBS or medium twice, and the cell number is then determined. At this stage, cells should be counted on a hemocytometer (not a coulter counter) because the condition of the cells can be seen while counting. Separated lymphocytes are seeded at a density of 2×10^5 cells in 9.9 mL medium in a suitable flask or tube.

Human lymphocytes (from both separated and whole blood) are initiated and cultured in lymphocyte medium.

Whole blood cultures are initiated by addition of 0.5 mL whole blood to 9.4 mL of medium in 25-cm^2 flasks and placed upright in an incubator set at 37 °C and, if medium is not HEPES-buffered, in an atmosphere containing 5% carbon dioxide.

Forty-four hours after initiation, whole blood and separated lymphocyte cultures are treated with test compound or vehicle control and simultaneously with the addition of cytochalasin B 6 µg/mL [25].

Sixty-eight hours following initiation, whole blood cultures are harvested by separation of lymphocytes. Seventy-two hours following initiation, separated lymphocyte cultures are harvested. Slides from both culture methods are prepared by cytocentrifuge (600 rpm 5 min) and air-dried. Slides are then fixed in 100% methanol for 8 min and stored at room temperature.

A more detailed human lymphocyte protocol for problem-solving can be found in *Nature Methods* [26].

6.5.3.5 Staining and analysis

Slides are dipped in fresh phosphate buffer (0.66% w/v potassium phosphate monobasic plus 0.32% w/v sodium phosphate dibasic; pH, 6.4−6.5) and stained in a solution of AO (12 mg AO/100 mL buffer) for 1 min. Slides are then placed in buffer for 10 min, followed by a another 15 min in a fresh batch of buffer. After staining, slides are air-dried and stored protected from light.

6.5.3.6 Coding of slides

All slides are coded prior to being scored for micronuclei as described in the previous section on mononuclear slide preparations.

6.5.3.7 Analysis of slides

1. Slides are wet-mounted (carefully avoiding air bubbles) prior to scoring with phosphate buffer and a glass coverslip. Microscopic analysis is performed using a fluorescence microscope−appropriate triple bandpass filter.
2. The cells are identified by the following staining properties of AO: nuclei and micronuclei (DNA) are stained yellow/green and the cytoplasm is stained red. Micronuclei are identified according to criteria reported elsewhere [5, 27].
3. Scoring is performed on electronic digital counters and data are recorded on paper.
4. Relative proportions of micronuclei are determined in a total of 1000 binuclear cells per culture to give a total of 2000 binucleates per dose.
5. Two thousand binucleate cells are scored for each dose. The number of mononuclear and multinucleated cells are scored along with the binucleate count to

calculate the replicative index. In addition, the number of necrotic and apoptotic cells are noted.

6. In the event of an equivocal result, analysis may be extended up to 4000 binucleate cells.

7. To resolve equivocal data, the number of cells scored may be extended; however, the number to score should be determined with statistical assistance regarding the cell type used and with reference to the historical control data for the individual laboratory. If the result remains borderline, then supplementary testing may be required.

6.5.3.8 Evaluation of results (acceptance criteria and statistics)

There are several criteria for determining a positive result, such as a concentration-related increase or a reproducible increase in the number of cells containing micronuclei. The biological relevance of the results should be considered first. Consideration of whether the observed values are within or outside of the historical control range can provide guidance when evaluating the biological relevance of the response. Appropriate statistical methods should be used to evaluate the test results [28,29], but they should not be the only determinant of a positive response. The experimental unit is the cell; reproducibility and biological relevance are paramount in evaluation of results [30].

6.5.3.9 Criteria for a valid assay

For a test to be considered valid, the following criteria should be fulfilled:

1. The mean concurrent vehicle control values fall within the acceptable limits as defined in the laboratory historical control data and should lie within the 95% control limits of the distribution of the laboratory's historical negative control database. The positive control group data clearly demonstrate a statistically and biologically significant increase when compared with the concurrent vehicle control group.

2. The test compound should be tested up to a dose level showing cytotoxicity of 50%, unless the top dose is based on other criteria (e.g., solubility in the culture medium or it is the standard limit dose).

6.5.3.10 Evaluation of data

The result of the test is assessed using the following criteria:

1. The test is regarded as clearly negative if there are no increases of either statistical or biological significance in the number of micronuclei at any dose compared with concurrent vehicle controls.

2. The test will be regarded as clearly positive if there is an increase in nuclei that is of statistical and biological significance and is above the higher acceptance limit (see historical control data in testing laboratory) and that clearly demonstrates a positive trend.

3. If an increase is seen that is statistically different from the concurrent control but does not fulfill the criteria for a positive result as defined, then further statistical and/or microscopic analyses may be performed. However biological relevance will remain the primary consideration.

6.5.4 Centromeric Labeling

6.5.4.1 FISH using a programmable hotplate such as HYBrite™ or Thermobrite™

Care should be taken at all stages of using the chromosome paints to minimize light exposure because they are photo-degraded.

Slides should be aged for at least 24 h at room temperature prior to centromeric labeling to dehydrate. The procedure is the same for human and mouse probes.

HYBrite™ (a programmable hotplate) is switched on prior to use to allow it to reach 42 °C (approximately 10 min). The slides to be painted are warmed by placing them on the hotplate surface prior to use. An important element of the programmable hotplate method is the humidified atmosphere that is achieved by placing water in the wells of the HYBrite machine. This water must never be allowed to seep onto the hotplate surface or a good contact between the hotplate and slide will not be obtained and the hybridization will fail.

The pan-centromeric paint (Cambio UK) is taken from the freezer to thaw prior to use (at least 15 min).

On each slide, 15–20 μL of mouse or human centromeric chromosome paint is added and a small coverslip is used. The coverslip is then sealed by adding rubber cement (glue) around the edges. When the glue has dried, the slides are placed on the HYBrite™ hotplate. The program has a denaturation step of 69 °C for 5 min, followed by hybridization at 42 °C for between 16 and 40 h.

Prepare 0.4X SSC with 0.3% Tween-20 in a glass Coplin jar and place in the waterbath with water covering approximately three-quarters of the height of the Coplin jar.

Heat to 73 ± 1 °C and allow approximately 1 h to get to temperature. Place 2X SSC 0.1% Tween-20 in a Coplin jar at room temperature.

Check the temperature of the water bath. The temperature of the water bath is the important temperature, not the temperature inside the Coplin jar.

Remove slides from Hybrite, remove glue, and gently slide off the coverslips. Place two slides only, at one time, in the Coplin jar in the water bath, agitate for 3–4 s, and leave in the Coplin jar for 1 min. Do not wash more than two slides at one time because each slide reduces the temperature of the Coplin jar by 1 °C. The water bath should be allowed to get back to temperature for at least 20 min prior to washing additional slides.

Transfer slides to a Coplin jar containing 2X SSC 0.1% Tween-20 for 2 min. Drain the slides (do not allow to dry), add antifade containing DAPI counterstain (Vectasheild™), add large (22 × 40 mm, or 22 × 50 mm) coverslip, place in card tray, and store flat in the dark prior to scoring on a suitable fluorescent microscope.

Allow temperature in the Coplin jar to return to the previous level (approximately 5−10 min) before washing the next two slides.

6.5.4.2 Alterative protocol for FISH

If a HYBrite™ machine is not available, then an alternative method must be used for probe hybridization (as described in "StarFISH™ Catalogue and Protocols," available from Cambio).

Initially, slides are dehydrated via serial ethanol washing in 70%, 70%, 90%, and 90% (v/v) ethanol for 2 min each, followed by 5 min in 100% ethanol.

Then, slides are denatured in prewarmed 70% formamide (70 mL formamide plus 30 mL 2X SSC solution) at 65 °C for 1.5−2 min.

Slides are then quenched in ice-cold 70% (v/v) ethanol for 4 min, followed by subsequent dehydration as described.

The whole chromosome probe, in hybridization buffer, should be warmed to 37 °C and denatured at 65 °C for 10 min.

The pan-centromeric probe in hybridization buffer is denatured at 85 °C for 10 min and then immediately put on ice.

Finally, the probes should be combined in proportions that depend on the probes and their age, applied to the slide, and then allowed to hybridize at 37 °C for approximately 16 h in an air-tight humidified box.

Following hybridization, slides should be washed twice for 5 min in 50% formamide/2X SSC at 37 °C and then twice in 2X SSC for 5 min.

6.5.4.3 Slide checking

Check slides after counterstain and antifade are added to determine the presence of centromeric signals (either red or green) under the microscope in any nucleated cells (blue from DAPI counterstain) to determine that the hybridization has taken place.

6.5.4.4 Slide scoring

Slides are scored using an appropriate fluorescence microscope with triple bandpass filter and individual single filters for CY3 and FITC. Scoring is performed on electronic digital counters. Data are recorded on paper.

One hundred micronuclei should be assessed. In control cultures or low levels of micronuclei induction, this may not be possible so stop scoring at 20,000 cells.

6.5.5 Nondisjunction Assay

6.5.5.1 FISH method

Slides are aged for at least 24 h at room temperature prior to centromeric labeling; alternatively, they may be aged artificially by baking them in an oven at 60 °C for 1 h prior to labeling to provide adequate dehydration.

Methods for FISH are the same as for centromeric labeling. However, concentrated probes are used to allow mixing of two (or three) probes specific to individual chromosomes. For example, a probe for centromere of Chromosome 2 labeled with FITC may be mixed with a probe for the centromere of Chromosome 7 labeled with CY3. The quantities of concentrated probe are approximately 3 μL per individual centromeric paint added to 10−12 μL hybridization buffer mix (supplied with paint and containing deionized formamide). The amounts of probe given are a starting place because batches of probes vary and it may be possible to reduce the amount of probe used. This should be tested on each new batch.

The program used for centromere-specific probes has a denaturation step at 72 °C for 2 min, followed by 16−40 h at 42 °C.

6.5.5.2 Slide checking

Check slides after counterstain and antifade have been added to determine the presence of centromeric signals (both red CY3 and green FITC) under the microscope in any nucleated cells (blue from DAPI counterstain) and to determine that the hybridization has taken place.

6.5.5.3 Slide scoring

One hundred binucleate cells in which all four signals (two for each paint) can be seen are selected for scoring and the distribution of centromeric signals in both nuclei are recorded. Any additional aberrant divisions with the distribution of signals are recorded on paper.

6.6 Flow Cytometric Method

The following section covers aspects of general study design and execution based on regulatory guidelines such as OECD 487 and ICH S2(R1). Depending on the information provided by these guidelines and the requirements of the regulatory bodies to which studies will be submitted, certain aspects of study design will have to be met. It is the responsibility of the user to understand these requirements, determine how they will be achieved, and manage their studies and reporting to ensure alignment with regulatory expectations.

As described, *in vitro* micronucleus formation can be assessed by visual observation using microscopy, but this indicator of chromosomal damage can also be studied using more automated approaches such as flow cytometry [31,32]. The assessment of micronuclei in cultured cells by flow cytometry is similar to manual microscopy in terms of general recommendations for treatment of cells and other guideline-driven requirements, but it differs mainly in how the samples are processed and how the samples are analyzed. Additionally, the cytokinesis block is not required.

The fundamental step to achieve analysis by flow is the liberation of nuclei and micronuclei via cell lysis. This is performed along with fluorescent staining of these two populations so they can be differentiated based on size and nucleic acid content. Analysis of the samples is accomplished via automated sample introduction and instrument software. It should be noted that all plating, processing and analysis of samples can be performed in the same 96-well plate, thus making this approach efficient and high-throughput. The method is also compatible with suspension [33] and attachment cell lines [34,35], and protocols for both are described here.

6.6.1 Equipment

The following is a list of equipment required for the flow cytometric method:

- 37 °C incubator or water bath
- Micropipettes (adjustable, repeating, and positive displacement)
- 8- or 12-channel pipettor
- Pipette aids
- Centrifuge with swinging bucket rotor
- 96-well plate carriers for centrifuge
- 2−8 °C refrigerator
- −10 to −30 °C freezer
- Vortex mixer

(*Continued*)

(Continued)

- Flow cytometer equipped with 488 nm laser and a high-throughput sampler (HTS) capable of working with 96-well plates
- Light source to photoactivate nucleic acid dye A—fluorescent or incandescent; fluorescent is preferred because it is cooler
- 8-channel aspirator manifold (V&P Scientific, cat. no. 180B)
- 8-channel aspirator bridge (V&P Scientific, cat. no. 180S)
- Plate shaker (optional)

© Litron Laboratories.

6.6.2 *Consumables*

The following is a list of consumables required for this method (sterile where appropriate):

- Suspension cell lines L5178Y or TK6; approximate doubling times for these cells is 12—14 h. Additional cell lines are undergoing review, and information can be found in the literature.
- Attachment cell lines V79 or CHO-K1; approximate doubling times for these cells is 12—14 h. Additional cell lines are undergoing review, and information can be found in the literature.
- Flaked/chipped ice
- 15 mL polypropylene centrifuge tubes
- Flow cytometry tubes
- Disposable sterile pipettes, sizes 5, 19, 25, 50 mL
- Heat-inactivated, filter-sterilized fetal bovine serum (FBS)
- 6-micron fluorescent latex microspheres, "counting beads" (Invitrogen cat. no. P14828)
- 96-well plates (U-bottom plates are recommended for suspension cells; flat bottom plates are recommended for attachment cells)

Advance preparation of specific reagents and software templates is advised to facilitate easier sample processing. Label all necessary tubes and plates with sample IDs prior to beginning sample processing.

© Litron Laboratories.

6.6.3 *Reagents and recipes*

As indicated, many of the reagents and materials required for flow cytometric scoring of micronuclei in cultured cells are provided with *In Vitro* MicroFlow® kits available from Litron Laboratories (Rochester, NY). Additional materials and supplies that are required, but not supplied with the kits, are specifically noted in Section 6.

Individual reagents supplied with in vitro MicroFlow kit:

> Incomplete lysis solution 1
> Incomplete lysis solution 2
> Nucleic acid dye A
> Nucleic acid dye B
> RNase solution
> 10X buffer

Solution and Materials Preparation

The following solutions are made fresh daily (with the exception of the cell culture media) under sterile conditions. The volumes provided here are shown as the amounts required for one 96-well plate. Determine the number of samples you plan to process in a single day and scale the volumes accordingly.

1X Buffer Solution

Combine 18 mL deionized water (dH$_2$O) with 2 mL 10X buffer and 0.4 mL FBS. Filter-sterilize and store on ice until ready for use.

Nucleic Acid Dye A Working Solution

Combine 6.5 mL 1x buffer solution with 65 μL nucleic acid dye A. Protect from light and keep on ice.

Complete Lysis Solution 1

Combine 1 mL incomplete lysis solution 1 with 44 μL nucleic acid dye A and 55 μL RNase solution. Protect from light and keep at room temperature until use.

Complete Lysis Solution 2

Combine 11 mL incomplete lysis solution 2 with 44 μL nucleic acid dye B. Protect from light and keep at room temperature until use.

Medium for TK6 cells

Combine RPMI 1640 (Mediatech, Manassas, VA) with 200 mg/mL sodium pyruvate, 2 mM L-glutamine, 50 units/mL penicillin, 50 mg/mL streptomycin, and 10% v/v heat-inactivated horse serum. Store at refrigerated temperatures and warm to 37 °C prior to use.

Medium for CHO-K1 cells

Combine Ham's F12 with L-glutamine (Mediatech, Manassas, VA), 1.5 g/L sodium bicarbonate, 50 units/mL penicillin, 50 mg/mL streptomycin, and 10% v/v heat-inactivated FBS. Store at refrigerated temperatures and warm to 37 °C prior to use.

6.6.4 Suspension Cell Protocol

6.6.4.1 Treatment, preliminary assessments

In general, exposure of cells will be similar for both manual and flow cytometric approaches. Thus, test article—treated cells should be allowed to incubate with compound for the duration of time that is approximately equal to 1.5—2.0 normal cell cycle lengths: cell cycle time for cell lines in the exponential stage of growth is, for all practical purposes, equal to the doubling time. A general starting point recommended for TK6 cells is 20,000 cells per well, with exposure occurring immediately. Depending on the cell line being used, each laboratory should empirically determine the appropriate plating densities for their culture system.

At the time of harvest, it is useful to place the 96-well plate(s) under an inverted microscope and examine the cultures. Through this preliminary assessment, the user may be able to eliminate some overly cytotoxic concentrations from MN scoring. Additionally, in some cases test articles may have precipitated out of solution. Caution should be exercised if wells with precipitate are analyzed because precipitate may interfere with reliable flow cytometric analysis.

6.6.4.2 Cell harvest

1. Remove 96-well plate(s) containing treated cells from the incubator.
2. Collect cells via centrifugation at $300 \times g$ for 5 min.
3. Slowly and carefully aspirate the supernatants. The 8-channel manifold recommended can greatly simplify aspiration steps and ensure consistent and effective removal of supernatants. If this device is not available, then be very careful during aspiration steps to avoid disturbing the cell pellet.
4. Loosen cells by gentle tapping or place plates on a plate shaker. Ensure that the speed is low enough so that the well contents do not spill.
5. Place samples on wet ice for approximately 20 min before continuing to the next section.

6.6.4.3 Complete nucleic acid dye A staining

1. Add 50 μL complete nucleic acid dye A solution to each well. Gently pipette up and down, making sure all cells come into contact with this solution.
2. Place plates on wet ice.
3. Leave the plate cover off and place a light source approximately 6 inches above the plates (see Section 15). With plates on ice, expose the samples to visible light for 30 min.
4. Turn off the visible light source and add 0.15 mL of cold 1X buffer solution to each sample. From this point forward, limit the exposure of samples to light.
5. Collect cells via centrifugation at $300 \times g$ for 5 min.
6. Slowly and carefully aspirate the supernatants (with manifold if available), taking care not to disturb the pellet.
7. Loosen cells by gentle tapping or place plates on a plate shaker. Ensure that the speed is low enough so that the well contents do not spill. Proceed immediately to Section 8.4.

(Continued)

(Continued)

6.6.4.4 Simultaneous cell lysis and nucleic acid dye B staining
1. Add 100 μL complete lysis solution 1 to the first row using a multichannel pipette. Immediately pipette the samples up and down to make sure all cells come into contact with the reagents.
2. Change tips and repeat steps 1 and 2 for all remaining rows.
3. Incubate the samples for 1 h in the dark at 37 °C.
4. Add 100 μL complete lysis solution 2 to the first row using a multichannel pipette. Immediately pipette the samples up and down to make sure all cells come into contact with the reagents.
5. Repeat step 4 for all remaining rows.
6. Incubate the samples for 30 min in the dark at room temperature.
7. Store samples at room temperature and protect from light for up to 24 h before flow cytometric analysis. Use of adhesive film that prevents evaporation should be considered.

© Litron Laboratories.

6.6.5 Attachment Cell Protocol

6.6.5.1 Treatment, preliminary assessments
Test article—treated cells should be allowed to incubate for the duration of time that is approximately equal to 1.5–2.0 normal doubling times. As a generally recommended starting point for an attachment cell line like CHO-K1, an initial plating density of approximately 7500 cells per well followed by a 24-h attachment period and then initiation of exposure are recommended. Depending on the cell line being used, each laboratory should empirically determine the appropriate plating densities for their culture system. At the time of harvest, there is merit to placing the 96-well plate(s) under an inverted microscope. Through this preliminary assessment, it may be possible to eliminate some overly cytotoxic concentrations from MN scoring. Additionally, in some cases test article may have precipitated out of solution. Caution should be exercised if wells with precipitate are analyzed, because precipitate may interfere with reliable flow cytometric analysis.

6.6.5.2 Cell harvest
1. Remove 96-well plate(s) containing treated cells from the incubator.
2. Place plates on wet ice for 20 min.
3. Slowly and carefully aspirate the supernatants. The 8-channel manifold recommended can greatly simplify aspiration steps and ensure consistent and effective removal of supernatants. If this device is not available, then be very careful during aspiration steps to avoid disturbing the cell monolayer. Immediately proceed to Section 9.3.

(Continued)

(Continued)

6.6.5.3 Complete nucleic acid dye A staining
1. Carefully add 50 μL of complete nucleic acid dye A solution to each well. Make sure that the entire cell surface is covered with this solution.
2. Leave the plate cover off and place a light source approximately 6 inches above the plates (see Section 16). With plates on ice, expose the samples to visible light for 30 min.
3. Turn off the visible light source and add 0.15 mL of ice-cold 1X buffer solution to each sample. From this point forward, limit the exposure of samples to light by covering the plate with aluminum foil if not actively working with the samples.
4. Carefully aspirate supernatants. Immediately proceed to Section 9.4.

6.6.5.4 Simultaneous cell lysis and nucleic acid dye B staining
1. Add 100 μL of complete lysis solution 1 to each well. Gently mix the plate for 5 s on a plate shaker set low enough not to splash the solution out of the wells.
2. Incubate the samples for 1 h in the dark at 37 °C.
3. Add counting beads to complete lysis solution 2. Do this by briefly sonicating and vortexing a stock bead suspension, then add approximately one drop of bead suspension per 10 mL of complete lysis solution 2. Mix the bead/lysis solution well after addition of the beads and just prior to use. Protect these solutions from light, and ensure they are at room temperature before adding the solutions to samples.
4. Vortex or resuspend complete lysis solution 2 and add 100 μL to each well. Gently rock the plate.
5. Incubate the samples for 30 min in the dark at room temperature.
6. Store samples at room temperature and protect from light for up to 24 h before flow cytometric analysis. Use of adhesive film that prevents evaporation should be considered.

© Litron Laboratories.

6.6.6 Flow Cytometric Data Acquisition

1. Before analyzing samples, ensure that the flow cytometer is working properly. Follow the manufacturer's instructions for the appropriate setup and quality control procedures. Templates for CellQuest™ Pro and FACSDiva™ users are available from the Litron Laboratories website. Otherwise, users will need to create a template following recommendations found in Section 12. Because these templates are relatively complex, this should be done prior to cell harvest.
2. The plots, hierarchical gating, and statistics shown here were taken from a FACSCanto II running FACSDiva software. These examples will not translate across other machines running different software, but they should provide sufficient information to understand gating and sample analysis.
3. For FACSDiva™ users, an experimental template can be downloaded from the Litron Laboratories website (www.litronlabs.com) that needs to be placed in the appropriate

folder on the flow cytometer computer. Place the .xml file in BDExport > Templates > Experiment > General. When opening the template, go up to the tabs and select "new experiment," go to the general tab, and select the template.

4. For BD-brand HTS systems, we recommend replacing BD-brand sheath solutions with a blood bank saline solution or filtered distilled water. Note that for core facilities or other similar situations in which you do not directly control the instrument, this substitution should be approved by the staff in charge of maintaining the flow cytometer. HTS users should set their loader settings as follows:

Throughput = Standard
Sample flow rate = 0.5 μL/s
Sample volume = 75 μL
Mixing volume = 100 μL
Mixing speed = 100 μL/s
Number of mixes = 2
Wash volume = 400 μL

5. Protect samples from light. Ensure samples have equilibrated to room temperature before data acquisition occurs.

6. The system should be primed at least three times before attempting analysis.

7. Prior to analyzing experimental samples, it is recommended that you analyze negative control and positive control samples first to verify that the template and instrument settings are appropriate.

8. Just prior to analysis, resuspend the cells in all wells via pipetting each well sufficiently to mix. Place the plate on the flow cytometer. Using a negative control well for setup, acquire the sample in the "set-up mode." Adjust FSC and SSC voltages to bring nuclei into view as shown in Plot A (Figure 6.5).

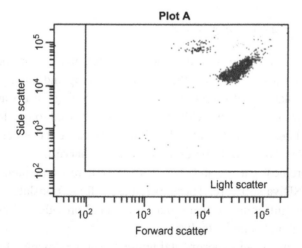

Figure 6.5
Plot A for light scatter.

9. Adjust FL3 PMT voltage (EMA fluorescence) as shown. This should result in nearly a log of fluorescent resolution between nuclei from healthy and dead cells. Representative plots showing EMA staining characteristics are shown in Figure 6.6.

   Locate the nuclei G1 peak in Plot B and adjust the FITC (FL1) PMT voltage until the peak is positioned at a high enough FITC (FL1) channel so that one one-hundredth of this fluorescence signal will still be on scale. It is important to set nuclei high in SYTOX-associated fluorescence because MN with one one-hundredth the intensity of G1 events need to be on scale (see Figure 6.7).

   Additionally, set the threshold parameter (also referred to as the acquisition trigger) to FITC (FL1) fluorescence (i.e., SYTOX Green). Adjust the threshold so that some

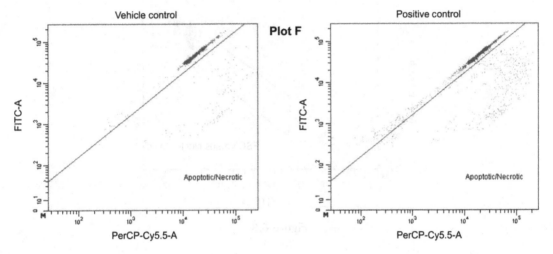

Figure 6.6
Plot F scatter plot for EMA.

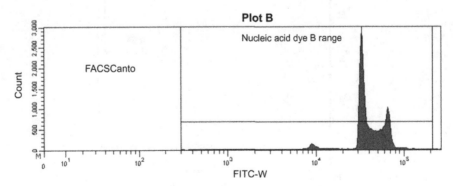

Figure 6.7
Plot B Histogram.

events are collected that fall just to the left edge of the FITC (FL1) range that is defined in Plot B. For those instruments that are capable of thresholding on two parameters, a second parameter (either SSC or FSC) is recommended. Note that when a light scatter secondary threshold is used, it is important not to set the value too high; otherwise, micronuclei will be excluded. Use the lower bounds of the "Light Scatter" region shown in Plot A (Figure 6.5) as a guide.

10. Adjust the position of the "FSC versus SYTOX" region until nuclei are positioned as shown in Plot D in Figure 6.8.

11. Adjust the position of the "SSC versus SYTOX" region until nuclei are positioned as shown in Plot E in Figure 6.9.

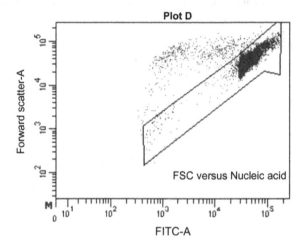

Figure 6.8
Plot D.

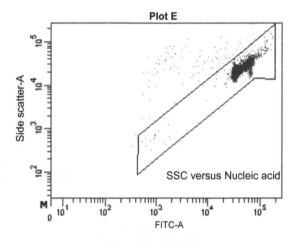

Figure 6.9
Plot E.

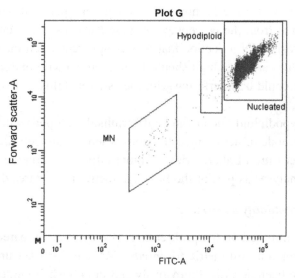

Figure 6.10
Plot G.

12. Ensure that nuclei are within the "Nucleated" region, as shown in Plot G in Figure 6.10.
13. It is preferable that the regions and instrument settings are not changed between experimental samples. This is why it is worth taking some extra time to carefully consider PMT voltage and threshold settings initially.
14. As explained in Section 12, configure collection criteria to store the desired number of events. Note that BD HTS users should include time in their gating logic so that the first several seconds of analysis for each well is omitted from the data files.
15. Acquire data for the plate in its entirety or select the wells you wish to process.

6.6.7 *Flow Cytometric Data Analysis*

1. MN values can be expressed as frequency percent by dividing the number of events that are within the "MN" region by the number of events that are within the "Nucleated" region and multiplying by 100. With properly defined gates, these measurements exclude debris and other spurious events that are identified by their anomalous light scatter profile and/or EMA-positive staining characteristic.
2. SYTOX-positive/EMA-negative Nuclei and Counting Beads are enumerated on a per well basis. By expressing these values as Nuclei-to-Bead ratios, it is possible to derive relative survival (RS) values. The advantage of these RS measurements is that they represent a multiparametric means of evaluating cell health.

3.   The number of EMA-positive events is determined on a per well basis. The health of cells can be inferred from the percentage of these particles. This statistic is particularly sensitive to apoptosis. MN induction that is only apparent when the percentage of EMA-positive values are very high should be interpreted with extreme caution, because overt cytotoxicity could be interfering with the assay's ability to evaluate cytogenetic damage potential.

4.   The number of hypodiploid nuclei can be determined on a per-well basis. This statistic can be useful for mode of action investigations when certain cell lines are used (e.g., CHO-K1). Contact Litron Laboratories for more information on the application of these mode of action analyses as part of the flow cytometric procedures described here.

6.6.7.1 Independent cytotoxicity assessment

Cytotoxicity assessment based on the proliferation of a culture compared to concurrent vehicle controls is often a useful metric for *in vitro* MN studies. Measurements such as RICC or RPD have been described previously and in published guidelines such as OECD 487.

One potential solution for obtaining this type of measurement by flow cytometry is to use a commercially available "absolute counting bead" (Thermo Fisher CountBrite™ Absolute Counting Beads, C36950) to obtain exact cell density values. The counting bead is added at a known concentration to an aliquot of cells taken initially at the time of treatment to determine a starting cell density. Similarly, aliquots from each well can be mixed with the same bead solution to generate cell density values for treated cultures. Comparison of the starting values with those obtained at the time of harvest for MN assessment will yield the desired values for the calculation of the desired proliferation metric.

6.6.7.2 Criteria for a valid assay

For the flow cytometric *in vitro* MN assay in TK6 cells, the criteria for a valid assay include a baseline MN frequency of <1% and a baseline frequency of EMA(+) events of <4%. In addition, the population doubling in the solvent control should be between 1.5 and 2.0 ×. Finally, the negative and positive control MN frequencies should be within the expected distribution as defined by historical data (e.g., within the 90−95% tolerance interval). If these criteria are not met, then the assay should be repeated. Similar criteria may be used for attachment cells such as CHO-K1. Each laboratory should develop its own specific criteria for what comprises a valid assay.

6.6.7.3 Criteria for positive/negative outcomes

Assessment of genotoxicity in the flow cytometric *in vitro* MN assay is primarily based on the level of induction of MN in cultures that are exposed to high enough concentrations of test article to either induce a predefined level of cytotoxicity (e.g., $\geq 45 \pm 5\%$) or reach established limit concentrations based on recommendations in specific guidelines. For those concentrations where appropriate cytotoxicity is achieved, the data should be reviewed for any treatments that resulted in an appreciable increase in MN frequency over the solvent control average (e.g., $\geq$ threefold). If conditions are identified with sufficient MN induction, then these concentrations should be qualified further by confirming that the mean percentage of EMA(+) events are less than fourfold over the solvent control mean. A positive response is also frequently characterized by dose-related induction of MN that achieves values above historical control baseline values (e.g., exceeding 95% tolerance interval).

These criteria are provided as an example of what can be applied to make an assessment of positive or negative genotoxicity. Each laboratory is responsible for generating and interpreting its own historical database and rationally adjusting the MN and EMA(+) cut-off values to appropriately calibrate the assay to meet its assay performance requirements [36,37]. Conducting appropriately designed and executed internal validation studies is an important part of establishing and demonstrating proficiency with the assay.

6.6.8 Creating an Analysis Template

CellQuest™ Pro v5.2 and FACSDiva™ 6.1 template files can be downloaded from the Litron Laboratories website (www.litronlabs.com). This template is used for all the protocols described in this manual, and the following pages show actual screen images of the plots found on the FACSDiva™ template (six bivariate graphs and two histograms). The various gates utilized for these analyses are described here. Flow cytometry operators who are not using BD software should find these pages valuable for constructing their own data acquisition and analysis templates.

1. Create plots and regions as shown here.
2. Define gates based on the following regions. These will be arranged into a hierarchical gating as shown in Figure 6.11.
   Gate no./region(s) that comprise the gate
   "Light scatter" in Plot A
   "Nucleic acid dye B range" in Plot B
   "Apoptotic/necrotic" in Plot F
   "SSC versus nucleic acid dye B" in Plot D
   "FSC versus nucleic acid dye B" in Plot E
   "Beads" in bead plot
   "Time" in time histogram
   "MN," "Nucleated," and "Hypodiploid" (optional) in Plot G
3. Set a stop mode in the FACSDiva software based on the number of events in the healthy nuclei region defined in Plot G. This number is typically set for the nuclei of at least 5000 healthy cells.

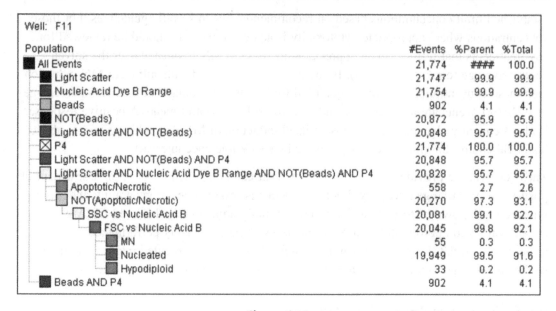

Population	#Events	%Parent	%Total
All Events	21,774	####	100.0
Light Scatter	21,747	99.9	99.9
Nucleic Acid Dye B Range	21,754	99.9	99.9
Beads	902	4.1	4.1
NOT(Beads)	20,872	95.9	95.9
Light Scatter AND NOT(Beads)	20,848	95.7	95.7
P4	21,774	100.0	100.0
Light Scatter AND NOT(Beads) AND P4	20,848	95.7	95.7
Light Scatter AND Nucleic Acid Dye B Range AND NOT(Beads) AND P4	20,828	95.7	95.7
Apoptotic/Necrotic	558	2.7	2.6
NOT(Apoptotic/Necrotic)	20,270	97.3	93.1
SSC vs Nucleic Acid B	20,081	99.1	92.2
FSC vs Nucleic Acid B	20,045	99.8	92.1
MN	55	0.3	0.3
Nucleated	19,949	99.5	91.6
Hypodiploid	33	0.2	0.2
Beads AND P4	902	4.1	4.1

Well: F11

Figure 6.11
Hierarchical gating scheme.

4. Set the storage gate to G9. In conjunction with the time histogram shown, this gating logic excludes the first few seconds of data from each well. This strategy is important for BD-brand HTS users, because fluorescence signals tend to require several seconds before they stabilize.

5. It is important not to be too restrictive with the "light scatter" region because MN could be excluded based on their small size. Therefore, the lower bounds of the region should be approximately 2 logs lower in FSC and SSC than the bottom left edge of the nuclei events, as shown in Figure 6.10.

6. The "nucleic acid dye B range" region should include nuclei as well as sub-$2n$ chromatin that exhibit up to one one-hundredth the nucleic acid dye B fluorescence signal as $2n$ nuclei (Figure 6.7).

7. Much of the chromatin associated with dead/dying cells is above an appropriately located "FSC versus nucleic acid dye B" region (Figure 6.8).

8. Much of the chromatin associated with dead/dying cells is above an appropriately located "SSC versus nucleic acid dye B" region (Figure 6.9).

9. A gate based on an appropriately positioned "apoptotic/necrotic" region is used to exclude the chromatin of dead/dying cells (Figure 6.12).

10. The bead count plot allows for the resolution of the counting beads used for the nuclei-to-bead ratio calculation (Figure 6.13).

11. Only the nuclei of healthy cells, hypodiploid nuclei, and micronuclei that meet the multiple characteristics associated with the hierarchical gating described are used to calculate MN frequency (Figure 6.10).

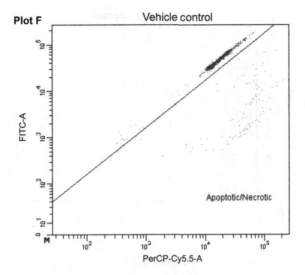

Figure 6.12
Plot F.

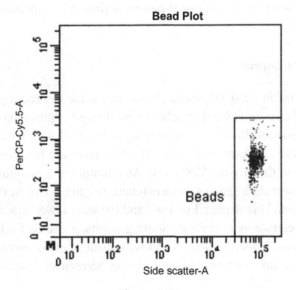

Figure 6.13
Bead plot.

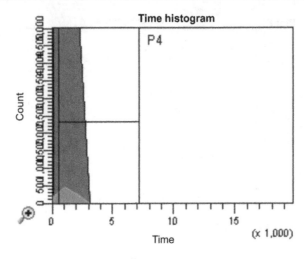

Figure 6.14
Time histogram.

12.   When analyzing 96-well plates using BD-brand HTS equipment, a "time" marker should be set and used in the data acquisition logic so that the first approximately 10 s of data are not saved. Over this initial period of time, FL1 fluorescence is not stable (Figure 6.14).

6.6.9 Example Plate Layout

A typical dose range for *in vitro* MN studies is to start at the desired top concentration and use a half-dilution scheme downward to achieve the desired exposure conditions. One advantage of the plate-based flow cytometric assay is the ease with which one can examine many doses over a large concentration range. This is a rationale for closely spacing test article concentrations in the *in vitro* MN assay. An example of a recommended plate layout that addresses a narrower dose spacing is shown here (Figure 6.15). In this example, the top concentration of test article is depicted as 1×, and the next lower concentration is 0.75×. Using these two concentrations as separate starting points, a one-half dilution scheme skipping every other row is used as shown and will result in good coverage of the dose range. In this case, each concentration is studied in quadruplicate (except for solvent control).

The plate layout that is ultimately used depends on numerous factors specific to each laboratory. In the case of screening studies, a laboratory may perform single well treatments and cover many concentrations and several compounds per plate. In the case of a more definitive study, three to four replicates per condition and only one compound with concurrent positive and negative controls at several concentrations may be examined.

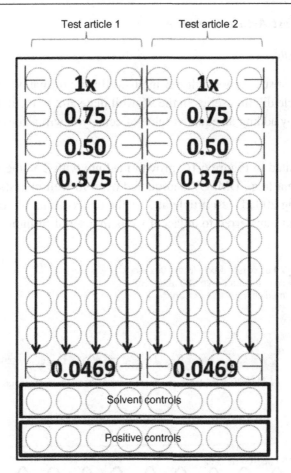

Figure 6.15
Sample plate layout.

6.6.10 *Example Results Table*

See Table 6.5. Based on the data obtained from the flow cytometer, similar tables can be generated and used to obtain information on endpoints such as fold increase in MN from baseline and percentage of relative nuclei.

Table 6.5: Example Results Table

Specimen Name	Well Name	Concentration (μg/mL)	#Beads	Apoptotic/ Necrotic (%)	Nucleated #Events	MN #Events	MN (%)	EMA (%)	Nuclei: Bead	MN Fold	EMA fold	RNC (%)
MMS	E11	100.0	1447	11	10000	293	2.93	11	6.91	4.12	3.46	46.72
MMS	E12	50.0	895	4.1	10000	110	1.10	4.1	11.17	1.55	1.29	75.54
DMSO	G11	0.0	711	3.2	10000	57	0.57	3.2	14.06	0.80	1.01	95.08
DMSO	G12	0.0	859	3.1	12000	100	0.83	3.1	13.97	1.17	0.98	94.44

6.6.11 Advice for Test Article Exposure

6.6.11.1 Suspension cells

To most efficiently treat suspension cultures in 96-well plate format, we suggest first preparing the test article dilution series in the 96-well plate at 2 × the desired final concentration. Then, by adding an equal volume of cells, you will achieve the desired final concentrations.

In the example illustrated in Figure 6.16, growth medium with 2 × the desired final concentration of solvent (e.g., DMSO) is aliquoted over 96-well plates(s) at 100 μL/well. From a well containing 200 μL test article at 2 × the desired final top concentration, 100 μL is removed and transferred to adjacent wells in a serial fashion. The last

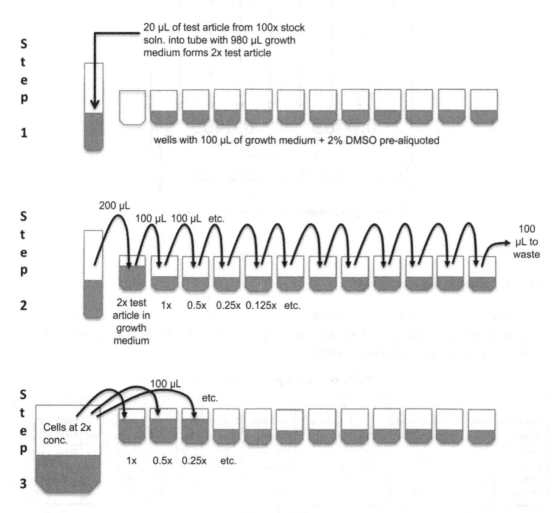

Figure 6.16
Plating and treatment scheme for suspension cells.

concentration requires 100 µL to be removed and discarded. When an equal volume of cells is added to each well, the desired final concentration of test article is achieved. Following this dilution scheme will achieve a "broader" dose range than the one described in the example plate layout.

6.6.11.2 Attachment cells

To most efficiently treat attachment cultures in a 96-well plate format, we suggest first allowing cells to attach overnight. On the day of treatment, prepare the test article in growth medium at the desired final top concentration. Then, by performing serial dilutions, the desired final concentration is achieved. See example in Figure 6.17.

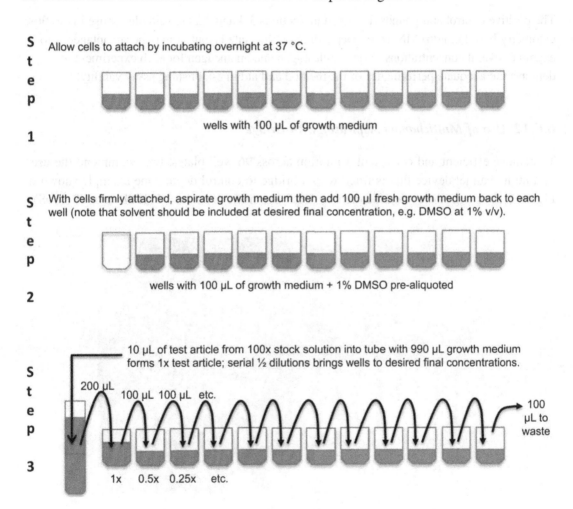

Figure 6.17
Plating and treatment scheme for attachment cells.

6.6.11.3 *Metabolic activation*

Compounds that require bioactivation can be investigated via the application of an exogenous metabolic system such as rat liver S9. Typically, this is accomplished with a short-term treatment of 4 h in the presence of S9, followed by washout of the treatment medium, replacement with fresh medium, and incubation for an additional period of time to achieve the desired 1.5–2 population doublings. S9 mix can be quite toxic, so it is recommended to not exceed 3% during treatment. Exact conditions for various cell types and experimental designs should be determined empirically by each laboratory.

6.6.11.4 *Positive controls*

The positive control compounds described in Sections 3.4 and 3.5 are suitable for use in the flow cytometry-based *in vitro* MN assay. Depending on the plate layout, it may be advantageous to examine several concentrations of both a clastogen and an aneugen for each experiment to demonstrate adequate performance of the method and aid in establishing assay validity.

6.6.12 *Use of Multichannel Aspirator with Bridge*

To achieve efficient and consistent aspiration across 96-well plates, we recommend the use of a multichannel device that is fitted with a bridge to control depth. One example shown in Figure 6.18 is a product manufactured by V&P Scientific (cat. no. VP 180B and VP 180S).

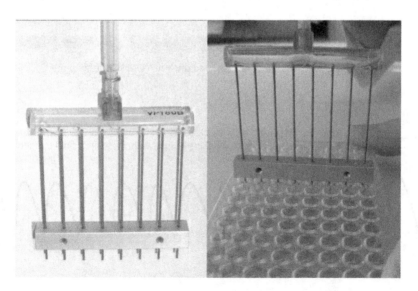

Figure 6.18

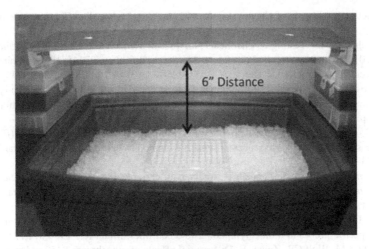

Figure 6.19

6.6.13 Plate Placement During Nucleic Acid Dye B Photoactivation

See Figure 6.19.

6.6.14 Updates and Future Work

Litron Laboratories continues to investigate the application of our flow cytometric *in vitro* micronucleus detection method, so please refer to our website www.litronlabs.com for any additional updates or modifications to the method that occurred after publication of this book. Current studies are investigating the benefits of additional biomarkers associated with DNA damage to assess mode of action to enhance the assessment of genotoxicity using the *in vitro* micronucleus assay.

References

[1] Evans HJ, Neary CJ, Williamson FS. The relative biological efficiency of single doses of fast neutrons and gamma rays on *Vicia faba* roots and the effect of oxygen, Part II. Chromosome damage: the production of micronuclei. Int Jnl Rad Biol 1959;3:216–29.

[2] Klein G, Klein E. The viability and the average desoxypentosenucleic acid content of micronuclei-containing cells produced by colchicine treatment in the Ehrlich ascites tumor. Cancer Res 1952;12:484–9.

[3] Matter B, Schmid W. Trenimon-induced chromosomal damage in bone-marrow cells of six mammalian species, evaluated by the micronucleus test. Mutat Res 1971;12:417–25.

[4] Heddle JA. A rapid *in vivo* test for chromosomal damage. Mutat Res 1973;18:187–90.

[5] Countryman PI, Heddle JA. The production of micronuclei from chromosome aberrations in irradiated cultures of human lymphocytes. Mutation Res 1976;41:321–32.

[6] Fenech M, Morley AA. Measurement of micronuclei in lymphocytes. Mutat Res 1985;147:29–36.

[7] Carter SB. Effects of cytochalasins on mammalian cells. Nature 1967;213(5073):261–4.

[8] OECD Guideline for Testing of Chemicals. No. 473: *In Vitro* Mammalian Chromosome Aberration Test; 1997.

[9] OECD Guideline for the Testing of Chemicals No. 487: *In Vitro* Mammalian Cell Micronucleus Test 26 September 2014, <http://www.oecd-ilibrary.org/docserver/download/9714561e.pdf?expires = 1418124182 &id = id&accname = guest&checksum = 8CD943AC6BC1A014AD28C9EA8E36AA11>.

[10] Migliore L, Bocciardi R, Macri C, Lo Jacono F. Cytogenetic damage induced in human lymphocytes by four vanadium compounds and micronucleus analysis by fluorescence in situ hybridization with a centromeric probe. Mutat Res 1993;319:205−13.

[11] Marshall RR, Murphy M, Kirkland DJ, Bentley KS. Fluorescence *in situ* hybridization (FISH) with chromosome-specific centromeric probes: a sensitive method to detect aneuploidy. Mutat Res 1996;372:233−45.

[12] Zijno P, Leopardi F, Marcon R, Crebelli R. Analysis of chromosome segregation by means of fluorescence *in situ* hybridization: application to cytokinesis-blocked human lymphocytes. Mutat Res 1996;372:211−19.

[13] Doherty AT, Ellard S, Parry EM, Parry JM. A study of aneugenic activity of trichlorofon detected by centromere-specific probes in human lymphoblastoid cell lines. Mutat Res 1996;372:221−31.

[14] Ong T, Mukhtar M, Wolf CR, Zeiger E. Differential effects of cytochrome P450-inducers on promutagen activation capabilities and enzymatic activities of S-9 from rat liver. J Environ Pathol Toxicol 1980;4:55−65.

[15] Elliott BM, Combes RD, Elcombe CR, Gatehouse DG, Gibson GG, Mackay JM, et al. Alternatives to Aroclor 1254-induced S9 in *in-vitro* genotoxicity assays. Mutagenesis 1992;7:175−7.

[16] Fellows MD, O'Donovan M, Lorge E, Kirkland D. Comparison of different methods for an accurate assessment of cytotoxicity in the in vitro micronucleus test. II. Practical aspects with toxic agents. Mutat Res 2008;655:4−21.

[17] Lorge E, Hayashi M, Albertini S, Kirkland D. Comparison of different methods for an accurate assessment of cytotoxicity in the in vitro micronucleus test. Theoretical aspects. Mutat Res 2008;655:1−3.

[18] Hozier J, Sawyer J, Moore M, Howard B, Clive D. Cytogenetic analysis of the L5178Y/TK$^{+/-}$ mouse lymphoma mutagenesis assay system. Mutat Res 1998;84:169−81.

[19] Varga D, Johannes T, Jainta S, Suchuster S, Schwarz-Boeger U, Kiechle M, et al. An automated scoring procedure for the micronucleus test. Mutagenesis 2004;19:391−7.

[20] Schunck C, Johannes T, Varga D, Lörch T, Plesch A. New developments in automated cytogenetic imaging: unattended scoring of dicentric chromosomes, micronuclei, single cell gel electrophoresis, and fluorescence signals. Cytogenet Genome Res 2004;104:383−9.

[21] Lorge E, Thybaud V, Aardema MJ, Oliver J, Wakata A, Lorenzon G, et al. SFTG International collaborative study on in vitro micronucleus test. I. General conditions of the study. Mutation Res 2006;607:13−36.

[22] Clare G, Lorenzon G, Akhurst LC, Marzin D, van Delft J, Montero R, et al. SFTG International collaborative study on the in vitro micronucleus test. II. Using human lymphocytes. Mutation Res 2006;607:37−60.

[23] Miller B, Potter-Locher F, Seelbach A, Stopper H, Utesch D, Madle S. Evaluation of the in vitro micronucleus test as an alternative to the in vitro chromosomal aberration assay: position of the GUM Working Group on the in vitro micronucleus test. Gesellschaft fur Umwelt-Mutations-forschung. Mutation Res 1998;410:81−116.

[24] Bonassi S, Fenech M, Lando C, Lin YP, Ceppi M, Chang WP, et al. Human MicroNucleus Project: international database comparison for results with the cytokinesis-block micronucleus assay in human lymphocytes. I. Effect of laboratory protocol, scoring criteria and host factors on the frequency of micronuclei. Environ Mol Mutagen 2001;37:31−45.

[25] Ellard S, Parry EM. A modified protocol for the cytochalasin B in vitro micronucleus assay using whole human blood or separated lymphocyte cultures. Mutagenesis 1993;4:317−20.

[26] Fenech M. Cytokinesis-block micronucleus cytome assay. Nat Protoc 2007;2:1084−104.

[27] Fenech M. The in vitro micronucleus technique. Mutat Res 2000;455:81−95.

[28] Hoffman WP, Garriott ML, Lee C. *In vitro* micronucleus test. In: Chow S, editor. Encyclopedia of biopharmaceutical statistics. New York, NY: Marcel Dekker, Inc; 2003, p. 463−7.

[29] Garriott ML, Phelps JB, Hoffman WP. A protocol for the in vitro micronucleus test I. Contributions to the development of a protocol suitable for regulatory submissions from an examination of 16 chemicals with different mechanisms of action and different levels of activity. Mutat Res 2002;517:123−34.

[30] Kirsch-Volders M, Sofuni T, Aardema M, Albertini S, Eastmond D, Fenech M, et al. Report of the in vitro micronucleus assay working group. Mutat Res 2003;540:153−63.

[31] Avlasevich S, Bryce SM, Cairns SE, Dertinger SD. In vitro micronucleus scoring by flow cytometry: differential staining of micronuclei versus apoptotic and necrotic chromatin enhances assay reliability. Environ Molec Mutagen 2006;47:56−66.

[32] Avlasevich S, Bryce S, De Boeck M, Elhajouji A, Van Goethem F, Lynch A, et al. Flow cytometric analysis of micronuclei in mammalian cell cultures: past, present and future. Mutagenesis. 2011;26 (1):147−52.

[33] Bryce SM, Avlasevich SL, Bemis JC, Tate M, Walmsley RM, Saad F, et al. Flow cytometric 96-well microplate-based in vitro micronucleus assay with human TK6 cells: protocol optimization and transferability assessment. Environ Mol Mutagen 2013;54(3):180−94.

[34] Bryce SM, Avlasevich SL, Bemis JC, Dertinger SD. Miniaturized flow cytometry-based CHO-K1 micronucleus assay discriminates aneugenic and clastogenic modes of action. Environ Mol Mutagen 2011;52(4):280−6.

[35] Bryce SM, Shi J, Nicolette J, Diehl M, Sonders P, Avlasevich S, et al. High content flow cytometric micronucleus scoring method is applicable to attachment cell lines. Environ Mol Mutagen 2010;51 (3):260−6.

[36] Shi J, Bezabhie R, Szkudlinksa A. Further evaluation of a flow cytometric in vitro micronucleus assay in CHO-K1 cells: a reliable platform that detects micronuclei and discriminates apoptotic bodies. Mutagenesis 2010;25:33−40.

[37] Thougaard AV, Christiansen J, Mow T, Hornberg JJ. Validation of a high throughput flow cytometric in vitro micronucleus assay including assessment of metabolic activation in TK6 cells. Environ Mol Mutagen 2014;55(9):704−18.

The In Vitro Chromosome Aberration Test

Marilyn Registre[1] and Ray Proudlock[2]

[1]Department of Genetic Toxicology, Charles River Laboratories Montreal ULC, Canada
[2]Boone, North Carolina, USA

Chapter Outline

7.1 Introduction   208
7.2 History   209
7.3 Fundamentals   211
7.4 Equipment   212
7.5 Consumables and Reagents   214
7.6 Reagents and Recipes   215
  7.6.1 Colcemid 10 µg/mL in PBS   216
  7.6.2 Fix   216
  7.6.3 F-12 Complete   216
  7.6.4 Freezing Medium 10% (CHO Cells)   216
  7.6.5 Hypotonic Solution (0.075 M KCl)   217
  7.6.6 Heparin Sodium 1000 U/mL   217
  7.6.7 G6P 1 M: Glucose-6-Phosphate   217
  7.6.8 KMg   217
  7.6.9 NADP 0.1 M   217
  7.6.10 PHA M Form (Phytohemagglutinin)   217
  7.6.11 Phosphate Buffer 0.2 M, pH 7.4   218
  7.6.12 Positive Control Solutions   218
  7.6.13 RPMI Complete   218
  7.6.14 S9 Fraction   218
  7.6.15 S9 Mix   219
7.7 Phases in Development of the Test   219
7.8 Cell Characterization   221
  7.8.1 Modal Chromosome Number   222
  7.8.2 Mycoplasma   224
  7.8.3 Cell-Cycle Time   224
7.9 Routine Testing   225
  7.9.1 General Considerations   225
  7.9.2 Dose Regimens   225
  7.9.3 Metabolic Activation System   226
  7.9.4 Test Substance Considerations   226
  7.9.5 Vehicle Selection and Dose Volume   227

Genetic Toxicology Testing.
DOI: http://dx.doi.org/10.1016/B978-0-12-800764-8.00007-0
© 2016 Elsevier Inc. All rights reserved.

7.9.6 Dose Level Selection   227
7.9.7 Positive Controls   230
7.10 Standard Test Procedures   230
7.10.1 Experimental Design Spreadsheet   231
    7.10.1.1 CHO cells: routine maintenance   231
7.10.2 CHO Cells: Test Procedures   233
7.10.3 HPBL Test Procedures   238
7.10.4 Slide Staining: All Cell Types   241
7.10.5 Selection of Slides for Detailed Examination   242
    7.10.5.1 Cell lines   242
    7.10.5.2 HPBL selection of slides for provisional detailed examination   243
7.10.6 Slide Coding   243
7.10.7 Preliminary Slide Reading   243
7.10.8 Slide Scoring   244
    7.10.8.1 Basics   244
    7.10.8.2 Understanding the normal karyotype   245
    7.10.8.3 Routine scoring   247
    7.10.8.4 Classification   248
7.11 Interpretation of Results   253
7.11.1 Evaluation of Toxicity   253
7.11.2 Validity of the Study   253
7.11.3 Criteria for Negative/Positive/Equivocal Outcome   253
7.11.4 Interpretation of Numerical Aberrations   257
7.11.5 Unexpected and Borderline Results   257
7.11.6 Follow-up *In Vivo* Testing   257
7.11.7 Reporting   258
    7.11.7.1 Results tables   260
7.11.8 Historical Control Results   262
7.11.9 Testing of Volatile and Gaseous Compounds   262
7.12 Screening Versions of the Test   263
7.13 Automation   264
References   264

7.1 Introduction

The chromosome aberration test involves treatment of mammalian cells in culture with the test substance in the absence and in the presence of an exogenous metabolic system (S9 mix). Double-stranded DNA damage can be induced directly or, in the case of most genotoxins, indirectly as a result of errors in replication or repair of DNA lesions, leading to double-strand breaks (DSB), which are the major cause of structural chromosome aberrations [1]. Many aberrations are lethal or lost during subsequent cell divisions, so they are best observed at the first metaphase after induction. Various cultured cell lines (including CHL and CHO) can be used to test for chemical induction of DNA damage and are suitable for regulatory testing. However, cell lines are genetically unstable and tend to lose and gain chromosomes or parts of chromosomes spontaneously, so they show a higher and more variable spontaneous rate of chromosome aberrations compared with primary diploid cell cultures such as mitogen-stimulated lymphocytes. Therefore, some laboratories prefer to use primary lymphocytes for routine testing, although these have their own practical drawbacks in terms of ease of culturing, assessment of toxicity, and slide reading (Chinese hamster cell lines have fewer and larger chromosomes than human lymphocytes). This chapter focuses on the description of the two most widely used systems: those using Chinese hamster fibroblast cell lines and those using human peripheral blood lymphocyte (HPBL) cultures, in which lymphocytes are stimulated into division using phytohemagglutinin (PHA). For the lymphocyte culture system, many laboratories use a density gradient technique to separate white blood cells from erythrocytes prior to culture; however, we describe the whole-blood technique here because it is simpler and provides a high yield of mitotic cells.

In all systems, cells are arrested at metaphase (when chromosome morphology is clearest) using colchicine or colcemid, swollen in hypotonic solution, and then fixed before being dropped onto slides, air-dried, and then stained. In this way the chromosomes of metaphase cells are well-spread in a single plane and show clear morphology. Chromosome breakage is evident in the form of various structural aberrations that are scored using high-resolution light microscopy. Increases in the proportion of aberrant metaphase cells (i.e., those showing at least one chromosome aberration) as a result of treatment are indicative of genotoxicity. In routine experiments, cells are treated with the test agent using short (3−6 h) and long exposure times (equal to 1.5 cell-cycle times). Because cell lines and lymphocytes have limited ability to metabolize xenobiotics, cultures are treated in the absence and presence of an exogenous metabolic activation system, usually S9 mix, which consists of a chemically induced rat liver S9 fraction with appropriate cofactors. Treatment in the presence of S9 is performed using only the short exposure period because S9 is somewhat toxic and rapidly loses metabolic activity after addition to the test system.

The main endpoints scored in the test are gross (i.e., observable with standard staining methods) structural aberrations. Polyploidy and any evidence of other forms of aneuploidy are recorded as incidental observations, but increases in these are not necessarily considered indicative of genotoxicity. More subtle chromosomal aberrations including translocations between chromosomes or rearrangements within a chromosome can also occur as a result of treatment with genotoxic agents, but these generally need special staining methods and/or more lengthy analysis to be recognized and therefore are not scored routinely.

7.2 History

Structural and numerical aberrations are associated with adverse health effects, including congenital abnormalities and neoplasia, and approximately 50% of human miscarriages show chromosomal abnormalities [2]. It has been known for more than a century that chromosome aberrations can be used as a marker of exposure for both radiation and genotoxic chemicals. Early cytogenetic studies studied the effect of radiation in various meiotic and somatic tissues with limited success because of the poor quality of the preparations. Progress in the field included examination of giant salivary gland chromosomes in the F1 generation of *Drosophila* as described by the Nobel prize winner Hermann Muller in the 1920s [3]. Later, aberrations were noted at anaphase in plant root tip squash preparations soon after exposure [4], as described in reviews of the theory and history of the test by Kirkland [5] and Natarajan [2].

In the 1950s and 1960s, various technical improvements made examination of chemically induced aberrations in mammalian cells feasible. In particular, use of colchicine to accumulate cells in metaphase, hypotonic treatment to spread chromosomes, and fixation of cells in suspension were described by Ford and Hamerton in 1956 [6], while a modified method involving air-drying of fixed preparations further enhanced preservation of chromosome morphology [7]. Plant lectins including PHA were found to stimulate lymphocyte division in cultures, allowing chromosome analysis of a large number of diploid cells from human donors after simple and minor invasive sampling of peripheral blood [8]; a combination of these techniques was used to demonstrate the clastogenic (chromosome-breaking) effect of the cross-linking agent mitomycin C (MMC) in dividing lymphocytes [9,10]. Sources of exogenous metabolic activation were introduced in later studies using CHO cells to evaluate indirect acting carcinogens [11,12]. These improved methodologies enable the assay to be used in various screening studies on chemical mutagens or carcinogens in the environment, as well as food additives [11,13−18]. In approximately 1990, many laboratories, particularly in Japan, moved from using CHO to CHL cells because the latter seemed to show increased sensitivity [19] and the background rate of aberrations in some CHO cell lines was unstable. Both CHO and CHL are similar transformed Chinese hamster fibroblast cell lines, so it seems that differences in sensitivity were probably due to procedural differences; however, some CHO sublines were found to be unstable in terms of rates of aberration [5,20,21]. These points emphasize the importance of obtaining cell lines from a reliable laboratory and then ensuring they are pure and appropriately characterized before using them for testing.

More recently, many works have been published proposing standard protocols for the test [22−25], including the original (1983) OECD guidelines for the test. However, discussions continued concerning the appropriate cell type, harvest times, limits of toxicity, and indirect effects resulting from departures from physiological conditions in terms of pH and osmolality [18,26a,b,−29]. In 1994, an International Workshop on Genotoxicity Testing working group discussed various previously unresolved or controversial aspects of the study design/evaluation aspects of the then current OECD test guidelines, including metabolic activation, exposure concentrations, number of replicates, treatment and harvest times, analysis/evaluation of results, and repeat testing [30], and reached a consensus on most of these items. Important points raised by the group included the poor reproducibility of toxicity between testing occasions and the need to delay the main sampling until approximately 1.5 cell cycles after exposure because of the cytostatic (cycle delaying) effects of clastogens at higher dose levels. In the 2000s, there was a growing concern over the lack of specificity of the mammalian cell tests in general following a series of publications that addressed the assay's performance in terms of discriminating rodent carcinogens and noncarcinogens and apparent oversensitivity. In particular, oversensitivity could be explained by much higher and more toxic concentrations being used in the *in vitro* systems than could be realistically achieved in the *in vivo* situation [31−33], which was a key point in the discussion of how to determine the relevance of *in vitro* findings to human health [34]. In an attempt to reduce these "misleading" positive results, and to allow conditions that would still maintain the element of hazard identification, new upper limits have recently been set by ICH and OECD in the two documents most often cited in justification of chromosome aberration test studies designed for regulatory submission [35,36]. At the same time, the parallel OECD test guidelines for the *in vitro* micronucleus test were similarly updated [37].

7.3 Fundamentals

Treatment of cells with DNA-damaging agents (*in vitro* or *in vivo*) can result in unrepairable lesions in both strands of DNA. This leads to chromosome breakage that can be seen on microscopic examination of metaphase preparations (Figure 7.1).

In the *in vitro* test, cultures of established mammalian cell lines or primary cultures of human or rodent cells are grown before addition of the test substance to three sets of cultures. An exogenous metabolic activation system (S9) is added to one set of cultures at the same time as the test substance. One set of cultures without S9 and one with S9 are washed free of the test substance 3−6 h later. All cultures are then incubated for a total period equivalent to 1.5 cell cycles after initiation of treatment. The third set of cultures is treated in the absence of S9 only for a continuous period equivalent to 1.5 cell cycles. About two hours prior to harvesting, all three sets of cultures are treated with an agent that arrests cells in the metaphase stage of cell division (e.g., colcemid or colchicine) when the structure of the chromosomes is most clear. The most commonly used primary cells are human peripheral blood lymphocytes (HPBL), which, like other lymphocytes, must be exposed to a plant lectin/mitogen and cultured for approximately 48 h before they are actively dividing and most sensitive to DNA-damaging agents.

The cells are then harvested, separated by centrifugation, and resuspended in hypotonic potassium chloride solution. This causes the cells to swell and enhances eventual separation of the chromosomes to facilitate analysis. The cells are fixed and washed in a mixture of methanol and acetic acid and then dropped onto glass microscope slides. Slides are stained (typically with Giemsa), mounted with coverslips, and examined by light microscopy.

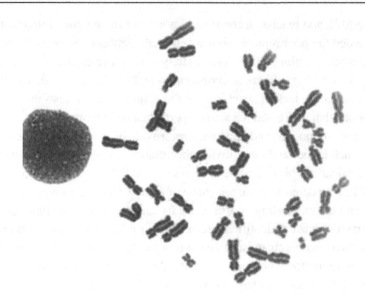

Figure 7.1
Human lymphocyte in metaphase showing a chromosome break with fragment.

The various types of structural chromosome aberration observed are tabulated; however, these all result from chromosome breakage. The main parameter used to assess genotoxicity is the percentage of cells showing structural aberrations. Apparent gaps in chromatid or chromosome structure are also observed occasionally; these are recorded but are not included in assessment of genotoxicity because they do not necessarily involve chromosome breakage.

High-quality metaphase preparations, a trained and experienced observer who is familiar with the karyotype, together with appropriate acceptance, and evaluation criteria are essential for producing reliable results [38].

A test substance formulation that causes a substantial increase in the proportion of metaphases showing chromosome aberrations is regarded as clastogenic and therefore genotoxic.

7.4 Equipment

The following is a list of specialized equipment expected to be found in a laboratory performing tests on a routine basis:

1. Autoclave
2. Binocular light microscope with high-quality, flat-field achromatic optics and parfocal objectives: medium-power plan objective (16× or similar) and high-power oil-immersion

(100✕). The oil immersion lens should be plan apochromat (Planapo), although plan fluorite may be preferred if the microscope will also be used for fluorescence work. Investment in a high-quality microscope is critical to facilitate accurate assessment of chromosome damage and minimize operator fatigue. Most good modern microscopes use infinity-corrected extra-low dispersion glass lenses and Köhler illumination to optimize image quality. If you have a limited budget, then consider buying a second-hand microscope, because a good microscope will last a lifetime if properly cared for; in this case, ensure the lenses are not damaged (scratched or with deterioration of the cement between components of compound lenses). Carl Zeiss Axio Scope, Leica DM, Nikon Labophot II, and Olympus BX all have good reputations and are, arguably, the only makes worth considering

3. Vibration-proof bench for the microscope
4. Biological containment cabinet class II (externally vented)
5. Büchner funnel and Büchner vacuum flask with adapter ring (with clamp stand) connected to an aspirator or vacuum pump via vacuum tubing for vacuum filtration of diluted Giemsa stain
6. Cell maintenance log[1]
7. Centrifuge—bench-top, low-speed swing-out with adapters for 15 mL tubes. The speeds of centrifugation indicated in this chapter are for guidance and may need adjusting depending on the particular centrifuge rotor.
8. CO_2 incubator with gas supply
9. Electronic cell counter,[1] such as a Coulter counter; other electronic cell counting systems may also be suitable and much less expensive, such as Millipore Scepter™ 2.0
10. Fume hood/cupboard
11. General laboratory equipment: balances, glassware refrigerator, purified water, timer, pipette aids, and others
12. Hemocytometer with coverslips
13. Inverted microscope[1]
14. Liquid nitrogen cell storage system[1]
15. Micropipettes (adjustable, repeating, and positive displacement types; range 2–1000 μL)
16. Microscope slides with a frosted end. Plain slides can be used if an automated slide labeling/etching system is available
17. Pump for aspirations, with receiving flask/bottle
18. Racks for culture tubes
19. Slide storage system for archiving slides—cardboard systems are most economical and least liable to damage the slides

---

[1] Mainly for use with cell lines.

20. Stainless steel slide racks and staining dishes—cleaned by washing in 50% acetic acid and then dried before each use
21. Two-channel bench-top tally counter, such as Denominator-type or electronic
22. Vortex mixer
23. Waterbath

7.5 Consumables and Reagents

Consumables typically used in a testing laboratory (sterile where appropriate) include:

1. Blood collection tubes with sodium heparin[2]
2. Centrifuge tubes, 15 and 50 mL polypropylene with caps
3. Colchicine or colcemid
4. Coverslips, 22×50 mm
5. Culture medium. RPMI 1640 is used for lymphocytes and is available commercially in various forms: powder, $10\times$ and $1\times$ liquid, and as an autoclavable solution. The $1\times$ liquid can usually be used as is, but other forms will need supplementing with sodium bicarbonate and/or glutamate if these are not already present. Some forms of RPMI (Dutch modification) include HEPES as a buffering agent, but this tends to be inhibitory and is best avoided. (Ham's) F-12 medium is used for CHO cells
6. Culture vessels: 25 and 75 cm^2 vented flasks (used for adhesive cell lines)[3]; vials, tubes, or plates as appropriate, such as 4 mL clear, glass, flat-bottom, screw cap vials or flat-sided culture tubes (Nunc or equivalent) for 1 and 5 mL blood cultures, respectively[2]
7. Dulbecco's phosphate-buffered saline (DPBS) without calcium or magnesium[3]
8. Fetal calf serum (FCS)/fetal bovine serum (FBS)
9. Filter papers, Whatman No. 1 to fit Büchner funnel (or cotton wool)
10. Filters units, 0.2 or 0.22 μm Luer-Lok syringe-fitting for aqueous solutions and solvents, such as Millex®
11. Fix—3 volumes methanol:1 volume glacial acetic (ethanoic) acid prepared just before each use
12. Gentamicin, aqueous 10 mg/mL (commercially available)
13. Hypotonic—0.075 M potassium chloride
14. Immersion oil for microscopy
15. Isoton II diluent for cell counting with the Coulter counter[3]
16. Labels, self-adhesive printed with code number—code numbers can be generated in Excel using the random function and then printed onto sheets of adhesive labels with

[2] HPBL.
[3] For attached cell lines including CHO.

an appropriate number of replicate labels per culture. The slide code should be printed and saved electronically to decode results later.

17. Medical wipes, such as Kimwipes
18. Microcentrifuge tubes
19. Micropipette tips, sterile
20. Pasteur pipettes—the polypropylene ones are most convenient
21. Phosphate buffer, 0.2 M, pH 7.4
22. Pipettes, sterile plastic disposable
23. Positive control agents
24. Purified water
25. Results sheets/forms
26. S9 fraction and cofactors
27. Slide mountant (Cytoseal, DPX, Permount, or similar permanent nonaqueous type)
28. Slide trays, cardboard
29. Solvents including appropriate anhydrous organic solvents; DMSO in particular is hygroscopic and can develop mutagenic impurities in the presence of small amounts of water. Pure organic solvents should be maintained in an anhydrous condition by addition of a small quantity of a compatible predried molecular sieve (type 4A in the case of DMSO) and stored well-sealed over anhydrous silica gel.
30. Stain, Giemsa solution in methanol/glycerol (see recipe in the rodent micronucleus chapter). Giemsa stain Gurr solution can also be purchased from VWR and Fisher.
31. Syringes, disposable
32. Trypan blue, 0.4% solution in DPBS
33. Trypsin 0.25% in DPBS (with or without 1 mM EDTA)[3]

Gas syringes or metering equipment, 24 mL glass anaerobic culture tubes (Bellco Glass), gas-impermeable injectable butyl rubber septum, gas bags, sealable vials, and other specialist equipment or components will be needed to test gases.

See the next section (Reagents and Recipes) for additional components and reagents that may be needed.

7.6 Reagents and Recipes

The following reagents may be purchased from commercial suppliers such as Sigma-Aldrich, Moltox, or manufactured in-house, in which case we suggest that each recipe should be prepared using a form (an appendix to the standard operating procedure) so that appropriate details including supplier, batch number, and amounts of components can be maintained. It is convenient to create a template for each class of reagent (e.g., solution, medium, etc.).

In the following recipes, water refers to deionized reverse-osmosis purified water; other forms of purified water including distilled water may be used. Volumes of each component mentioned should be adjusted in proportion to the total volume of reagent required. Filter-sterilization normally involves the use of a 0.22 μm filter. Reagents should be labeled with identity, preparation date (or batch number), and expiry date.

Expiry dates are based on the date of preparation and should take into account the expiry dates of individual components. Expiry dates can be extended provided that results are available in the laboratory to prove the reagent is still fit for its purposes.

7.6.1 Colcemid 10 μg/mL in PBS

Colcemid 10 μg/mL in PBS is available commercial and is used to arrest cells in metaphase. Colchicine 12.5 μg/mL may also provide satisfactory results.

7.6.2 Fix

Add 750 mL of methanol to a measuring cylinder. Make up to 1 L with glacial acetic acid. Transfer to an appropriate container, seal, and mix by hand. Store at room temperature and use on the day of preparation.

7.6.3 F-12 Complete

This medium is used for culturing the CHO cells. Note that Eagle's minimum essential medium is also often used for CHL cells (e.g., [19]).

Completely thaw 100 mL of FCS in a 37°C waterbath and then mix by swirling or inversion. Add the serum and 5 mL gentamicin 10 mg/mL to 1 L of sterile (Ham's) F-12 medium by filter-sterilization and then mix well. The medium can be stored in the refrigerator for up to 2 months. Any medium that develops a precipitate should be discarded.

7.6.4 Freezing Medium 10% (CHO Cells)

Filter-sterilize one volume of DMSO into nine volumes of F-12 complete in a sterile container. Store at room temperature and use on the day of preparation. Note that this medium is diluted with an equal volume of cell suspension in normal growth medium, so the final concentration of DMSO is 5% v/v at freezing.

7.6.5 Hypotonic Solution (0.075 M KCl)

Prepare a 0.75 M potassium chloride (KCl; formula weight, 75) stock solution in advance by dissolving 56 mg of KCl per 1 mL of water and store in the refrigerator for up to 1 year. On the day of use, dilute one volume of the stock with nine volumes of water and mix well.

7.6.6 Heparin Sodium 1000 U/mL

Heparin is incorporated into RPMI complete as an anticoagulant and is commercially available as a sterile solution in saline.

7.6.7 G6P 1 M: Glucose-6-Phosphate

The solution is prepared by dissolving G6P at 260 mg/mL of water; if the sodium salt is used, then it should be dissolved at the rate of 282 mg/mL. Filter-sterilize and then store in a freezer; this expires after 1 year.

7.6.8 KMg

Potassium chloride (KCl; formula weight 75) 124 mg and magnesium chloride ($MgCl_2.6H_2O$; formula weight, 203)   81 mg comprise KMg.

Each 1 mL of solution contains 124 mg Potassium chloride (KCl; formula weight 75) and 81 mg Magnesium chloride hexahydrate ($MgCl_2.6H_2O$; formula weight 203). Dissolve the salts in water (80% of the final volume) and then make the volume with water. Autoclave or filter-sterilize the solution and then store it at room temperature in ambient light for up to 1 year.

7.6.9 NADP 0.1 M

Dissolve β-nicotinamide adenine dinucleotide phosphate sodium salt (formula weight 765) at 76.5 mg/mL of water. Filter-sterilize, store refrigerated in the dark, and use on the day of preparation.

7.6.10 PHA M Form (Phytohemagglutinin)

This is a crude extract in the form of an aqueous solution and is used for stimulating T lymphocytes into division. It is available commercially and is used at a final concentration of approximately 2% v/v in the culture medium (final concentration approximately $2-10$ µg/mL in terms of solid PHA M).

7.6.11 Phosphate Buffer 0.2 M, pH 7.4

This solution is used to make the S9 mix. Mix the following two solutions in the proportions shown: sodium dihydrogen phosphate (NaH$_2$PO4) 0.2 M 146 mL and disodium hydrogen phosphate (Na$_2$HPO4) 0.2 M 854 mL.

Confirm that the pH is in the range of 7.3—7.5, and then autoclave or filter-sterilize it. Store at room temperature in ambient light. This expires after 1 year.

7.6.12 Positive Control Solutions

Stock solutions of MMC can be prepared in DMSO before use and then aliquoted in convenient amounts before storing in the freezer for up to 18 months. Frozen solutions should be completely thawed. Solutions of cyclophosphamide monohydrate (CP) are made on the day of use. Volatile positive controls should be avoided because of potential contamination of the incubator. On thawing any stored solution, ensure the material is completely dissolved before use.

7.6.13 RPMI Complete

This medium is used for culturing the HPBL. Completely thaw 100 mL of FCS in a 37°C waterbath and then mix by swirling or inversion. Filter-sterilize the serum, 5 mL of gentamycin 10 mg/mL and 4 mL of heparin sodium 1000 U/mL into 1 L of sterile RPMI 1640 medium (with NaHCO$_3$ and L-glutamine) and mix well. The medium can be stored in the refrigerator for up to 2 months.

7.6.14 S9 Fraction

The S9 fraction routinely used is identical to that described for the bacterial mutation test. It is prepared from the liver of rats that have been induced by intraperitoneal injection of Aroclor 1254 at 500 mg/kg bodyweight on one occasion or by multiple administrations of a mixture of phenobarbital with β-naphthoflavone either orally or by intraperitoneal injection to promote the levels of xenobiotic metabolizing enzymes [39—45]. S9 fraction is conventionally prepared by homogenization of liver in isotonic potassium chloride (0.15 M KCl) at a rate of 1 g wet tissue per 3 mL and then separated by centrifugation at 9000 g. S9 fraction may also be prepared using a lower proportion of 0.15 M KCl and then diluted to a standardized protein concentration (typically 40 mg/mL) based on biochemical estimation of protein content. Rarely, S9 preparations from other species (e.g., pooled human liver when testing compounds with known human-specific metabolism) or even other tissues may be included when appropriate and justified [46].

Most laboratories purchase precertified S9 fraction from a commercial source to avoid issues with handling animals and Aroclor (polychlorinated biphenyls are banned by some countries and some individual companies) and additional biochemical assays. Commercial S9 fraction can be obtained in frozen or lyophilized form in appropriately sized aliquots; alternatively, lyophilized preformulated S9 mix is available from Moltox. The quality control certificate supplied with commercial S9 should be retained with the raw study data. Frozen S9 should be stored below $-70°C$, thawed entirely immediately before use, and mixed well. Thawed S9 degrades fairly rapidly, so any excess should be discarded and not refrozen for later use.

7.6.15 S9 Mix

S9 mix may be prepared in the same way as for the bacterial mutation test, although some laboratories use different buffers/diluents. The concentration of S9 fraction in the S9 mix depends on the laboratory and test system. We suggest 15% and 10% v/v for CHO and HPBL, respectively, which both yield a final concentration of 2% v/v after dilution in culture medium. Typically, the final concentration of S9 fraction in the culture medium is 1−2%; higher concentrations may inhibit cell growth. In addition, S9 mix contains the following cofactors: 8 mM $MgCl_2$, 33 mM KCl, 100 mM sodium phosphate buffer pH 7.4, 5 mM glucose-6-phosphate, and 4 mM NADP [40]; therefore, each 1 mL of S9 mix contains:

	10%	15%
Water	0.335 mL	0.285 mL
Phosphate buffer 0.2 M pH 7.4	0.500 mL	0.500 mL
NADP 0.1 M	0.040 mL	0.040 mL
G6P	0.005 mL	0.005 mL
KMg	0.020 mL	0.020 mL
S9 fraction	0.100 mL	0.150 mL

All components should be sterile and added aseptically in the proportions and order listed here to a sterile container on ice, kept on ice or refrigerated, and used on the day of preparation.

Unused S9 mix should be discarded and not frozen for future use because it rapidly loses activity.

7.7 Phases in Development of the Test

Development may be conveniently divided into phases as described for the bacterial reverse mutation test: research, setup, internal validation, routine maintenance, and testing. Particular attention should be given to achieving a good mitotic index (MI) (in the case of lymphocytes) and the quality of slide preparations in terms of spreading of metaphases, morphology, and staining. Colcemid or colchicine may be used to arrest cells in metaphase at concentrations of approximately 0.1 μg/mL and 0.25 μg/mL, respectively. Many laboratories may prefer colcemid for *in vitro* studies because it seems less toxic; during the setup phase, we recommend that you test a range of concentrations of each to determine the optimal concentration for producing a large number of well-spread readable metaphases. Note that optimized and standardized culture conditions will result in mitotic indices routinely in excess of 5% in the case of HPBL. Metaphases should be sufficiently spread so that the chromosomes do not overlap, but without bursting some of the cells (in that case, individual chromosomes will be released from the boundaries of the cells and will be found floating free), chromatids should be separated with a clear outline and fairly deeply stained with the centromeres being identifiable; the cytoplasm should be only vaguely evident in the background and lightly stained. Readable metaphases will show all these characteristics and have a chromosome number very close to the diploid (HPBL) or modal (cell lines). Particular attention should be given to standardizing conditions of fixation and slide "dropping" so that excellent preparations can be made regularly with little "fine tuning"; this especially applies to temperature and, most importantly, to humidity [22,41−44], which is usually not controlled and subject to high seasonal variations in the laboratory. You will find it useful to monitor and record the temperature and humidity (using a hygrometer) in the slide-making area for reference purposes.

Unlike cell lines, the mitotic activity of lymphocyte cultures depends on:

- the culture vessel size and shape of the bottom of the vessel; flat-bottomed vessels tend to give the best results
- the depth and volume of the culture medium
- the density of the cells

In particular, if the MI during exposure and cell harvesting is high, then this will be expected to maximize sensitivity to mutagens and it will greatly reduce time and effort involved in slide reading. We recommend that each laboratory experiments with different culture vessels as well as the density and culture volume to maximize the MI at harvest using the conditions described in this chapter as a starting point. Note that assessment of the MI in lymphocytes is not straightforward because, unlike cell lines in culture, a proportion of the cells are undergoing necrosis (see Assessment of Toxicity later). The flat-sided culture vessels that we describe for lymphocyte culture are convenient for examination and because cells can be processed and fixed *in situ*.

Once the test methodology is standardized, your laboratory will need to establish an adequate negative and positive control database; these will be regularly updated and summarized in future reports. The negative control database is particularly important because vehicle control and test substance results in all future studies will be compared with it to confirm assay validity and help interpret any apparent increases in the incidence of aberrant cells. Initially, the negative control database should include an absolute minimum of 10, and preferably 20, experiments [36] (see also the General Recommendations chapter in this book). Incidences of aberrant cells in the negative/untreated control groups are normally similar between treatment regimes and should be pooled within one database unless there is any substantial difference. For cell lines in particular, special attention should be given to any apparent upward shifts in the incidences of aberrant metaphases and the database should only cover the past 2 or 3 years.

Consideration should be given to validating the *in vitro* versions of the chromosome aberration and micronucleus test in tandem because there is a very large overlap in culture and dosing requirements. This has the added benefit that the results of the two test systems can be compared directly.

7.8 Cell Characterization

Cell lines should be obtained from a reliable genetic toxicology laboratory that has maintained and characterized them appropriately as described here. Some cultivars (sublines) may be inappropriate for genetic toxicology testing because of genetic instability; the WBL clone of CHO cells has given good results in several laboratories and appears to be stable [47]. Appropriate characteristics of cells should be determined as listed by OECD TG473 before conducting GLP experiments. On arrival or after being rederived, cell lines should be assessed for stability of the modal chromosome number and the absence of mycoplasmal contamination, purified by cloning, characterized, and stored for later use. Once test methods have been optimized and standardized, the cell-cycle time of all cell types used in the test should be determined under typical negative control conditions in the laboratory; values obtained should be consistent with the published values. It is useful to establish representative karyotypes of cell lines on arrival for comparative purposes (e.g., with other laboratories and to check for potential shift over time); this can be performed using G-banding or related techniques [48]. Human lymphocytes have the same karyotype as other diploid human cells, and organized karyotypes showing grouping by size and centromere location are freely available online (e.g., http://www.web-books.com/MoBio/Free/Ch1C3.htm). A printed copy of the normally stained (unbanded) karyotype ideogram should be retained for training purposes and should be available in the slide reading area for potential reference.

Appropriate stocks of cell lines should be stored in the vapor phase of liquid nitrogen and appropriate clones should be used to generate frozen permanents, which are divided into two categories: master and test batch frozen permanents. Master frozen permanents are frozen cell aliquots set aside for long-term storage and generation of new test batches. Test batches are used to inoculate cultures for routine experiments.

Details of cell line maintenance, characterization, storage, and passage (number and details of subculturing) should be maintained in the cell maintenance log book.

7.8.1 Modal Chromosome Number

Normal diploid human cells all contain 23 pairs of chromosomes (including XX or XY pairs) at metaphase, which show high consistency between cells. However, cell lines have a variable and less stable number of chromosomes. The distribution of the number of chromosomes is characteristic of a particular clone; however, especially in less stable cell lines and those grown under inappropriate conditions, this and the karyotype in general will change over the course of multiple subculturings. Cell lines used for cytogenetic studies should have a relatively stable chromosome complement and, to help achieve this, should be subcultured as little as possible (i.e., the passage number should be low) and never grown beyond log phase. To demonstrate stability on initial acceptance for use and over time, the chromosome number distribution and modal number of cell lines should be established in each laboratory and monitored. Although Chinese hamsters themselves have a stable karyotype with 22 chromosomes, CHO and CHL cell lines show a varied number of chromosomes around the modal number, with the modal number being the most common number of chromosomes. For CHO-K1 cells, this can be 20 (ATCC cell line grown at CRL) or 21 [26b], whereas a value of 21 has been reported for CHO-WBL cells [19,49], and a value of 25 is considered normal for CHL cells [13,12,14,19,26b].

Prior to routine use and as part of routine maintenance, cells should be cultured and metaphase preparations should be made and stained as described later. One hundred metaphases should be examined and the distribution of chromosome numbers should be plotted and recorded (e.g., using the distribution function in Excel) to establish the modal chromosome number. An appropriate form for recording the original results is shown here (Figure 7.2).

Note that all forms used to collect results should be appendices to SOPs and should include appropriate information in the footer, such as version date and complete electronic directory path.

If a departure from the established modal chromosome number or a more variable chromosome number is seen over time, then the cell line should be discarded and rederived. Importantly, the modal number is used to help define which metaphases are considered readable during routine testing, and a centromeric count can help distinguish structural aberrations from preparation artifacts.

Modal Chromosome Count Sheet

Exp. number:			Culture ID:			Microscope number:	

Cell number	Number of chromosomes	Cell number	Number of chromosomes	Cell number	Number of chromosomes	Cell number	Number of chromosomes
1		26		51		76	
2		27		52		77	
3		28		53		78	
4		29		54		79	
5		30		55		80	
6		31		56		81	
7		32		57		82	
8		33		58		83	
9		34		59		84	
10		35		60		85	
11		36		61		86	
12		37		62		87	
13		38		63		88	
14		39		64		89	
15		40		65		90	
16		41		66		91	
17		42		67		92	
18		43		68		93	
19		44		69		94	
20		45		70		95	
21		46		71		96	
22		47		72		97	
23		48		73		98	
24		49		74		99	
25		50		75		100	

Slide reader (init./date): _____

Distribution

No. of chromosomes											
No. of cells											

Modal No.:_____   Calculated by init./date:_____

Reviewed by (init./date): _____   Page 1 of 1

Figure 7.2
Modal chromosome number scoring sheet.

7.8.2 Mycoplasma

All cell lines used in genotoxicity should be checked for mycoplasmal infection on arrival and regularly afterwards, for example, on generation of each new batch of frozen stock. Mycoplasma infection will result in unhealthy cells that grow more slowly than usual, but low-level infections can be difficult to detect. Cells should be checked for infection following two subculturings in antibiotic free medium. Mycoplasma can then be tested for in a number of ways, including PCR (e.g., Venor® GeM Mycoplasma Detection Kit), ELISA, immunostaining, autoradiography, or by growth in selective microbiological media, although none of these methods is infallible. The most straightforward and practical technique for most laboratories involves fluorescent staining with Hoescht, which allows direct visual identification of the DNA of mycoplasma in the cytoplasm [50,51].

7.8.3 Cell-Cycle Time

In exponentially dividing cell lines, the doubling time is a reasonable approximation of the cell-cycle time. However, lymphocytes do not greatly increase in number during culture because only a proportion of them divide, and a proportion of the dividing cells dies during the culture period. Therefore, especially in the case of lymphocytes, cell-cycle time needs to be quantified using a more appropriate technique. The most widely used method for lymphocytes (which is also appropriate for other cultured cells) involves examining the degree and pattern of quenching in cells labeled with 5-bromo-2'-deoxyuridine (BUDR) and then stained with Hoechst 33258 [52–54]. In the usual continuous labeling technique, BUDR is added to actively dividing cells (at the 48-h time point in the case of HPBL) at a final concentration of 25 μM, cells are harvested 24 h later (2 h after colcemid addition), and metaphase preparations are made in the same way as in the standard chromosome aberration test (see later). After staining with Hoescht 33258, the metaphases show distinctive patterns of fluorescence that depend on how many S-phases they have passed through in the presence of BUDR [38,53]. Note that some laboratories use Giemsa in combination with Hoescht, in which case the various metaphase populations can be distinguished by light rather than fluorescence microscopy. The proportions of first, second, and third division metaphases are determined and used to calculate the proliferative index (PI), calculated as:

$$(1 \times M1 + 2 \times M2 + 3 \times M3) \div 100\%$$

Where M1, M2, and M3 indicate the % of metaphases in the first, second, and third division stages after incorporation of BUDR in the S-phase.

The average cell-cycle time is calculated as:

$$\text{Number of hours in BUDR} \div \text{PI}$$

Using this differential staining technique, laboratories report a cell-cycle time of approximately 14.5 h for HPBL [55]. When using other cell types, it is advisable to investigate a range of concentrations of BUDR to obtain optimal staining results and minimize cytostatic effects at excessive concentrations of BUDR.

7.9 Routine Testing

7.9.1 General Considerations

Studies of nonpharmaceuticals for regulatory submission generally should follow the guidance of the latest OECD test guideline 473, whereas testing of pharmaceuticals should also take into account ICH S2 [35]; all such studies should be performed in compliance with GLP when possible. Some additional guidance on test performance is given in the FDA Redbook 2000 [56]. As in other tests, any planned deviation from these practices should be described and scientifically justified in the protocol and report; the potential impact of any unplanned deviation should be addressed in the report.

7.9.2 Dose Regimens

The test substance is usually evaluated under three different exposure conditions (regimens):

- *Short exposure 0S9.* Cultures are treated with the test substance in the absence of an exogenous metabolic activation system for 3−6 h and then washed; culture is continued for a total period of 1.5 normal cell-cycle lengths after the initiation of treatment.
- *Short exposure +S9.* Cultures are treated with the test substance in the presence of an exogenous metabolic activation system for 3−6 h and then washed; culture is continued for a total period of 1.5 normal cell-cycle lengths after the initiation of treatment.
- *Long exposure 0S9.* Cultures are treated continuously with the test substance in the absence of an exogenous metabolic activation system for 1.5 normal cell-cycle lengths after the initiation of treatment.

The three dosing regimens are illustrated graphically in the example for HPBL here. In the case of CHO cells, the initial incubation period is routinely 20 h. The total incubation period of 21 h after dosing is based on the cell-cycle time of HPBL and CHO cells in our experiments (i.e., 1.5 cell-cycle times = 21 h for untreated cultures) and may need to be adjusted depending on the cycle time determined in your laboratory under standardized conditions.

Set	Incubate	Dose	Incubate	Wash	Incubate	Colcemid	Incubate	Harvest
1	48 h	Test formulation	4 h	Wash	15 h		2 h	
2	48 h	S9 + test formulation	4 h	Wash	15 h		2 h	
3	48 h	Test formulation	Incubate 19 h without washing				2 h	

The reader should be aware that some classes of chemical, such as nitrosamines, nucleoside analogues, and other cytostatic drugs, may require inclusion of an even longer exposure time in the absence of S9 for optimal detection of clastogenic activity, in which case a fourth exposure regime may need to be included in the study. It is most efficient to test all exposure regimes in parallel rather than using sequential testing.

7.9.3 Metabolic Activation System

The metabolic activation system used for routine testing consists of S9 mix containing induced rat liver S9 fraction at 5–30% v/v (typically 10% or 15%) and is usually diluted in culture medium to a final 1% or 2% in terms of S9 fraction. The S9 mix contains NADP and G6P cofactors but does not necessarily need to include the inorganic cofactors used in for the bacterial mutation test because these are automatically incorporated in the culture medium.

Most laboratories never experience problems with S9 fraction; however, if your laboratory finds that a particular batch of S9 inhibits mitotic activity (or causes other technical problems such as particulate), you should consider prequalifying a batch of S9 fraction sufficient to cover, for example, 1 year of routine testing.

7.9.4 Test Substance Considerations

The chromosome aberration test is used to evaluate a wide range of chemicals, impurities, and biological materials. Medical devices are usually extracted and tested as per ISO standards series 10993 (in particular, Part 3 Tests for genotoxicity, carcinogenicity, and reproductive toxicity and Part 12 sample preparation and reference materials; see https://www.iso.org for current details).

It is important to gather relevant physical and chemical information regarding the nature of the test substance in advance so that appropriate methods of sample preparation and testing are used. At the same time, the chemist involved in the project may be able to give you useful information about potential solvents. Despite the efforts of ICH, OECD, ISO, and others, there are national variations and preferences in test requirements, so it is useful to consider the final use of the test substance and which regulatory bodies will be involved when designing the study. The reader should also consult the General and Formulation chapters of this book for additional guidance.

7.9.5 Vehicle Selection and Dose Volume

The test substance will normally require dissolving, diluting, or suspending in an appropriate liquid for dosing, taking into account chemical stability and compatibility of the vehicle with the test system. The same type of formulation will normally be used for the bacterial mutation test that is often performed in parallel to the chromosome test (refer to the Formulations chapter for more details). Aqueous solvents such as water and saline are preferred vehicles and can be used at levels up to approximately 20% v/v. If solubility is slightly lower, then it may be possible to dissolve the material directly in culture medium and dose the cells (at the high dose at least) by performing a change of medium. If the test substance has low aqueous solubility (i.e., less than 5 mg/mL), then organic solvents are often used at a maximal dose of 10 μL/mL (1% final concentration in culture). Relatively nontoxic miscible organic solvents include dimethyl sulfoxide, dimethylformamide, ethanol, methanol, propanone (acetone), and acetonitrile.

Appropriate volumes of relatively nontoxic solvents are not expected to affect the background % aberrant cells substantially; nevertheless, inclusion of an untreated control group is advisable if a novel solvent is used. When working with novel solvents, it may be appropriate to perform a preliminary compatibility test using the long exposure in the absence of S9 and the short exposure with S9 ahead of study. We suggest you evaluate a range of likely solvents during the validation phase of the assay to facilitate vehicle selection later.

When, for practical reasons, the dose volume is variable and the solvent is not expected to have a significant effect on the background percentage of aberrant cells, it is justifiable to use only the maximal dose volume for the concurrent vehicle control. A different solvent and dose volume may be used for the positive control articles and will normally be standardized for that laboratory. There is no need to include a separate vehicle control for the positive control; instead, comparison of results is normally made with the (test substance) vehicle control.

7.9.6 Dose Level Selection

Prior to finalizing the protocol and performing the chromosome aberration test, solubility testing will normally be required to decide or confirm an appropriate maximum dose level for the test (see later and Formulation chapter).

Based on these guidelines, the maximum concentration of test substance assessed in the test should be the limit of toxicity, solubility, or the standard upper limit of 10 mM, 2 mg/mL, or 2 μL/mL (or 1 mM or 0.5 mg/mL in the case of pharmaceuticals), whichever is the lowest. Doses higher than the standard upper limit may be justifiable in some cases, such as when testing mixtures or when qualifying a pharmaceutical with a suspect impurity.

ICH defines the limit of toxicity as a reduction of approximately 50% in cell growth, however, OECD is apparently more restrictive, indicating that the high dose should cause inhibition of growth by 55±5%. The measures of toxicity indicated by OECD are also appropriate for pharmaceuticals and are based on reduction in the relative rate of growth of the treated cells compared with the negative control cells, such as MI in the case of lymphocytes and relative increase in cell count (RICC) or relative population doubling (RPD) in the case of cell lines (see Assessment of Toxicity section). In practice, these measures tend to vary as a result of experimental variation, so the ±5% limits mentioned by OECD should not be too strictly applied. In particular, MI can vary quite widely between cultures. Whatever the situation, apparent effects seen only at the limit of toxicity should be interpreted with caution.

In the case of nontoxic compounds with limited solubility in culture medium, the highest concentration analyzed should produce turbidity or precipitate at the end of the treatment period. An inverted microscope should be available to facilitate observation of precipitation. It may also be useful to treat a parallel set of mock cultures without cells in those cases where precipitate might be expected to be obscured by the cells and/or the S9. In cases where precipitation is observed, the lowest concentration showing precipitate should be the highest dose selected for detailed examination of aberrations because precipitate can be carried over with the cells during washing and other procedures and cause physical or chemical toxicity or interfere with cell spreading and staining. The guidelines do not provide guidance on testing of materials that have very low aqueous solubility (e.g., many polyaromatic hydrocarbons). In these cases, every reasonable effort should be made to expose the cells to solubilized material or, in the case of mixtures or environmental samples, extracts of the material. Then, the highest dose selected for examination should not be excessively toxic or interfere with the quality of the metaphase spreads.

We suggest a standard dose interval between each concentration of approximately 2. A smaller interval may be used when the test substance is suspected of having a steep toxicity curve and is often appropriate in the case of confirmatory testing. In the following example, the test substance showed reasonable solubility in the culture medium in a preliminary assessment and therefore could be dosed at the standard limit suggested by the guidelines. Note that in the case of a test substance with a low molecular weight (MW), the dose levels should be proportionately lower, i.e., for pharmaceuticals the highest dose should be reduced to 1 mM if MW is <500 daltons, and for nonpharmaceuticals the highest dose should be reduced to 10 mM if MW is <200 daltons. However, ICH also indicates "For pharmaceuticals with unusually low molecular weight (e.g., less than 200) higher test concentrations should be considered," implying that the high dose of 0.2 mg/mL would be appropriate when the MW of a drug is <200 daltons. For compounds with solubilities below these limits, the high dose should show slight precipitation in the culture medium.

Suggested default standard study design: main test

Dose Level/ Treatment	Final Concentration, $\mu g/mL^a$		Number of Replicates		
	ICH	OECD	Short Exposure 0S9	Short Exposure + S9	Long Exposure 0S9
Vehicle	0	0	2	2	2
1/Test substance	1	4	2	2	2
2/Test substance	2	8	2	2	2
3/Test substance	4	16	2	2	2
4/Test substance	8	32	2	2	2
5/Test substance	16	64	2	2	2
6/Test substance	32	128	2	2	2
7/Test substance	64	256	2	2	2
8/Test substance	128	512	2	2	2
9/Test substance	256	1024	2	2	2
10/Test substance	500	2000	2	2	2
1/Positive control	b	b	2	2	2
2/Positive control	b	b	2	2	2
3/Positive control	b	b	2	2	2

0S9   without S9.
+ S9   with S9.
[a]Dose levels should be proportionately lower if the test substance has a low molecular weight or if more than one of the dose levels mentioned is above the limit of solubility (see previous paragraph).
[b]Standard positive control chemicals and dose levels as determined during set-up and validation work. Three dose levels of each positive control are dosed and processed to slides later for each regimen, but only a single dose showing low to slightly toxicity is subjected to detailed examination for chromosome aberrations.

Based on the aforementioned study design, you would expect the study to consist of a total of:

14 formulations $\times$ 3 regimens $\times$ 2 replicate cultures = 84 cultures.

In addition, a few untreated control cultures should be initiated to act as potential replacements in the event of a technical error and to check the suitability of slide-dropping conditions later. Although this can be mentioned in the protocol, no results will be reported for these cultures.

In the unlikely event that results are not available for an adequate number of dose levels due to toxicity, a supplementary test will be necessary.

In the case of extracts of medical devices where no significant amount of material is expected to be extracted from the device, some laboratories test only the extract undiluted (i.e., a single dose level); however, this does not comply with the OECD requirement to test at least three dose levels. In the case of medical devices, normally two extracts are tested, one in a polar (aqueous) solvent and one in a nonpolar organic solvent, using appropriate solvent controls for comparative purposes.

7.9.7 Positive Controls

Positive controls are used to confirm the sensitivity of the test system and the effectiveness of the S9 mix; examples given in OECD TG473 are listed here:

S9 Conditions	Chemical	CAS Number
0	Methyl methanesulfonate	66-27-3
0	Mitomycin C	50-07-7
0	4-nitroquinoline N-oxide	56-57-5
0	Cytosine arabinoside	147-94-4
+	Benzo[a]pyrene[a]	50-32-8
+	Cyclophosphamide[b]	50-18-0

[a]We do not recommend use of benzo[a]pyrene as a positive control for HPBL because its low solubility in culture media can result in weak clastogenic effects, lack of a clear dose-response, and carry-over with the cells after washing. The aqueous solubility of this chemical is listed as 1.6 μg/L by PubChem.
[b]Note that cyclophosphamide (MW 261) is usually supplied and used in genotoxicity tests in the monohydrate form (CAS 6055-19-2, MW 279) and should be reported as such.

To account for variability in toxicity shifts between experiments, it is recommended that three dose levels should be tested, but only one should be selected for evaluation based on observed toxicity and/or preliminary examination of the slides.

Suggested routine positive controls and guidance dose levels are listed here:

Exposure	Cell Type	Compound	Abbreviation	Concentration, μg/mL	S9
Short and long	HPBL	Mitomycin C[a]	MMC	0.05–0.20	0
Short	HPBL	Cyclophosphamide	CP	4.0–8.0	+
Short	CHO	Mitomycin C[a]	MMC	0.05	0
Short	CHO	Cyclophosphamide	CP	1.5–4.5	+
Long	CHO	Mitomycin C	MMC	0.10	0

[a]OECD TG473 and ICH indicate that the direct genotoxin (mitomycin C) may be omitted for the short treatment if the cyclophosphamide treatment and the treatment in the presence of S9 are performed at the same time as the short treatment. This may be problematic if there is a technical issue with the +S9 regime so we do not recommend it.

7.10 Standard Test Procedures

Note that procedures, media, and reagents are performed/used at room temperature unless otherwise stated. The incubator should have a stainless steel tray containing water in the bottom to maintain high humidity (important if multiwell cultures are used). Centrifugations are performed using a bench-top centrifuge; speeds and timing should be adequate to pellet the cells but are not considered critical, and the speeds given here are for guidance and may need adjusting depending on the particular rotor. The harvest times and the long exposure time indicated in the procedures are based on the cell-cycle time estimate for CHO and HPBL cells at Charles River Laboratories, Montreal, and should be adjusted according to cell-cycle determinations in your own laboratory. However, 21 h = 1.5 cell cycles is fairly typical for these cell types (see Henderson et al. [55] for example). Longer cell-cycle times may be indicative of suboptimal growth conditions.

7.10.1 Experimental Design Spreadsheet

The experimental design spreadsheet should be generated prior to the study from a standard template file with cultures numbered sequentially to specify the treatment conditions for each culture and who did what and when. The example in Table 7.1 includes the vehicle and positive controls and all dose levels of a single substance in one test regimen (i.e., short exposure in the absence of S9). The comment column allows documentation of incidental observations such as changes in medium color and precipitation at the various phases of culture processing. The sheet also includes appropriate space to document the staff involved and dates. The design can be separated into sections:

1. The first column and second column identify the treatment regimen
2. Culture number identification is provided in the third column
3. The next columns provide information on the dose number associated with the formulated material to be dosed, as well as the amount to be administered to each culture
4. The last columns are provided for comments and staff identification for procedure accountability
5. These steps are repeated for the two remaining dose regimens (short exposure in the presence of S9 and long exposure in the absence of S9). With a design of 10 dose levels of test substance, a total of $3 \times 28 = 84$ cultures would be needed for a complete experiment.

7.10.1.1 CHO cells: routine maintenance

CHO cells are grown using standard techniques for attached cell lines, such as described by Freshney [57]. All media including DPBS and trypsin should be warmed to room temperature before use. Approximately 6 days to 2 weeks prior to the planned day of dosing, rapidly thaw a frozen vial of cells ($1.0 - 2.0 \times 10^6$ cells/mL/vial in complete medium with 5% DMSO) in a 37°C water bath while agitating by hand. Lay a 75 cm^2 vented flask labeled with today's date and other appropriate details (e.g., cell type, passage

Table 7.1: Experimental design spreadsheet example

Regime	Culture No.		Material	Dose No.	Dose Volume µL	Final Concentration µg/mL	Comments and Observations			
							Before Dose	After Dosing	After Exposure	At Harvest
4 h 0S9	01	02	Water	0	50	–				
Set 1	11	12	X	1	50	1				
	21	22	X	2	50	2				
Prefix*	31	32	X	3	50	4				
1	41	42	X	4	50	8				
	51	52	X	5	50	16				
	61	62	X	6	50	32				
	71	72	X	7	50	64				
	81	82	X	8	50	128				
	91	92	X	9	50	256				
	101	102	X	10	50	500				
	111	112	MMC	M1	50	0.05				
	121	122	MMC	M2	50	0.10				
	131	132	MMC	M3	50	0.20				
Performed by (initial/date)										

Explanation: Prefix prior to the culture number indicates dose regime (set number): 1 indicates 4 h without S9 (4 h 0S9); 2 indicates 4 h with S9 (4 h + S9); and 3 indicates long exposure without S9. In this case the test substance has been given the code letter X. The final concentrations shown here are typical for a relatively high-molecular-weight pharmaceutical when not limited by solubility. In similar situations, a nonpharmaceutical would be dosed at levels four-times higher. Although this study design includes duplicate vehicle control cultures, inexperienced laboratories in particular (i.e., those with a limited historical control database) should consider inclusion of an untreated pair of cultures or quadruplicate control cultures to produce more reliable results and to build their own historical control database.

number, and density or split ratio) on its side and then transfer the contents of the thawed vial before gradually adding 12 mL F-12 complete while gently agitating. Incubate the culture under standard conditions (37°C in an atmosphere containing 5% v/v CO_2). Check the condition and degree of confluence of the cells regularly and before harvesting. The cells must be subcultured before approaching confluence: if a one-tenth split is used for subculturing (i.e., one-tenth of the cells at harvest are used to inoculate another 75-cm² flask), then the cells will multiply by a factor of approximately 10 over the course of 3 days and therefore will need further subculturing every 3 days. To harvest the cells, remove the supernatant medium from the flask completely using a pipette, rinse the cell monolayer very gently with 10 mL DPBS (add the buffer to the side of the flask), remove the DPBS completely, and then add 5 mL trypsin 0.25% in the same way. Leave the trypsin in contact with the cells for approximately 20 seconds, stand the flask upright to drain before removing the trypsin using a pipette. Incubate the culture for approximately 10 min until the cells appear rounded when viewed under the microscope. Knock the cells into suspension by tapping the flask gently against the side of the bench and then add 12 mL

F-12 complete before dissociating the cells by repeated aspiration using a 10 mL pipette ("rough pipetting"). Transfer the cell suspension to a sterile centrifuge tube, pellet the cells by centrifugation at 500 g for 5 min, discard the supernatant, knock the cells into suspension, resuspend them in 12 mL F-12 complete, and then rough pipette to disperse any clumps. At this point the cell density can be accurately quantified, if desired, and cells can be frozen for future use, as summarized in the next paragraph. Add an appropriate volume of cells to F-12 complete to achieve the desired split (e.g., 1.2 mL cell suspension is added to 10.8 mL medium in a 75-cm^2 flask). The new culture is labeled and incubated as before. At each subculture, the passage number is increased by one and an appropriate note is made in the cell maintenance log or raw study data, as appropriate.

To perform a live ("viable") cell count (i.e., to determine cell density), dilute 100 μL of cell suspension with 100 μL trypan blue 0.4%, mix, and load a hemocytometer with the diluted suspension before counting those cells that appear bright (i.e., exclude trypan blue). Note that a normal healthy culture will contain very few dead cells. To freeze CHO cells in suspension, determine the cell density of a freshly harvested culture after dilution in complete medium and adjust the density to 2×10^6 cell/mL by dilution in F-12 complete. Dilute the suspension 1:1 with freezing medium. Dispense the cell suspensions in 1 mL aliquots into prelabeled cryovials and freeze them slowly (at 1°C/min) to avoid large ice crystal formation. This can be achieved by placing the cells in a partly insulated polystyrene foam container (e.g., manufactured in-house or Mr. Frosty™ from Thermo Scientific) before transfer to a −70°C freezer or by using a special cell-freezing insert placed inside the neck of a liquid cell storer. After overnight freezing, the ampoules should be rapidly transferred (within 2 min) to canes for storage in the gaseous phase of the liquid nitrogen cell store. Note that if ampoules are stored in the liquid nitrogen phase, shrinkage of the seal can allow liquid nitrogen to enter the vial; some makes of ampoule seem much more prone to this than others. The depth of liquid nitrogen should be monitored continually, such as by using an electronic alarm system and by performing weekly checks using a wooden 1-meter rule or similar. The insulating insert in the lid of a liquid nitrogen cell store should be replaced if it shows signs of deterioration to minimize losses of liquid nitrogen.

7.10.2 CHO Cells: Test Procedures

Refer to the experimental design to determine the number of cultures required, remembering to include some extra to act as potential replacements and for counting and slide-making checks.

Day −4 (4 days prior to dosing). Grow a sufficient number of cells in flasks as described above (see Section 7.10.1.1). These flasks would normally be inoculated 3 days prior to initiation of cultures to be used in the study.

Day −1 (1 day prior to dosing). After incubation for 3 days, once the cells have grown to approximately 50% confluence, remove the flask(s) from the incubator and record the inoculation date, passage number, percentage of confluence, and any comments appearing in the study raw data file. To harvest the cells, remove the supernatant medium from the flask completely using a pipette, rinse the cell monolayer gently with 10 mL DPBS (add the buffer to the side of the flask), remove the DPBS completely, and discard it; then, add 5 mL trypsin 0.25% in the same way. Leave the trypsin in contact with the cells for approximately 20 s by leaving the flask flat on the work surface. Remove the trypsin from the flask using a pipette and then incubate the culture for 5−10 min until the cells appear rounded when viewed under the microscope. Knock the cells into suspension by tapping the flask gently against the side of the bench and add 12 mL F-12 complete before dissociating the cells by repeated aspiration using a 10 mL pipette (rough pipetting). Transfer the cell suspension to a sterile centrifuge tube, pellet the cells by centrifugation at 500 g (1000 rpm) for 5 min, discard the supernatant, knock the cells into suspension by flicking with the fingers, resuspend them in 12 mL F-12 complete, and then rough pipette to disperse any clumps before adding enough F-12 complete to bring the suspension to the same volume as was in the original cultures (i.e., number of cultures × 12 mL). Perform a live (viable) cell count by diluting 100 μL of cell suspension with 100 μL trypan blue 0.4%, mix, and load a hemocytometer with the diluted suspension before counting those cells that appear bright (i.e., live cells exclude trypan blue).

1. *Day 1 Initiation*
   a. Prepare a sufficient volume of cell suspension by diluting an appropriate volume of the aforementioned cell suspension with F-12 complete to give a final density of 0.08×10^6 cells/mL in a sterile bottle. While continually agitating the suspension to ensure a similar number of cells are dispensed to each flask, dispense 5 mL per flask into 25-cm^2 culture flasks that have been prelabeled in accordance with the experimental design sheet. You should have three sets of culture flasks plus a few spare flasks to act as potential replacements to measure cell density at the start of treatment and to act as procedural controls during slide-making.
   b. Incubate all cultures for 20 h. Note all incubations are at 37°C in a humid atmosphere containing 5% v/v CO_2.
2. *Day 0 Dosing*
   a. Remove the flasks from the incubator approximately 20 h after initiation and, using an inverted microscope, check that the cells appear healthy and have started to grow.
   b. Harvest the cells from one of the flasks to perform a live cell as described for Day −1. In this case, however, the final cell pellet should be suspended and mixed in 500 μL of F-12 complete before diluting 100 μL with an equal volume of trypan blue 0.4% and counting. The cell count should indicate a density of approximately 0.8×10^6 cells per flask (i.e., approximately double the density at initiation).

This number is important because it represents the density of live cells at the start of treatment and will be used in the calculation of toxicity later. The cells from this culture can be discarded after the count.

   c. Remove 0.650 mL of medium from the flasks for S9 treatment and then add 0.650 mL of 15% S9 mix to them immediately prior to addition of the test formulation.

   d. Add vehicle and test compounds to cultures as described in the experimental design sheet. Gently swirl each flask after dosing.

   e. Check medium color and precipitation in all cultures.

   f. Incubate all cultures as before.

3. *Day 0 Washing: Sets 1 and 2 only*

   a. After 4 h, remove Sets 1 and 2 cultures from the incubator and make a note of color and precipitation.

   b. Completely remove the medium from each culture and add 5 mL fresh F-12 complete to each and gently agitate to resuspend any precipitate.

   c. Completely remove the medium from each culture and add 5 mL fresh F-12 complete to each.

   d. Incubate the cultures for another 15 h.

4. *Colcemid*

   a. Remove Set 3 cultures (and any remaining spare cultures) after 19 h of continuous exposure to the test formulations. Sets 1 and 2 should be removed 15 h after the start of reincubation following washing. Add 50 μL of colcemid 10 μg/mL to all cultures to achieve a final concentration of 0.1 μg/mL and mix. Slightly loosen caps (if using unvented flasks) to facilitate gas exchange and immediately return the cultures to incubator for another 2 h.

5. *Harvest*

   a. Remove the cultures from the incubator after 2 h of incubation in the presence of colcemid.

   b. Record medium color and absence or presence of precipitation and its appearance. Record the appearance of the cells as a preliminary indication of toxicity. *Note that dead cells will often slough off into the supernatant medium.*

   c. Remove the medium from the flasks.

   d. Rinse cells once with 5 mL DPBS per flask. Remove and discard the DPBS.

   e. Add 1 mL of Trypsin 0.25% to the monolayer of cells in each flask.

   f. Incubate the flasks for 5−10 min.

   g. When the cells are rounded, knock each flask to detach the cells and then stand them in an upright position to allow the cells to drain to the bottom. Add 9 mL of F-12 complete to rinse the growth surface of each flask.

   h. Transfer the suspensions to prelabeled 15 mL centrifuge tubes.

   i. Pellet cells using a centrifuge at 500 g (1000 rpm) for 5 min.

j. Discard the supernatant and then flick the cells to resuspend them in the residual medium.

k. Resuspend each culture in 7 mL F-12 complete and then mix the suspension prior to sampling as described below.

l. To determine the limit of toxicity, remove a 1.0 mL sample from each tube and place into an appropriate container; then, use this sample to perform cell counts using a Coulter counter if available. Perform a live cell count for cultures from dose levels with a count of 45–55% of the vehicle control and at least two or three lower dose levels (i.e., those cultures that might be subject to detailed examination for aberrations later). To perform a live cell count, take 100 μL of the 1.0 mL sample and dilute it with an equal volume of trypan blue 0.4%; mix and load a hemocytometer with the diluted suspension before counting those cells that appear bright (i.e., exclude trypan blue). Record the density of live and dead cells for each to calculate percentage of viability and absolute density of live cells. Perform similar live counts on the vehicle control and at least one low or slightly toxic dose level of the positive control.

m. If a Coulter counter system is not available, then live cell counts should be performed using a hemocytometer as described in the previous paragraph. In this case, the dose(s) selected for counting should be selected based on the preliminary visual assessment of toxicity performed when the cultures were removed from the incubator. Again, live/dead cell counts should be performed for all cultures for which a detailed assessment of aberrations might be performed later.

n. Cultures that show severe toxic effects (all cells dead) do not need processing beyond this point and can be discarded. Otherwise, process each tube as indicated below.

o. Pellet cells using a centrifuge at 500 g (1000 rpm) for 5 min.

p. Discard the supernatant and flick the cells to resuspend them in the residual medium.

q. Add 1 mL Hypotonic solution to each tube and mix by gentle flicking.

r. Leave the tubes at room temperature for 10 min

6. *Fixation*

a. Add 1 mL Fix to the cells suspended in Hypotonic solution while gently agitating.

b. Pellet the cells by centrifugation at 900 g (1500 rpm) for 5 min.

c. Remove the supernatant and resuspend the cells in the residual solution by gentle flicking.

d. Add 1 mL Fix to the suspended cells while mixing continuously.

e. Leave tubes at room temperature for at least 30 min or overnight in the refrigerator.

f. Pellet the cells by centrifugation at 900 g (1500 rpm) for 5 min.

g. Remove the supernatant and resuspend the cells in the residual Fix by gentle flicking.

h. Add 1 mL Fix to the suspended cells while mixing continuously.

i. Cells should be stored refrigerated at least overnight, but they may be stored for several months. If stored for an extended period, then check for evaporation and deterioration of the plastic tubes.

j. Pellet the cells by centrifugation at 900 g (1500 rpm) for 5 min.

k. Carefully remove the supernatant to avoid disturbing the pellet and resuspend the cells in the residual Fix by gentle flicking.

l. Add 1 mL Fix to each tube. At this point cells can be stored refrigerated for several months, if necessary.

7. *Slide preparation*

a. Select appropriate cultures for slide preparation and potential detailed examination based on live cell counts. In this case, slides will need to be prepared from each of the three sets of cultures for the vehicle control, at least one nontoxic or slightly toxic dose level of the positive control and at least three dose levels of the test substance. If in doubt about the level of toxicity, it is best to prepare slides from one or two additional dose levels for potential examination. *Only those cultures that are needed for examination need to be processed to slides as detailed here.* Fixed preparations from the remaining cultures should be returned to the refrigerator in the event they are needed for examination later (e.g., to clarify borderline results).

b. Prelabel the microscope slides with a unique identifier (e.g., experiment or study number with culture number underneath). In the case of frosted slides, this is best performed using a 2H pencil.

c. Pellet the cells by centrifugation at 900 g (1500 rpm) for 5 min.

d. Remove the supernatant carefully to avoid disturbing the pellet.

e. Add at least two drops of Fix to each tube. If necessary, add additional drops of Fix to adjust the density as judged by eye; the suspension should appear slightly cloudy.

f. Put a drop of cell suspension from a spare culture onto a clean slide using a fresh Pasteur pipette.

g. Allow the slide(s) to air-dry and then check the degree of metaphase spreading using a microscope (phase contrast, if available). If the degree of metaphase spreading is appropriate, then continue with slide preparation until enough slides are obtained per culture to ensure an adequate number of readable metaphases (at least two slides per culture should be made). If necessary, metaphase spreading can be aided using a humid atmosphere (e.g., expose slides to vapor from a 70°C water bath during the dropping procedure).

h. Once slide preparation is complete, add 5 mL Fix to all tubes and store refrigerated in case additional slides need to be made later (e.g., in case the required number of readable metaphases is not available from any of the original slides).

7.10.3 HPBL Test Procedures

HPBL are normally grown as 5 mL cultures in prelabeled Nunc polystyrene flat-sided culture tubes incubated with the flat side down and placed in a rack. Refer to the experimental design to determine the number of cultures required, remembering to include some extra to act as potential replacements and for slide-making checks. You will need at least 0.5 mL blood per culture plus a small amount to allow for waste. All incubations described here are at 37°C in a humid atmosphere containing 5% CO_2.

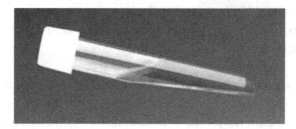

HPBL 5 mL culture. *Photograph courtesy of Fisher Scientific.*

HPBL can also be successfully grown in 1 mL cultures, but this may limit the number of metaphases available for analysis later; therefore, this method is more suited to screening studies when the test substance is in limited supply. In this case, dispense 1.0 mL aliquots of the blood-medium-PHA mixture described below into clear, flat-bottom, 4 mL glass vials with screw caps for treatment in the absence of S9 and dispense 0.8 mL aliquots into vials for treatment in the presence of S9.

Day −2 (2 days prior to dosing). Initiate cultures 2 days prior to dosing using sodium-heparinized fresh blood samples obtained by venipuncture (usually from the median cubital vein on the inside of the elbow) from healthy (normally male) human volunteers; donors should be nonsmoking individuals of approximately 18−35 years of age with no known illness, recent viral infection, or recent exposure to drugs or radiation that might increase the background incidence of chromosomal aberrations. OECD TG473 indicates that there is a slight trend for increased background rates of aberration with age, which is more marked in females than males. The blood can be taken from a single donor or pooled (after dilution in culture medium) from more than one donor if a larger volume is needed. The number of donors used should be indicated in the eventual study report. Some individual donors seem to provide blood that results in higher MI cultures than others; subsequently, these donors are generally preferred.

Dilute the whole blood with RPMI complete (1 volume of blood per 9 mL medium) in a sufficiently large sterile bottle and add 1 mL PHA M solution per 50 mL of diluted blood. For reference purposes, white cell counts can be made at this point or later during culture process by dilution of 100 μL of suspension with an equal volume of white cell counting fluid (WCF; consists of 1 mg crystal violet per 1 mL of aqueous 1.5% v/v acetic acid), which fixes and stains white cells while lysing red cells. White cells can then be counted with the aid of a hemocytometer.

Note the instructions that follow apply to 5 mL cultures; volumes of additions described here should be adjusted proportionately for 1 mL cultures (i.e., by a factor of one-fifth). We routinely include a 24-well plate containing 1 mL RPMI complete per well that is dosed and incubated in parallel with the other cultures to facilitate checks for precipitation at the start and end of each treatment period because it can be very difficult to see this in the presence of cells in the standard culture tubes.

1. *Day −2 Initiation.* Prelabel the culture tubes as per the experimental design. Dispense aliquots of the blood-medium-PHA mixture into each flat-sided culture tube while stirring the mixture regularly. Divide cultures into three sets (one for each treatment regimen) plus a 24-well plate as follows:
   a. Set 1: 5 mL/tube
   b. Set 2: 4 mL/tube
   c. Set 3: 5 mL/tube
   d. 24-well plate: 1 mL medium (without cells) per well
   e. Spare cultures: 5 mL/tube, not dosed with formulation (unless needed as replacements) but dosed with colcemid and harvested alongside Set 3 to act as a procedural control at the slide preparation stage.
   Incubate all cultures with the flat side down in racks for 48 h.
2. *Day 0 Dosing.* Remove the cultures from the incubator without disturbing them 48 ± 0.5 h after initiation.
   a. Add 1 mL of S9 mix to Set 2 cultures.
   b. Add vehicle and test compounds to cultures in accordance with the experimental design sheet. Mix the cultures well after treatment.
   c. Check medium color and precipitation in all cultures. Check the 24-well plate under a microscope for precipitate.
   d. Incubate all cultures as before.
3. *Washing.* After 4 h, remove the 24-well plate and Sets 1 and 2 from the incubator and make a note of color and precipitation.
   a. Return the 24-well plate to the incubator.
   b. Pellet the cells in culture Sets 1 and 2 by centrifugation at 500 g (1000 rpm) for 5 min.
   c. Discard the supernatant and flick the tube to resuspend the cells in the residual medium.
   d. Resuspend each culture in 5 mL fresh RPMI complete (without PHA) and mix. Slightly loosen tube caps to allow gas exchange.
   e. Incubate the cultures for another 15 h (±30 min).

4. *Day 1. Colcemid.* Remove Set 3 cultures after 19 h of continuous exposure to the test formulations. Sets 1 and 2 should be removed 15 h after the start of reincubation after washing. Add 50 μL colcemid 10 μg/mL to each culture to achieve a final concentration of 0.1 μg/mL and mix. Slightly loosen caps to allow gas exchange and immediately return the cultures to the incubator for another 2 h.

5. *Day 1 Harvest.* After 2 h of incubation in the presence of colcemid:

    a. Remove the cultures from the incubator.

    b. Check medium color in Sets 1, 2, and 3, and check precipitation in the 24-well plate using an inverted microscope. Discard the multiwell plate after recording observations.

    c. Pellet the cells by centrifugation at 500 g (1000 rpm) for 5 min.

    d. Remove the supernatant and resuspend the cells in residual supernatant by flicking (striking the side of the tubes with the fingers).

    e. Add 1 mL Hypotonic solution to each tube and mix by gentle flicking; then, add an additional 4 mL Hypotonic solution and mix gently.

    f. Put the tubes in a 37°C water bath for 10 min

6. *Fixation.* Add 1 mL Fix to the cells suspended in Hypotonic solution and mix.

    a. Pellet the cells by centrifugation at 900 g (1500 rpm) for 5 min. Note that after fixation, the cell pellet will be very small because any remaining erythrocytes will have lysed (the supernatant will have a brown coloration).

    b. Remove the supernatant and resuspend the cells in the residual solution by gentle flicking.

    c. Add 5 mL Fix to the suspended cells while mixing continuously.

    d. Leave tubes at room temperature for at least 30 min or overnight in the refrigerator.

    e. Pellet the cells by centrifugation at 900 g (1500 rpm) for 5 min.

    f. Remove the supernatant and resuspend the cells in the residual Fix by gentle flicking.

    g. Add 5 mL Fix to the suspended cells while mixing continuously.

    h. Cells should be stored refrigerated at least overnight, but they may be stored for several months. If stored for an extended period, then check for evaporation and deterioration of the plastic tubes.

    i. Pellet the cells by centrifugation at 900 g (1500 rpm) for 5 min.

    j. Carefully remove the supernatant to avoid disturbing the pellet and resuspend the cells in the residual Fix by gentle flicking.

    k. Add 5 mL Fix to each tube. Cells can be stored refrigerated for several months, if necessary.

7. *Slide preparation.* Prelabel the microscope slides with a unique identifier (e.g., experiment or study number with culture number underneath). In the case of frosted slides, this is best done using a 2H pencil.

a. Pellet the cells by centrifugation at 900 g (1500 rpm) for 5 min.

b. Remove the supernatant carefully to avoid disturbing the pellet and place the tubes upside down in a rack for at least 2 min.

c. Add at least two drops of Fix to each tube. If necessary, add additional drops of Fix to adjust the density as judged by eye; the suspension should appear slightly cloudy.

d. Put a drop of cell suspension from a spare culture onto a clean slide using a clean Pasteur pipette.

e. Allow the slide(s) to dry and then check the degree of metaphase spreading using a microscope (phase contrast, if available). If the degree of metaphase spreading is appropriate, then continue with slide-making until enough slides are obtained per culture to ensure an adequate number of readable metaphases (at least two slides per culture should be made). If necessary, metaphase spreading can be aided using a humid atmosphere (e.g., slide exposure to hot water vapors from a 70°C water bath).

f. Once slide preparation is complete, add 5 mL Fix to all tubes and store refrigerated in case additional slides need to be made later, for example, in case the required number of readable metaphases is not available from any of the original slides.

7.10.4 Slide Staining: All Cell Types

1. Place all the slides in clean stainless steel slide racks.

2. Within 1−2 h of staining, dilute neat Giemsa (Gurr's Improved R66) with 9 parts purified water and filter it through cotton wool (absorbent cotton), or, when using a Büchner filtration system, through Whatman no. 1 filter paper.

3. Pour the filtered dilute stain into a staining trough and, immediately prior to use, remove any oxide film from the surface using paper tissue.

4. Rinse the slides in three changes of purified water for at least 1 min/change.

5. Stain all the slides for 15 min in Giemsa 10% staining solution. Remove the film at the surface of the stain before removing slides.

6. Rinse the slides in one change of purified water (in-house) for at least 1 min.

7. Wash the slides in running tap water for 2 min.

8. Rinse the slides in one change of purified water (in-house) for at least 1 min.

9. Drain the slides and allow them to air-dry.

10. Working in a fume hood, mount all the stained slides permanently with 50 mm coverslips using nonaqueous mountant (e.g., Cytoseal, DPX, Permount). There is no need to clear the slides in xylene prior to mounting.

11. Allow the mountant to harden at least overnight. The slides can be transferred to a warm cabinet at approximately 50°C at this point to accelerate further hardening of the mountant.

12. Slides should be subjected to a preliminary microscopic examination to determine which dose levels from each regimen will be examined for MI.

7.10.5 Selection of Slides for Detailed Examination

To ensure that appropriate cultures are chosen for detailed examination and results are produced for vehicle and positive controls, and that at least three dose levels of the test substance are examined for each dose regimen without having to examine an unnecessary number of slides, we recommend you use the following procedures.

7.10.5.1 Cell lines

Estimates of toxicity are based primarily on reductions in the expected increase in live cell numbers compared to the concurrent vehicle control over the period between dosing (start) and cell harvest (final). In accordance with OECD guidelines for the chromosome aberration test [36] and the closely related *in vitro* micronucleus test [37], either of two formulae can be used to calculate relevant values that are termed RICCs and RPD. These are calculated as:

$$RICC\ (\%) = [(\text{Increase in number of cells in treated cultures (final} - \text{starting))}$$
$$\div (\text{Increase in number of cells in control cultures (final} - \text{starting))}] \times 100\%$$

$$RPD\ (\%) = (\text{No. of Population doublings in treated cultures})$$
$$\div\ (\text{No. of Population doublings in control cultures}) \times 100$$

where:

$$\text{Population Doubling} = [\log(\text{Post} - \text{treatment cell number} \div \text{Initial cell number})] \div \log 2$$

Although OECD is rather strict in its definition that, in the case of toxicity, the highest dose examined should cause a $55 \pm 5\%$ reduction in one of these, the two calculations will yield somewhat different results, so you may find it convenient to report both. Note that OECD indicates that RPD may not be appropriate for prolonged exposures (greater than the standard 1.5 cell cycles).

For each dosing regimen, the highest test substance dose chosen for detailed examination should show moderate toxicity (i.e., approximately 55 [OECD G473] or 50% [ICH S2] reduction in RICC or RPD). In that case, the two adjacent lower doses should also be selected for analysis unless the lowest dose also shows toxicity, in which case the lowest dose examined should be the highest dose not showing obvious toxic effects.

In the absence of toxicity (or any severe reduction in the density of mitotic figures), the highest dose chosen for each treatment regimen should be the lowest precipitating concentration or, in the absence of precipitate, the highest dose level tested. The adjacent two lower dose levels should also be selected for detailed examination.

Slides from all vehicle control slides should be selected for potential analysis. One dose level of the positive control from each regimen should also be selected for examination that shows no or a slight reduction in RICC or RPD. This dose should cause a moderate, but not immediately obvious, increase in the incidence of aberrant cells.

7.10.5.2 HPBL selection of slides for provisional detailed examination

For HPBL, although the MI is later determined upon slide reading, slides for encoding and examination must be chosen prior to coding by preliminary screening under the microscope. When toxicity is seen, the highest test substance dose chosen for detailed examination should show approximately 50% reduction in the MI when compared to the vehicle. In that case, one dose higher and two doses lower that that target dose should be selected to ensure the appropriate range of toxicity is covered and should include one nontoxic dose. One dose level of the positive control should also be selected for examination that does not cause a substantial reduction in the density of mitotic cells. Slides from all vehicle control slides should be selected for potential analysis.

In the absence of any substantial reduction in the density of mitotic figures, the highest dose chosen for each treatment regimen should be the lowest precipitating concentration or, in the absence of precipitate, the highest dose level tested. The adjacent two lower dose levels should also be selected for detailed examination.

7.10.6 Slide Coding

Slides are randomized and encoded by someone other than the slide reader to minimize potential operator bias. Slide code numbers can be generated using the random function in Excel and then printed onto adhesive labels. The labels should obscure the culture number but not the experiment/study number. Each slide from the same culture should be given the same code number. As the slides are read, the reader should use consecutive letters to indicate on the label and in the study records which results were obtained from which replicate slides to facilitate review. Although a label could also be placed or wrapped around the back of the slide, we do not recommend that because it makes focusing more laborious.

7.10.7 Preliminary Slide Reading

In the case of HPBL, the MI is determined by examination of at least 500 cells per culture. In this case, the following totals are scored using bench-top tally counters:

- number of nuclei (including mitoses)
- number of apparently diploid metaphases (mitoses)
- number of endoreduplicated metaphases
- number of polyploid metaphases

- number or comment on the proportion of metaphases that might not be readable due to apparent test substance effects (e.g., centromeric disruption)
- comments on slide quality that might prohibit reading, such as if the total number of readable metaphases on the slide appears low (likely test substance effect) or if there is a large number of free chromosomes (preparation artifact)

The MI is calculated as the total number of metaphases÷number of nuclei (including mitotic nuclei).

Note that lymphocyte cultures contain a proportion of dead and degrading cells. To help standardize assessment of MI between different slide readers, small pyknotic (condensed and structureless) or faintly stained nuclei should not be included in the count of normal nuclei.

The responsible scientist should review these results before deciding which slides need to be subjected to detailed examination for chromosome aberration. At this point, it may be appropriate to remove or replace some dose levels in each treatment regimen. Occasionally, the test substance will affect the quality of the metaphase spreads or reduce the absolute number of readable metaphases without causing a substantial reduction in MI. In this case, the highest dose level subjected for detailed analysis may need to be lowered accordingly; detailed and appropriate justification for this course of action should be noted in the raw data by the study director and presented in the report, with representative photographic evidence if possible.

7.10.8 Slide Scoring

7.10.8.1 Basics

To produce reliable results, the slide reader should understand the basics of chromosome morphology and how aberrations are formed. Structural aberrations fall into two main categories:

- breaks (including deletions) result from double-strand breaks (DSB) in the DNA that are not repaired
- exchanges result from two or more DSBs with inappropriate rejoining/repair of the "sticky ends" within a single chromosome ("intrachanges") or between chromosomes ("interchanges")

The majority of clastogenic chemicals cause single-strand lesions that, during the course of DNA repair, can be converted to a DSB. If the DSB persist through the S phase, then it will be replicated and becomes evident as a chromatid break at metaphase [1]. In turn, if the chromatid break is not repaired, then it can be replicated, resulting in formation of a chromosome break. However, chromatid lesions are the major type of chemically induced damage seen using the standard sampling time of 1.5 cell cycles because they become evident at the first metaphase following induction [58]. Radiation and a few radiation-like chemicals can cause double-strand breakage directly; if this occurs after the S phase, then it will lead to chromatid lesions (breaks and exchanges); however, if it occurs prior to the S phase and is not repaired, then it will lead to chromosomal lesions involving both sister chromatids. Certain types of radiation-induced chromosome exchanges (notably dicentrics and centric rings) are accompanied by a paired fragment; in the case of chemicals, these derived aberrations are usually seen at the second metaphase after induction of damage and are not usually accompanied by fragments because acentric fragments tend to be lost during the first anaphase.

Gaps are achromatic lesions smaller than the width of one chromatid with minimum misalignment of the chromatid(s). Gaps are recorded but not scored as structural aberrations because they do not necessarily involve chromosome breakage. Note that identification criteria for gaps can vary between laboratories and countries. In addition, the width of the chromatids will depend on the degree of condensation, whereas not all chromatids have an equally clear outline. So, in a few cases, lesions classified as gaps may, in fact, be true breaks or even intrachanges.

Numerical aberrations (endoreduplication and polyploidy), if observed, are recorded and reported but are not necessarily indicative of genotoxicity. Apparent losses (in particular) or gains of one or two chromosomes in most metaphase figures are usually an artifact of slide preparation and therefore are not usually recorded or reported (i.e., the standard chromosome aberration test is not generally considered appropriate for detection of aneugenic events other than polyploidy).

Chemicals may have other observable effects on chromosomes (e.g., disruption of the centromere resulting in partial dissociation of the sister chromatids), which can be noted and reported as incidental observations. Although these may result in cytostatic or cytotoxic effects, they are not considered indicative of genotoxicity.

7.10.8.2 *Understanding the normal karyotype*

It is important to understand the structure of the individual chromosomes to facilitate identification of aberrations (e.g., chromosome breaks) and to avoid misclassification (e.g., secondary constrictions can appear similar to chromosome gaps); associations (attraction) of chromosomes via satellite bodies can give chromosome arrangements that appear similar to chromosome exchanges.

At metaphase, each pair of chromatids is joined by a constriction point called the centromere, which divides the chromosome into two arms. The short arm of the chromosome is termed the p (petite) arm and the longer arm is referred to as the q arm. The relative length of the chromosome and the ratio of the length of the p:q arms help identify the chromosome or the group of chromosomes.

- Metacentric chromosomes have the centromere near the center of the chromosome.
- Submetacentric means that the centromere is slightly off-center.
- Acrocentric means that the centromere is distant from the center.
- Telocentric means that the centromere is near one end of the chromosome.

The following descriptions refer primarily to diploid human metaphases (e.g., HPBL), but each laboratory should establish similar details (i.e., a chromosome map/karyotype) for any cell lines they use in the chromosome aberration test.

Diploid human cells contain 22 pairs of the autosomal chromosomes and a pair of sex chromosomes (XX for females and XY for males). Chromosomes are primarily identified and classified by size, with number 1 being the largest and chromosomes 22 and 21 being the smallest (they are approximately one-fourth the size of chromosome 1). The chromosomes are further classified into groups A to G:

- Group A (1−3): Large metacentrics; individually identifiable by size and p/q ratio
- Group B (4 and 5): Large submetacentrics
- Group C (6−12 and X): Medium-sized metacentrics and submetacentrics
- Group D (13−15): Medium-sized acrocentrics with satellites
- Group E (16−18): Shorter metacentric/submetacentrics
- Group F (19−20): Short metacentrics
- Group G (21, 22, and Y): Short acrocentrics with satellites on 21 and 22.

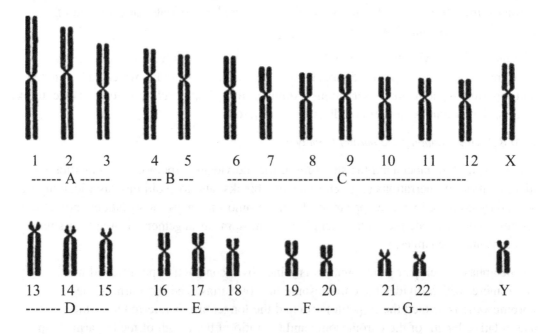

Some chromosomes often have associated morphological characteristics:

- Chromosomes 1, 9, and 16 secondary constrictions
- D and G group chromosomes satellite associations
- X and Y loss of centromeric activity
- Y chromosome is often slightly distorted

The slide reader needs to aware of these features (particularly secondary constrictions and satellite associations) to avoid misidentification of aberrations.

7.10.8.3 Routine scoring

If microscopes are equipped with a vernier scale stage, then slides should be placed on the stage in a standard orientation each time as defined in the SOP (e.g., label to the left).

The coded slides should be methodically scanned at medium power (e.g., 16× objective). Metaphase spreads that are unbroken and show good morphology are subjected to detailed analysis. Under high power (100× oil-immersion objective), the chromosomes should be well defined and should not be in an early C-anaphase state with completely separated chromatids. To avoid the analysis of cells with random chromosome loss due to preparation artifacts, only cells with the modal (cell lines) or diploid number of centromeres ±2 in a single stage of condensation should be scored. During counting of the chromosomes, any structural aberrations or gaps should be recorded. The vernier reading of aberrant metaphases should be recorded against the aberration details. Especially during training, it can greatly facilitate review of results and correction of any misidentification if the slide reader draws a simple diagram for each recorded aberrant metaphase, indicating the approximate location within the cell of the lesion together with a stick drawing of the lesion.

Readable metaphases are identified by the following criteria:

- chromosome/centromere number within ±2 of diploid (44−48 for HPBL) or modal number (for cell lines) in a single stage of condensation
- well-spread with minimal overlap of chromosomes and chromosome arms
- chromatids separate with centromere intact
- structure of chromosomes clear and well-defined

If, for any reason, the required total of 150 readable metaphases is not obtained, then additional slides should be prepared and examined from the reserved fixed material from that culture. Sometimes, due to technical problems with slides from a particular culture, it may be necessary to read additional metaphases from the other duplicate culture to reach the desired total of 300 readable metaphases per experimental point. In that case, this should be mentioned and justified in the report.

7.10.8.4 Classification

Metaphases are classified into the three following categories.

1. Normal metaphase (may have chromosome or chromatid gaps)
2. Those with structural aberrations
3. Numerical aberrations (polyploid, endoreduplicated, or hyperdiploid cells); these cells are not included in the readable metaphase totals

The main purpose of slide examination is to determine the proportion of metaphases with structural aberrations. A total of 300 readable metaphases (usually 150 per each of two cultures) per experimental point is examined for the presence of chromosome aberrations. Scoring less than this (e.g., when a clear positive response is evident) should be justified in the report and, ideally, the protocol.

The International System for Chromosome Aberration Nomenclature [59] is used to help classify structural aberrations into three main groups:

1. Chromosome
    a. breaks/deletions
    b. exchanges
2. Chromatid
    a. breaks/deletions
    b. exchanges
3. Other (complex damage)
    a. multiple (multiple aberrations in a single cell, e.g., >5)
    b. pulverized chromosome
    c. pulverized metaphase where some or all the chromosome is pulverized

The chromatid and chromosome categories are divided into two subcategories: breaks (result of a single DNA break) and exchanges (result of two or more breaks with inappropriate rejoining). These subcategories can be further subdivided, but that does not seem to provide any useful additional information in the case of routine testing. Representative examples of lesions in human lymphocytes are shown in Figure 7.3.

Although much of the theory of how the various aberrations are formed was developed early during the development of the test, recent technical advances including the use of specific chromosome paints have helped confirm the details [1]. An excellent review of the mode of formation of chromosome lesions, their identification, and artifacts that might be misinterpreted as aberrations was presented by Natalie Danford in 2012 [58], whose company offers training and outsourced slide reading for cytogenetic toxicology tests (see http://www.microptic.com/).

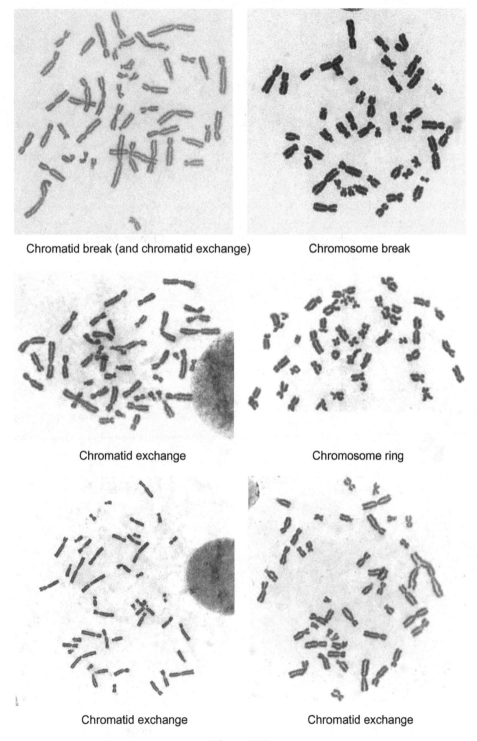

Figure 7.3
Structural aberrations and other lesions in human lymphocytes.

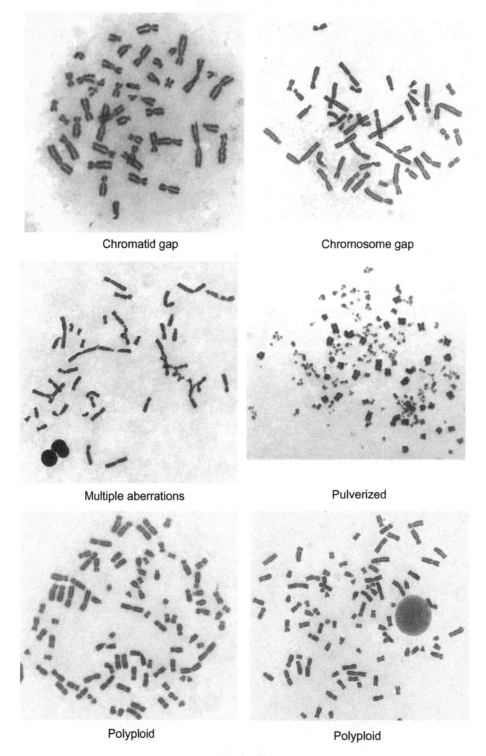

Chromatid gap

Chromosome gap

Multiple aberrations

Pulverized

Polyploid

Polyploid

Figure 7.3
(Continued).

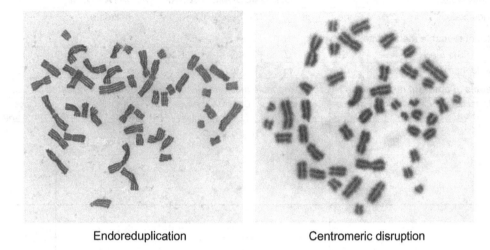

Endoreduplication   Centromeric disruption

Figure 7.3
(Continued).

Cytogenetic analysis has a subjective component, with even highly experienced analysts differing in their interpretation of the same cell. However, there are a number of instances in which misinterpretation can occur, most commonly resulting in a normal configuration being scored as aberrant, thus indicating the importance of recognizing secondary constrictions, satellites and satellite associations, and overlapping chromatids. There are also easily missed aberrations. Analysts need to be aware of these potential situations. Unfortunately, there is no substitute for experience.

Following is a list of potential misinterpretations analysts should be aware of:

Cause	Confused With
Crossing-over of sister chromatids	Dicentric
Satellite association: two chromosomes attracted by satellite regions	Dicentric or exchange
Secondary constriction	Dicentric
Secondary constriction	Gap
Chromosomes overlapping near centromeres	Exchange (quadriradial)
Chromosome twisting and overlapping	Chromosome ring

Note that in the case of diploid cells, counting the centromeres can be a useful way of distinguishing artifacts from true lesions. Note that all these true lesions (with the exception of gaps) are relatively rare exchange events.

An example of a scoring sheet is illustrated in Figure 7.4. In this case, the standardized abbreviations for aberrations largely coincide with or are a simplification of those used by the ISCN.

CHROMOSOME ABERRATION DATA FORM

Slide code: Page ____ of ____   Microscope ID: Init./date:

No. of readable metaphases analysed:

Slide read	A	B	C	D	E	F	G	H
Metaphase No.	to	to	to	to	to	to	To	To

Details of aberrant metaphases *Read 200 readable metaphases per slide code unless indicated by SD.*

Metaphase No.	Vernier reading	No. of chromo-somes	Chromatid-type		Chromosome-type		Mult	Others			Gaps	
			ctb	cte	csb	cse		pvz cs	pvz cell		ctg	csg
Total, all slides this code												
Total aberrant cells all slides this code No., exclude cells with only gaps & numerical aberrations												

Ctb	chromatid break	cse	chromosome exchange	pvz cell	pulverized cell
cte	chromatid exchange	mult	>5 aberrations	ctg	chromatid gap
csb	chromosome break	pvz cs	pulverised chromosome	csg	chromosome gap

Numerical aberrations or potential evidence of cell cycle disruption & Total number seen

	Slide replicate and Vernier reading (first 10 observed)										Total
Endoreduplication											
Polyploidy											
Centromeric disruption											
Other _____											

Comments by slide reader:

Reviewed by/date:_____

Figure 7.4

Chromosome aberration scoring sheet example.

7.11 Interpretation of Results

7.11.1 Evaluation of Toxicity

Toxicity is expressed in terms of percentage of inhibition of cell division, such as reduction of RICC or RPD in the case of cell lines and reduction in MI relative to the concurrent control for lymphocytes. Where substantial toxicity is seen (e.g., >60%) any aberration values obtained (if any) would not normally be reported or, if used to support any other findings, would be reported in parentheses.

7.11.2 Validity of the Study

For an assay to be considered valid, the vehicle/negative control incidences of metaphases showing structural chromosome aberrations should lie within or close to the historical control range, whereas the positive controls should produce a statistically significant (see next section) and substantial increase in the incidence of aberrant cells with values above the 95% tolerance limits of the laboratory historical negative/vehicle control range. The dose level reported for the positive control in each regimen should not have caused excessive toxicity (>60%).

Valid results should have been obtained for at least three dose levels of the test substance for each treatment regimen. The high dose should be justifiable in terms of the standard limit, toxicity, precipitate, or obvious effect on the quality or absolute number of metaphases, whereas the lowest dose examined should show little or no toxicity. When valid results have not been obtained for a particular regimen, it would normally be appropriate to repeat that part of the experiment; in which case, the original results do not need to be reported in detail. For repeat tests, the number of dose levels can normally be reduced based on results obtained in the initial test. It may also be appropriate to consider modifying the dose interval for a repeat test to obtain appropriate levels of toxicity.

7.11.3 Criteria for Negative/Positive/Equivocal Outcome

Although OECD TG473 mentions the use of statistical analysis for interpretation of results, it does not give any firm guidance on how those methods should be applied. Statistical analysis, when used, should only be applied to the main endpoint of the test (i.e., the proportion of metaphases showing structural aberrations). The statistical methods used assume that the experimental unit of variance is the cell, which means that, with a minimum of 300 metaphases being examined per experimental point, even quite small increases above control levels can lead to calls of statistical significance. However, in reality, small differences can result from slight variations between cultures (e.g., somewhat lower than normal incidences of aberrations being obtained for the control group in a particular dose regimen). In addition, in a standard experiment, at least nine statistical comparisons can be made between the vehicle control and test substance groups. Therefore, applying an arbitrary critical *P*-value of 0.05 will result in at least one inappropriate call of statistical significance in approximately 50% of routine experiments as a result of chance variation. For more details, see the Statistical Analysis section of the General Recommendations chapter in this book. In summary, care should be taken to avoid inappropriate use of statistical methods and unreasonable conclusions. The interpretation criteria described here are suggested to avoid these situations.

- No statistical analysis will be performed unless the mean incidence of aberrant metaphases for any treatment with the test substance is above the expected range (i.e., beyond the upper 95% tolerance limit) for the laboratory vehicle/negative historical control database. If values are obtained beyond this limit at dose levels that are not excessively toxic, then the results from replicate cultures will be combined and compared to the results obtained for the concurrent vehicle control group from the same treatment regime using Fisher's exact test. A positive point is generally defined as a statistically significant increase ($P \leq 0.01$) in the incidence of aberrant cells for a treatment group compared with the concurrent control group, which is also above the laboratory historical negative control range (95% limits) and occurs at a dose that does not greatly exceed a 50% reduction in MI.
- The test substance is generally considered to have shown evidence of genotoxicity if there are at least two positive points. Evidence for a dose relation is also taken into account, although a dose-related response is not necessarily expected because higher doses of genotoxic agents can inhibit cell-cycle progression.
- A negative result is indicated where mean incidences of aberrant metaphase cells for the cultures treated with the test substance are within the historical control range or are not statistically significantly greater than the concurrent vehicle control.
- An equivocal response is obtained when the results do not meet the criteria specified for a positive or negative response.

Fisher's exact test can be performed in SAS or similar statistical package that has been approved by the test facility. Values should be entered in terms of absolute numbers of aberrant and nonaberrant metaphases. For example, for a control group with 3 aberrant and 297 nonaberrant metaphases and a treatment group with 13 aberrant and 287 nonaberrant metaphases, $P = 0.0098$ using a one-tailed Fisher exact test, which would be considered just significant provided the incidence for the treated group (4.3%), is above the upper tolerance limit for the laboratory historical vehicle/negative control. It may be convenient to produce a look-up table (which can be incorporated into an SOP) to avoid having to run the test on each occasion, as shown in Table 7.2 below.

Table 7.2: Fisher's exact test for 300 observations per group

		Incidences in the Control Group for 300 Observations													
	0	1	2	3	4	5	6	7	8	9	10	11	12	13	14
0	-	1.00000	1.00000	1.00000	1.00000	1.00000	1.00000	1.00000	1.00000	1.00000	1.00000	1.00000	1.00000	1.00000	1.00000
1	0.50000	0.75042	0.87563	0.93813	0.96927	0.98476	0.99246	0.99627	0.99816	0.99910	0.99956	0.99978	0.99989	0.99995	0.99997
2	0.24958	0.50000	0.68813	0.81355	0.89180	0.93860	0.96575	0.98117	0.98977	0.99449	0.99706	0.99845	0.99918	0.99957	0.99978
3	0.12437	0.31187	0.50000	0.65704	0.77481	0.85712	0.91180	0.94678	0.96849	0.98165	0.98946	0.99402	0.99665	0.99814	0.99897
4	0.06187	0.18645	0.34296	0.50000	0.63764	0.74775	0.83019	0.88888	0.92902	0.95560	0.97273	0.98352	0.99019	0.99423	0.99665
5	0.03073	0.10820	0.22519	0.36236	0.50000	0.62408	0.72749	0.80860	0.86922	0.91278	0.94306	0.96354	0.97704	0.98577	0.99130
6	0.01524	0.06140	0.14288	0.25225	0.37592	0.50000	0.61394	0.71160	0.79081	0.85221	0.89803	0.93112	0.95436	0.97028	0.98095
7	0.00754	0.03425	0.08825	0.16981	0.27251	0.38606	0.50000	0.60598	0.69871	0.77585	0.83736	0.88464	0.91986	0.94537	0.96341
8	0.00373	0.01883	0.05322	0.11112	0.19140	0.28840	0.39402	0.50000	0.59953	0.68799	0.76306	0.82427	0.87247	0.90930	0.93668
9	0.00184	0.01023	0.03151	0.07098	0.13078	0.20919	0.30129	0.40047	0.50000	0.59416	0.67890	0.75196	0.81263	0.86138	0.89942
10	0.00090	0.00551	0.01835	0.04440	0.08722	0.14779	0.22415	0.31201	0.40584	0.50000	0.58960	0.67106	0.74221	0.80221	0.85124
11	0.00044	0.00294	0.01054	0.02727	0.05694	0.10197	0.16264	0.23694	0.32110	0.41040	0.50000	0.58568	0.66422	0.73357	0.79281
12	0.00022	0.00155	0.00598	0.01648	0.03646	0.06888	0.11536	0.17573	0.24804	0.32894	0.41432	0.50000	0.58225	0.65817	0.72585
13	0.00011	0.00082	0.00335	0.00981	0.02296	0.04564	0.08014	0.12753	0.18737	0.25779	0.33578	0.41775	0.50000	0.57922	0.65279
14	0.00005	0.00043	0.00186	0.00577	0.01423	0.02972	0.05463	0.09070	0.13862	0.19779	0.26643	0.34183	0.42078	0.50000	0.57653
15	0.00003	0.00022	0.00103	0.00335	0.00870	0.01905	0.03659	0.06332	0.10058	0.14876	0.20719	0.27415	0.34721	0.42347	0.50000
16	0.00001	0.00011	0.00056	0.00193	0.00525	0.01203	0.02412	0.04345	0.07167	0.10981	0.15808	0.21571	0.28112	0.35204	0.42589
17	<.00001	0.00006	0.00030	0.00110	0.00313	0.00750	0.01566	0.02934	0.05021	0.07965	0.11845	0.16666	0.22349	0.28743	0.35642
18	<.00001	0.00003	0.00016	0.00062	0.00185	0.00461	0.01003	0.01952	0.03462	0.05682	0.08726	0.12654	0.17459	0.23061	0.29318
19	<.00001	0.00002	0.00009	0.00035	0.00108	0.00281	0.00634	0.01280	0.02352	0.03991	0.06325	0.09451	0.13413	0.18195	0.23717
20	<.00001	<.00001	0.00005	0.00019	0.00062	0.00169	0.00396	0.00829	0.01576	0.02763	0.04516	0.06949	0.10141	0.14125	0.18879
21	<.00001	<.00001	0.00002	0.00011	0.00036	0.00101	0.00245	0.00530	0.01042	0.01886	0.03178	0.05034	0.07551	0.10798	0.14796
22	<.00001	<.00001	0.00001	0.00006	0.00020	0.00059	0.00150	0.00335	0.00681	0.01271	0.02206	0.03595	0.05542	0.08133	0.11423
23	<.00001	<.00001	<.00001	0.00003	0.00011	0.00035	0.00091	0.00210	0.00439	0.00846	0.01511	0.02533	0.04011	0.06039	0.08693
24	<.00001	<.00001	<.00001	0.00002	0.00006	0.00020	0.00054	0.00130	0.00281	0.00556	0.01023	0.01762	0.02864	0.04423	0.06524
25	<.00001	<.00001	<.00001	<.00001	0.00004	0.00012	0.00032	0.00080	0.00177	0.00362	0.00684	0.01211	0.02020	0.03198	0.04831
26	<.00001	<.00001	<.00001	<.00001	0.00002	0.00007	0.00019	0.00048	0.00111	0.00233	0.00452	0.00822	0.01407	0.02283	0.03532
27	<.00001	<.00001	<.00001	<.00001	0.00001	0.00004	0.00011	0.00029	0.00069	0.00148	0.00296	0.00552	0.00969	0.01611	0.02551
28	<.00001	<.00001	<.00001	<.00001	<.00001	0.00002	0.00006	0.00017	0.00042	0.00093	0.00192	0.00367	0.00660	0.01123	0.01821
29	<.00001	<.00001	<.00001	<.00001	<.00001	0.00001	0.00004	0.00010	0.00026	0.00058	0.00123	0.00241	0.00444	0.00775	0.01285

Incidences in the Treated Group for 300 Observations

(Continued)

Table 7.2: (Continued)

					Incidences in the Control Group for 300 Observations										
	0	1	2	3	4	5	6	7	8	9	10	11	12	13	14
30	<.00001	<.00001	<.00001	<.00001	<.00001	<.00001	0.00002	0.00006	0.00015	0.00036	0.00078	**0.00157**	**0.00296**	**0.00529**	**0.00897**
31	<.00001	<.00001	<.00001	<.00001	<.00001	<.00001	0.00001	0.00004	0.00009	0.00022	0.00049	**0.00101**	**0.00196**	**0.00357**	**0.00619**
32	<.00001	<.00001	<.00001	<.00001	<.00001	<.00001	<.00001	0.00002	0.00006	0.00014	0.00031	0.00065	**0.00128**	**0.00239**	**0.00423**
33	<.00001	<.00001	<.00001	<.00001	<.00001	<.00001	<.00001	0.00001	0.00003	0.00008	0.00019	0.00041	0.00083	**0.00158**	**0.00286**
34	<.00001	<.00001	<.00001	<.00001	<.00001	<.00001	<.00001	<.00001	0.00002	0.00005	0.00012	0.00026	0.00053	**0.00104**	**0.00192**
35	<.00001	<.00001	<.00001	<.00001	<.00001	<.00001	<.00001	<.00001	<.00001	0.00003	0.00007	0.00016	0.00034	0.00068	**0.00127**
36	<.00001	<.00001	<.00001	<.00001	<.00001	<.00001	<.00001	<.00001	<.00001	0.00002	0.00004	0.00010	0.00021	0.00044	0.00084
37	<.00001	<.00001	<.00001	<.00001	<.00001	<.00001	<.00001	<.00001	<.00001	0.00001	0.00003	0.00006	0.00013	0.00028	0.00055
38	<.00001	<.00001	<.00001	<.00001	<.00001	<.00001	<.00001	<.00001	<.00001	<.00001	0.00002	0.00004	0.00008	0.00018	0.00035
39	<.00001	<.00001	<.00001	<.00001	<.00001	<.00001	<.00001	<.00001	<.00001	<.00001	<.00001	0.00002	0.00005	0.00011	0.00023
40	<.00001	<.00001	<.00001	<.00001	<.00001	<.00001	<.00001	<.00001	<.00001	<.00001	<.00001	<.00001	0.00003	0.00007	0.00014
41	<.00001	<.00001	<.00001	<.00001	<.00001	<.00001	<.00001	<.00001	<.00001	<.00001	<.00001	<.00001	0.00002	0.00004	0.00009
42	<.00001	<.00001	<.00001	<.00001	<.00001	<.00001	<.00001	<.00001	<.00001	<.00001	<.00001	<.00001	0.00001	0.00003	0.00006
43	<.00001	<.00001	<.00001	<.00001	<.00001	<.00001	<.00001	<.00001	<.00001	<.00001	<.00001	<.00001	<.00001	0.00002	0.00004
44	<.00001	<.00001	<.00001	<.00001	<.00001	<.00001	<.00001	<.00001	<.00001	<.00001	<.00001	<.00001	<.00001	<.00001	0.00002
45	<.00001	<.00001	<.00001	<.00001	<.00001	<.00001	<.00001	<.00001	<.00001	<.00001	<.00001	<.00001	<.00001	<.00001	0.00001
>45	<.00001	<.00001	<.00001	<.00001	<.00001	<.00001	<.00001	<.00001	<.00001	<.00001	<.00001	<.00001	<.00001	<.00001	<.00001

One sided *P*-values calculated using SAS versions 8.1 or 9.2. Values in bold are between 0.001 and 0.01.

7.11.4 Interpretation of Numerical Aberrations

Comments on any apparent treatment-related increases in polyploidy/endoreduplication should be made in the report. Although these may be indicative of disruption of cell-cycle progression or cell division, they are seen quite often in *in vitro* systems and are not usually indicative of genotoxic potential, so they should not be given any special weight; we suggest you include any comments about them under the title *Incidental observations* in the study report. Under some circumstances it may be appropriate to confirm the absence of related aneugenic effects *in vivo* using a rodent micronucleus test.

7.11.5 Unexpected and Borderline Results

In these cases the study director should always review the slides to check for potential artifacts and confirm the accuracy of slide reading. Borderline apparent increases in chromosome damage can occur as a result of chance variation or indirectly as a result of departures from normal physiological conditions.

The study director may consider various courses of action:

- Accept the results and report them accordingly
- Rereading of the slides by a second slide reader
- Making and reading of additional slides to clarify borderline results
- Performing a confirmatory test using the affected dose regimen, usually over a narrower dose range and using a narrower dose interval. If the original results does not fully meet the criteria for a positive result and the confirmatory test shows no evidence of clastogenicity, then the final conclusion would be negative (i.e., that the test substance is not considered to have shown evidence of genotoxicity in the test system). The study director should also consider the possibility of an error or event (unrelated to the test substance) that might have caused an unrepeatable result. Whatever the situation, it is not advisable to conclude that a test substance is genotoxic on the basis of apparent increases in the incidence of aberrant cells at a single experimental point without supporting evidence.

Usually the study director will discuss any proposed additional work (other than preliminary or standard checks) with the study monitor before producing a protocol amendment to describe the reasons for the additional work, the work itself, and the final decision criteria.

7.11.6 Follow-up In Vivo Testing

In cases where there is evidence of clastogenicity or induction of numerical aberrations, it may be appropriate to establish the relevance of the result using a rodent micronucleus test (provided systemic exposure is expected), sometimes in combination with examination of at least one other potential target and relevant organ (e.g., duodenum and liver using the comet assay).

7.11.7 Reporting

Readers should refer to the General Recommendations chapter of this book to establish the general layout and contents of the report. The experimental completion date is usually defined as the last day on which results were obtained directly from the test system; in the case of the chromosome aberration test, that would normally be the date of completion of slide reading. In accord with OECD TG473 and good practice, other specific details that should be mentioned include:

- methods used for assessing pH (not usually necessary unless indicator in the medium shows color change), osmolality, and precipitation following addition of test formulation to the culture medium
- any adjustment of test substance formulation to avoid pH changes
- Cells:
    - type and source of cells
    - karyotype features and suitability of the cell type used
    - modal number of chromosomes, for cell lines
    - methods of ensuring absence of mycoplasma for cell lines
    - information on cell-cycle time, doubling time, or proliferation index
    - number and sex of blood donors, age, whole blood or separated lymphocytes, mitogen used
    - number of passages, if available, for cell lines
    - methods for maintenance of cell lines
- Test conditions:
    - culture conditions, cell density at initiation, culture vessel
    - concentration of test chemical expressed as final concentration in the culture medium (e.g., μg or mg/mL or mM)
    - Rationale for selection of vehicle
    - Dose volumes
    - rationale for selection of concentrations and number of cultures, including, for example, toxicity results and solubility limitations
    - composition of media, CO_2 concentration if applicable, humidity level
    - incubation temperature
    - incubation time
    - duration of treatment
    - identity of the metaphase-arresting substance, concentration, and duration of exposure
    - harvest time after treatment

- cell density at seeding, if appropriate
- type and composition of metabolic activation system (source of S9, method of preparation of the S9 mix, the concentration or volume of S9 mix, and S9 in the final culture medium, quality controls of S9)
- positive and negative control substances, final concentrations for each condition of treatment
- methods of slide preparation and staining technique used
- criteria for acceptability of assays
- criteria for determining readability of metaphases
- classification system for aberrations and gaps
- number of metaphases analyzed
- methods for the measurement of toxicity
- any supplementary information relevant to cytotoxicity and method used
- criteria for considering studies as positive, negative, or equivocal
- Results:
  - cell density at start of treatment and at harvest (cell lines)
  - cytotoxicity measurements (e.g., RPD, RICC, MI) and other observations, if any
  - results of pH or osmolality checks, if any
  - change in color of medium, signs of precipitation, and point it was observed plus similar information on pH or osmolality, if assessed
  - results of chemical analysis (if performed) together with any other evidence supporting exposure of the cells to the test substance
  - rationale for selection of dose levels for analysis
  - changes in ploidy (polyploid cells and cells with endoreduplicated chromosomes, given separately), if seen
  - number of cells scored, number of cells with chromosomal aberrations, and type of chromosomal aberrations given separately for each treated and control culture, including and excluding gaps
  - statistical analysis (indicate one-tailed) and P-values, if any
  - concentration-response relationship, if any
  - concurrent negative (solvent) and positive control results (concentrations and solvents)
  - historical negative (solvent) and positive control data, with ranges, means, standard deviations, and 95% control limits for the distribution, as well as the number of experimental points
- Discussion of the results
- Conclusions
- References

Note that it is important to discuss any observations that support exposure of the cells to the test substance (e.g., precipitate and toxicity), especially when no supporting formulation analysis has been presented in the report.

7.11.7.1 Results tables

Aberrations and related values (incidental observations) are reported as integer values as in Table 7.3. Typically, MI and percentage of aberrations are reported to one decimal place, whereas RMI is reported to the nearest percentage (e.g., 83%). If statistical analysis is

Table 7.3: Report appendix: tabulated results for individual cultures

Treatment	Concentration, µg/mL	MI	No. of Cells Examined	No. of Aberrant Cells	b	e	B	E	Other	g	G	P	N	C
(No. of Aberrations)					b	e	B	E	Other	g	G	P	N	C
4-h treatment in the absence of S9 (0S9)														
Water	—	11.2	150	1	0	0	1	0	0	0	0	0	0	0
		11.0	150	1	1	0	0	0	0	1	0	0	0	0
Test item	128	12.6	150	1	0	0	1	0	0	2	0	0	0	0
		12.0	150	2	2	0	0	0	0	1	0	0	0	0
	256	11.8	150	2	2	0	0	0	0	0	0	0	0	0
		12.0	150	0	0	0	0	0	0	0	0	0	0	0
	500	5.8	150	3	2	0	1	0	0	1	0	0	0	0
		8.2	150	2	1	0	1	0	0	0	0	0	0	0
MMC	0.1	12.2	150	15	9	2	5	0	0	7	3	0	0	0
		10.0	150	13	9	1	3	1	0	8	2	0	0	0
4-h treatment in the presence of S9 (+S9)														
Water	—	9.6	150	0	0	0	0	0	0	2	0	0	0	0
		10.0	150	1	1	0	0	0	0	2	0	0	0	0
Test item	128	10.6	150	2	1	0	1	0	0	3	0	0	0	0
		9.2	150	0	0	0	0	0	0	2	0	0	0	0
	256	11.2	150	4	3	0	1	0	0	5	0	1	0	0
		11.0	150	2	1	0	1	0	0	1	0	0	0	0
	500	12.4	150	1	0	0	1	0	0	0	0	0	0	0
		11.8	150	3	3	0	0	0	0	2	0	0	0	0
CP	6	6.6	150	31	34	4	3	0	0	16	3	0	0	0
		5.2	150	23	27	2	4	1	0	10	2	0	0	1
21-h treatment in the absence of S9 (0S9)														
Water	—	12.4	150	3	2	0	1	0	0	2	0	0	0	0
		12.0	150	4	2	0	2	0	0	2	0	0	0	0
Test item	128	8.8	150	4	3	0	1	0	0	4	1	0	0	1
		11.0	150	3	0	0	3	0	0	7	1	0	0	1
	256	10.2	150	0	0	0	0	0	0	4	0	0	0	0
		12.0	150	1	1	0	0	0	0	3	0	0	0	0
	500	6.0	150	3	2	0	1	0	0	7	0	0	0	0
		5.8	150	5	2	0	3	0	0	9	0	0	0	0
MMC	0.05	12.4	150	12	6	1	5	0	0	12	3	0	0	0
		12.0	150	10	5	1	5	0	0	9	2	0	0	0

MI, Mitotic Index; b, e, g, Chromatid break, exchange, gap; B, E, G, Chromosome break, exchange, gap; Other, includes pulverized chromosomes and cells with >5 aberrations; P, Polyploidy; E, Endoreduplication; C, Centromeric disruption.
[a] g, G, P, and C are excluded from the calculation of % aberrant cells.

Table 7.4: Example summary table: HPBL

Treatment	Concentration, μg/mL	MI	RMI %	No. of Cells Examined	Aberrant Cells %	Aberrant Cells ρ	b	e	B	E	Other	g	G	P	N	C
4-h treatment in the absence of S9 (0S9)																
water	-	11.1	100	300	0.7		1	0	1	0	0	1	0	0	0	0
Test item	128	12.3	111	300	1.0		2	0	1	0	0	3	0	0	0	0
	256	11.9	107	300	0.7		2	0	0	0	0	0	0	0	0	0
	500[b]	7.0	63	300	1.7		3	0	2	0	0	1	0	0	0	0
MMC	0.1	11.1	100	300	9.3[c]	<0.01	18	3	8	1	0	15	5	0	0	0
4-h treatment in the presence of S9 (+S9)																
water	-	9.8	100	300	0.3		1	0	0	0	0	4	0	0	0	0
Test item	128	9.9	101	300	0.7		1	0	1	0	0	5	0	0	0	0
	256	11.1	113	300	2.0		4	0	2	0	0	6	0	1	0	0
	500	12.1	123	300	1.3		3	0	1	0	0	2	0	0	0	0
CP	6.0	5.9	60	300	18.0[c]	<0.01	61	6	7	1	0	26	5	0	0	1
21-h treatment in the absence of S9 (0S9)																
water	-	12.1	100	300	2.3		4	0	3	0	0	4	0	0	0	0
Test item	128	9.9	82	300	2.3		3	0	4	0	0	11	2	0	0	2
	256	11.1	92	300	0.3		1	0	0	0	0	7	0	0	0	0
	500[b]	5.9	49	300	2.7		4	0	4	0	0	16	0	0	0	0
MMC	0.05	12.2	101	300	7.3[c]	0.34	11	2	10	0	0	21	5	0	0	0

MI, Mitotic Index; RMI, Relative Mitotic Index (vehicle = 100%); b, e, g, Chromatid break, exchange, gap; B, E, G, Chromosome break, exchange, gap; Other, includes pulverized chromosomes and cells with >5 aberrations; P, Polyploidy; N, Endoreduplication; C, Centromeric disruption; P, 1-sided percentage probability using Fisher exact test where ≤ 1% is considered significant.

[a]g, G, P, N, and C are excluded from the calculation of % aberrant cells.

[b]Slight yellow precipitate seen at the end of the treatment period is consistent with appearance of the test substance.

[c]Substantial increase compared to concurrent vehicle control beyond 95% limits of the historical negative control range.

performed, then probability values may be reported to two significant figures; critical limits are expressed to one significant figure (e.g., $P = 0.058$ and $P < 0.01$).

It is useful to include a single table summarizing the most important results obtained in the test as well as the results of any statistical analysis, as in Table 7.4.

In this theoretical case, the test substance was a pharmaceutical; therefore, the top dose chosen for detailed analysis was the standard limit, although precipitation and toxicity were also seen at this level in the absence of S9 mix. The test substance has not shown any evidence of clastogenicity/genotoxicity, whereas the positive controls have caused substantial and highly significant increases in the incidence of metaphases with structural chromosome aberrations confirming the sensitivity of the test and the efficacy of the S9 mix.

Tables showing results in more detail are best presented as appendices, as shown in the corresponding Table 7.3.

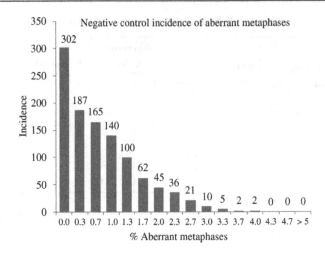

Figure 7.5

Example layout of theoretical laboratory historical control results. The laboratory historical mean incidence of aberrant metaphases for negative/vehicle control cultures is 0.83%, with a population standard deviation of 0.7; 95% of observed mean values lie within the range of 0−2.2%. These results are for 1077 groups of duplicate cultures with a total of 300 metaphases being analyzed for each group and they are taken from QA-audited experiments performed during the period from April 2014 to April 2016 and completed prior to the present study.

7.11.8 Historical Control Results

Relevant historical control results should be presented in the report to:

1. confirm the proficiency of the laboratory
2. demonstrate that negative and positive control results obtained for the present study are within normal limits and meet acceptance criteria specified in the protocol
3. help determine whether results for the test substance are within normal (tolerance) limits for unaffected cultures as defined in evaluation criteria specified in the protocol.

As indicated by OECD TG473, it is not sufficient to just list the upper and lower limits of the range of control values; the report must also show means, standard deviations, and 95% control limits for the distribution, as well as the number of experimental points (groups). It is particularly important to show the distribution for the negative/vehicle database because of evaluation criteria mentioned. The best way to summarize historical control data and their distribution is in a graphical form that can be included in an appendix to the report as per Figure 7.5.

7.11.9 Testing of Volatile and Gaseous Compounds

When testing volatile or gaseous chemicals, exposure should take place in sealed culture tubes to ensure adequate exposure. In the case of HPBL, this can be accomplished by transferring the cultures (with S9 mix where appropriate) to gas-tight 24 mL glass anaerobic culture tubes (Bellco Glass) immediately prior to dosing. Note that positive controls do not need to be transferred unless you decide to include gaseous or volatile positive controls. Seal the tubes with gas-impermeable, butyl rubber septum (injectable) stoppers and aluminum seals; when appropriate, perform subsequent procedures in a fume hood. Volatile liquids or dilutions of them can be injected directly through the septa.

In the case of gases, an adequate volume of gas should be transferred to a gas-tight (e.g., Tedlar®) bag with an injectable septum. An appropriate volume of air is then removed from each tube using a syringe fitted with a fine needle just prior to dosing. This volume of air is calculated as $19 \text{ mL} \times E\% \div (100\% - E\%)$, where E is the target concentration of gas and 19 mL is the approximate volume of air in the culture tube. A gas syringe fitted with a fine needle is used to remove the calculated required volume of gas (calculated as $19 \text{ mL} \times E\%$) from the gas bag via the injectable septum, and then this is injected directly into the culture tube. In the case of gases, we recommend a maximum dose of 50% v/v, in which case 19 mL air is removed (effectively half) and replaced by 9.5 mL gas.

In the case of volatiles and gases, culture tubes are then incubated at 37°C for the normal period and then vented in the fume hood before transferring back to standard culture tubes (i.e., after 4 h for Sets 1 and 2 and after 19 h and immediately prior to addition of colcemid in the case of Set 3). Cultures are then processed as usual.

7.12 Screening Versions of the Test

The methods described in the main body of this chapter largely relate to routine test performance using 5 mL cultures, although the HPBL test procedures section also describes the use of 1 mL cultures in 4 mL glass vials. Similarly, 1 mL cultures can be used with adherent cell lines like CHO; in this case, they can be grown in 24-well plates that make dosing and handling easier. The main advantage of these miniaturized versions is that they can meet all the requirements of the OECD test guidelines, including the specified upper concentration limit, while using one-fifth the amount of test substance and other components, including S9. The disadvantage is that the cell yield is proportionately lower, which may mean that the specified number of readable metaphases (300 per experimental point) is not always available for analysis, particularly at moderately toxic dose levels. Miniaturized versions are therefore suitable for non-GLP screening, especially when test substance supply is limited, but they are not necessarily suitable for routine regulatory testing. If you intend to set-up the HPBL in a different culture format, then you should optimize the cell density and culture volume to maximize the yield of mitotic cells.

7.13 Automation

Automatic (computerized robotic) metaphase finder systems that can capture images and stage locations of cells potentially suited for detailed analysis are available (e.g., Metafer http://www.metasystems-international.com/metafer/msearch). In this case, the slide reader reviews the images and selects those cells that appear suitable for analysis, and the system automatically moves the slide on the microscope to the appropriate location. Some systems can also automatically rank metaphases in terms of quality and can determine MI automatically. Therefore, they greatly reduce scanning and slide reading time. However, they are necessarily expensive, so they should only be purchased when throughput merits the expenditure.

References

[1]   Obe G, Pfeiffer P, Savage JR, Johannes C, Goedecke W, Jeppesen P, et al. Chromosomal aberrations: formation, identification and distribution. Mutat Res 2002;504(1−2):17−36.
[2]   Natarajan AT. Chromosome aberrations: past, present and future. Mutat Res 2002;504:3−16.
[3]   Muller HJ. The production of mutations by X-rays. Proc Natl Acad Sci USA 1928;14(9):714−16.
[4]   Sax K, Sax HJ. Radiomimetic beverages, drugs, and mutagens. Proc Natl Acad Sci USA 1966;55 (6):1431−5.
[5]   Kirkland D. Chromosome aberration testing in genetic toxicology-past, present and future. Mutat Res 1998;404(1−2):173−85.
[6]   Ford CE, Hamerton JL. A colchicine, hypotonic citrate, squash sequence for mammalian chromosomes. Stain Technol 1956;31(6):247−51.
[7]   Rothfels KH, Siminovitch L. An air-drying technique for flattening chromosomes in mammalian cells grown *in vitro*. Stain Technol 1958;33:73−7.
[8]   Moorhead PS, Nowell PC, Mellman WJ, Battips DM, Hungerford DA. Chromosome preparations of leukocytes cultured from human peripheral blood. Exp Cell Res 1960;20:613−16.
[9]   Nowell PC. Mitotic inhibition and chromosome damage by mitomycin in human leukocyte cultures. Exp Cell Res 1964;33:445−9.
[10] Shaw MW, Cohen MM. Chromosome exchanges in human leukocytes induced by mitomycin C. Genetics 1965;51:181−90.
[11] Natarajan AT, Tates AD, van Buul PPW, Meijers, de Vogel N. Cytogenetic effects of mutagens/carcinogens after activation in a microsomal system *in vitro*, I. Induction of chromosomal aberrations and sister chromatid exchanges by diethylnitrosamine (DEN) and dimethylnitrosamine (DMN) in CHO cells in the presence of rat-liver microsomes. Mutat Res 1976;37(1):83−90.
[12] Matsuoka A, Hayashi M, Ishidate Jr M. Chromosomal aberration tests on 29 chemicals combined with S9 mix. Mutat Res 1979;66(3):277−90.
[13] Ishidate Jr M, Odashima S. Chromosome tests with 134 compounds on Chinese hamster cells *in vitro*—a screening for chemical carcinogens. Mutat Res 1977;48(3−4):337−53.
[14] Ishidate Jr M, Sofuni T, Yoshikawa K, Hayashi M, Nohmi T, Sawada M, et al. Primary mutagenicity screening of food additives currently used in Japan. Food Chem Toxicol 1984; 22(8):623−36.
[15] Ivett JL, Brown BM, Rodgers C, Anderson BE, Resnick MA, Zeiger E. Chromosomal aberrations and sister chromatid exchange tests in Chinese hamster ovary cells *in vitro*. IV. Results with 15 chemicals. Environ Mol Mutagen 1989;14(3):165−87.

[16] Loveday KS, Lugo MH, Resnick MA, Anderson BE, Zeiger E. Chromosome aberration and sister chromatid exchange tests in Chinese hamster ovary cells *in vitro*: II. Results with 20 chemicals. Environ Mol Mutagen 1989;13:60–94.

[17] Loveday KS, Anderson BE, Resnick BE, Zeiger E, Holden HE. Chromosome aberration and sister chromatid exchange tests in Chinese hamster ovary cells *in vitro*. V: results with 46 chemicals. Environ Mol Mutagen 1990;16(4):273–303.

[18] Gulati DK, Witt K, Anderson B, Zeiger E, Shelby MD. Chromosome aberration and sister chromatid exchange tests in Chinese hamster ovary cells *in vitro*. III. Results with 27 chemicals. Environ Mol Mutagen 1989;13(2):133–93.

[19] Sofuni T, Matsuoka A, Sawada M, Ishidate Jr M, Zeiger E, Shelby MD. A comparison of chromosome aberration induction by 25 compounds tested by two Chinese hamster cell (CHL and CHO) systems in culture. Mutat Res 1990;241:175–213.

[20] Shelby MD, Sofuni T. Toxicology testing requirements and the US–Japan collaborative study on *in vitro* tests for chromosomal aberrations. Environ Health Perspect 1991;94:255–9.

[21] Galloway SM, Sofuni T, Shelby MD, Thilagar A, Kumaroo V, Kaur P, et al. Multilaboratory comparison of *in vitro* tests for chromosome aberrations in CHO and CHL cells tested under the same protocols. Environ Mol Mutagen 1997;29(2):189–207.

[22] Evans HJ, O'Riordan ML. Human peripheral blood lymphocytes for the analysis of chromosome aberrations in mutagen tests. Mutat Res 1975;31(3):135–48.

[23] Preston RJ, Au W, Bender MA, Brewen JG, Carrano AV, Heddle JA, et al. Mammalian *in vivo* and *in vitro* cytogenetic assays: a report of the U.S. EPA's gene-tox program. Mutat Res 1981;87(2):143–88.

[24] Galloway SM, Bloom AD, Resnick M, Margolin BH, Nakamura F, Archer P, et al. Development of a standard protocol for *in vitro* cytogenetic testing with Chinese hamster ovary cells: comparison of results for 22 compounds in two laboratories. Environ Mutagen 1985;7(1):1–51.

[25] Swierenga SH, Heddle JA, Sigal EA, Gilman JP, Brillinger RL, Douglas GR, et al. Recommended protocols based on a survey of current practice in genotoxicity testing laboratories, IV. Chromosome aberration and sister-chromatid exchange in Chinese hamster ovary, V79 Chinese hamster lung and human lymphocyte cultures. Mutat Res 1991;246(2):301–22.

[26a] Morita T, Watanabe Y, Takeda K, Okumura K. Effects of pH in the *in vitro* chromosomal aberration test. Mutat Res 1989;225(1–2):55–60.

[26b] Morita T, Nagaki T, Fukuda I, Okumura K. Clastogenicity of low pH to various cultured mammalian cells. Mutat Res 1992;268(2):297–305.

[27] Bradley MO, Taylor VI, Armstrong MJ, Galloway SM. Relationships among cytotoxicity, lysosomal breakdown, chromosome aberrations, and DNA double-strand breaks. Mutat Res 1987;189(1):69–79.

[28] Scott D, Galloway SM, Marshall RR, Ishidate Jr M, Brusick D, Ashby J, et al. International commission for protection against environmental mutagens and carcinogens. Genotoxicity under extreme culture conditions. A report from ICPEMC Task Group 9. Mutat Res 1991;257(2):147–205.

[29] Armstrong MJ, Bean CL, Galloway SM. A quantitative assessment of the cytotoxicity associated with chromosomal aberration detection in Chinese hamster ovary cells. Mutat Res 1992;265(1):45–60.

[30] Galloway SM, Aardema MJ, Ishidate Jr M, Ivett JL, Kirkland DJ, Morita T, et al. Report from working group on *in vitro* tests for chromosomal aberrations. Mutat Res 1994;312(3):241–61.

[31] Kirkland D, Aardema M, Henderson L, Müller L. Evaluation of the ability of a battery of three *in vitro* genotoxicity tests to discriminate rodent carcinogens and non-carcinogens I. Sensitivity, specificity and relative predictivity. Mutat Res 2005;584(1–2):1–256 Erratum in: Mutat Res 2005;588(1):70.

[32] Kirkland D, Aardema M, Müller L, Makoto H. Evaluation of the ability of a battery of three *in vitro* genotoxicity tests to discriminate rodent carcinogens and non-carcinogens II. Further analysis of mammalian cell results, relative predictivity and tumour profiles. Mutat Res 2006;608(1):29–42.

[33] Kirkland D, Speit G. Evaluation of the ability of a battery of three *in vitro* genotoxicity tests to discriminate rodent carcinogens and non-carcinogens III. Appropriate follow-up testing *in vivo*. Mutat Res 2008;654(2):114–32.

[34] Thybaud V, Aardema M, Clements J, Dearfield K, Galloway S, Hayashi M, et al. Strategy for genotoxicity testing: hazard identification and risk assessment in relation to *in vitro* testing. Mutat Res 2007;627(1):41−58.

[35] ICH (International Committee on Harmonisation). ICH S2(R1) Guidance on Genotoxicity Testing and Data Interpretation for Pharmaceuticals Intended for Human Use. Finalized November 2011. http://www.ich.org/products/guidelines.html

[36] OECD Guideline for the testing of chemicals, Genetic Toxicology No. 473, *In vitro* mammalian cell chromosomal aberration test, Organisation for Economic Co-Operation and Development, Paris, 26 September 2014. http://www.oecd-ilibrary.org/

[37] OECD Guideline for the testing of chemicals, Genetic Toxicology No. 487, *In vitro* mammalian cell micronucleus test, Organisation for Economic Co-Operation and Development, Paris, 26 September 2014. http://www.oecd-ilibrary.org/

[38] Clare G. The *in vitro* mammalian chromosome aberration test. In: Parry JM, Parry EM, editors. Genetic toxicology principles and methods. New York: Humana Press (part of Springer Science + Business Media); 2012. p. 69−91.

[39] Ong T, Mukhtar M, Wolf CR, Zeiger E. Differential effects of cytochrome P450-inducers on promutagen activation capabilities and enzymatic activities of S-9 from rat liver. J Environ Pathol Toxicol 1980;4(1):55−65.

[40] Maron DM, Ames BN. Revised methods for the Salmonella mutagenicity test. Mutat Res 1983;113(3−4):173−215.

[41] Spurbeck JL, Zinsmeister AR, Meyer KJ, Jalal SM. Dynamics of chromosome spreading. Am J Med Genet 1996;61(4):387−93.

[42] Claussen U, Michel S, Mühlig P, Westermann M, Grummt UW, Kromeyer-Hauschild K, Liehr T. Demystifying chromosome preparation and the implications for the concept of chromosome condensation during mitosis. Cytogenet Genome Res 2002;98(2−3):136−46.

[43] Deng W, Tsao SW, Lucas JN, Leung CS, Cheung AL. A new method for improving metaphase chromosome spreading. Cytometry A 2003;51(1):46−51.

[44] Callander RD, Mackay JM, Clay P, Elcombe CR, Elliott BM. Evaluation of phenobarbital/beta-naphthoflavone as an alternative S9-induction regime to Aroclor 1254 in the rat for use in *in vitro* genotoxicity assays. Mutagenesis 1995;10(6):517−22.

[45] García Franco S, Domínguez G, Pico JC. Alternatives in the induction and preparation of phenobarbital/naphthoflavone-induced S9 and their activation profiles. Mutagenesis 1999;14(3):323−6.

[46] Johnson TE, Umbenhauer DR, Galloway SM. Human liver S-9 metabolic activation; proficiency in cytogenetic assays and comparison with phenobarbital beta-naphthoflavone or Aroclor 1254 induced rat S-9. Environ Mol Mutagen 1996;28(1):51−9.

[47] Hilliard C, Hill R, Armstrong M, Fleckenstein C, Crowley J, Freeland E, et al. Chromosome aberrations in Chinese hamster and human cells: a comparison using compounds with various genotoxicity profiles. Mutat Res 2007;616(1−2):103−18.

[48] Bickmore W. Karyotype analysis and chromosome banding. eLS Encyclopedia of Life Sciences, 2001 Nature Publishing Group. http://onlinelibrary.wiley.com/doi/10.1038/npg.els.0001160/full *or* https://www.researchgate.net/publication/228017856_Karyotype_Analysis_and_Chromosome_Banding.

[49] Lynch AM, Robinson SA, Wilcox P, Smith MD, Kleinman M, Jiang K, et al. Cycloheximide and disulfoton are positive in the photoclastogencity assay but do not absorb UV irradiation: another example of pseudophotoclastogenicity? Mutagenesis 2008;23(2):111−18.

[50] Chen TR. *In situ* detection of mycoplasma contamination in cell cultures by fluorescent Hoechst 33258 stain. Exp Cell Res 1977;104(2):255−62.

[51] Battaglia M, Pozzi D, Grimaldi S, Parasassi T. Hoechst 33258 staining for detecting mycoplasma contamination in cell cultures: a method for reducing fluorescence photobleaching. Biotech Histochem 1994;69(3):152−6.

[52] Craig-Holmes AP, Shaw MW. Cell cycle analysis in asynchronous cultures using the BUdR-Hoechst technique. Exp Cell Res. 1976;99(1):79–87.

[53] Tice R, Schneider EL, Rary JM. The utilization of bromodeoxyuridine incorporation into DNA for the analysis of cellular kinetics. Exp Cell Res 1976;102:232–6.

[54] Alicata P, Castro A, Faro S, Motta S. Lymphocytes proliferation kinetics and SCE variation after rubella vaccination. Mutat Res 1988;198(1):215–19.

[55] Henderson L, Jones E, Brooks T, Chételat A, Ciliutti P, Freemantle M, et al. Industrial Genotoxicology Group collaborative trial to investigate cell cycle parameters in human lymphocyte cytogenetics studies. Mutagenesis 1997;12(3):163–7.

[56] FDA Redbook. U.S. Department of Health and Human Services, Food and Drug Administration, Center for Food Safety and Applied Nutrition, Guidance for Industry and Other Stakeholders, Toxicological Principles for the Safety Assessment of Food Ingredients, July 2000; Updated July 2007. http://www.fda.gov/Food/GuidanceRegulation/GuidanceDocumentsRegulatoryInformation/IngredientsAdditivesGRASPackaging/ucm2006826.htm#TOC

[57] Freshney RI. Culture of animal cells: a manual of basic technique and specialized applications. 7th ed Hoboken, New Jersey: Wiley-Blackwell; 2016.

[58] Danford N. The interpretation and analysis of cytogenetic data. In: Parry JM, Parry EM, editors. Genetic toxicology principles and methods. New York: Humana Press (part of Springer Science + Business Media); 2012. p. 92–120.

[59] (a) ISCN. An International System for Human Cytogenetic Nomenclature. Recommendations of the International Standing Committee on Human Cytogenetic Nomenclature, Memphis, Tenn., October 1994 Editor(s): Mitelman F. (Lund), Karger A.G., Basel. Note that a most recent version of the system is listed below. (b) ISCN. In: Shaffer LG, McGowan-Jordan J, Schmid M, editors. An international system for human cytogenetic nomenclature. Basel: S Karger; 2013.

CHAPTER 8

The In Vivo *Rodent Micronucleus Assay*

Laura Custer[1], Ann Doherty[2], Jeffrey C. Bemis[3] and Ray Proudlock[4]

[1]*Bristol-Myers Squibb, New Brunswick, NJ, USA* [2]*AstraZeneca Innovative Medicines and Early Development, Cambridge, UK* [3]*Litron Laboratories, Rochester, NY, USA* [4]*Boone, North Carolina, USA*

Chapter Outline

8.1 Introduction 270
8.2 History 271
8.3 Fundamentals 271
8.4 Test Substance Considerations 273
8.5 Study Design 273
    8.5.1 Animal Source, Housing, Maintenance, and Identification 274
    8.5.2 Animal Species, Strain, Age, and Sex 275
    8.5.3 Historical Negative/Vehicle and Positive Control Data 276
    8.5.4 Number and Size of Treatment Groups 277
    8.5.5 Acute and Repeat-Dose Schedules 278
    8.5.6 Dose Level Selection 279
    8.5.7 Dose Range-Finding Experiment 280
    8.5.8 Dose Administration 281
    8.5.9 Dose Volume 281
8.6 Manual Methods 282
    8.6.1 Equipment and Consumables 282
    8.6.2 Reagent Preparation 282
        8.6.2.1 Fetal calf serum 282
        8.6.2.2 Acridine orange 282
        8.6.2.3 Giemsa stain—Gurr's improved R66 283
    8.6.3 Sample Preparation 283
    8.6.4 Microscopic Methods 283
        8.6.4.1 Blood smears 283
        8.6.4.2 Mouse bone marrow smears 284
        8.6.4.3 Rat bone marrow smears 284
        8.6.4.4 Smear fixation and staining 284
        8.6.4.5 Giemsa staining 285
        8.6.4.6 Acridine orange staining 285
        8.6.4.7 Supravital staining of blood 286
        8.6.4.8 Microscopic evaluation 288
        8.6.4.9 Identification of micronuclei 290

Genetic Toxicology Testing.
DOI: http://dx.doi.org/10.1016/B978-0-12-800764-8.00008-2

8.6.5 Records   290
8.6.6 Identification of Aneugenic Agents   291
8.6.7 Centromeric Staining Using FISH   292
    8.6.7.1 Materials   292
    8.6.7.2 FISH method using programmable hotplate   292
    8.6.7.3 Alterative protocol for FISH   293
    8.6.7.4 FISH: slide checking   293
    8.6.7.5 FISH: slide scoring   294
8.6.8 Kinetochore Labeling   294
    8.6.8.1 Materials   294
    8.6.8.2 Methods   294
8.7   Automated Analysis and Flow Cytometry   297
8.7.1   Individual Reagents   297
8.7.2   Solution and Material Preparation   297
8.7.3   Flow Cytometry Method   299
8.7.4   Blood Collection   299
8.7.5   Bone Marrow Collection and Processing   299
    8.7.5.1 Prepare cellulose columns   299
8.7.6   Collect and Fractionate Bone Marrow Samples   300
8.7.7   Fixation of Blood and Bone Marrow Samples   300
8.7.8   Storage of Fixed Samples   303
    8.7.8.1 Wash samples out of fixative   303
8.7.9   Transfer Samples to LTSS   304
    8.7.9.1 Wash samples out of LTSS   304
8.7.10 Label Washed Samples for Flow Analysis   305
8.7.11 Flow Cytometric Analysis   306
    8.7.11.1 Flow cytometer calibration with biological standards   306
8.7.12 Analysis of Experimental Samples   311
8.7.13 Template Preparation for Flow Cytometric Analyses   312
8.8   Study Validity   314
8.9   Interpretation of Results and Statistical Analysis   315
8.9.1 MIE Values   315
8.9.2 Proportion of Immature Erythrocytes   316
8.10 Nongenotoxic Mechanisms of Induction of Micronucleated Erythrocytes   317
8.10.1 Causes   317
8.10.2 Avoiding and Recognizing Irrelevant Positives   317
8.11 Limitations of the Rodent Erythrocyte Micronucleus Test   318
References   319

8.1 Introduction

The rodent micronucleus test is routinely used to identify agents that induce chromosomal damage resulting in the formation of micronuclei in newly formed (immature) erythrocytes. It is particularly relevant to human risk assessment because it takes into account absorption, metabolism, DNA repair, and cell cycle control mechanisms that are poorly represented by *in vitro* systems. Micronuclei, also known as Howell-Jolly bodies, are round, membrane-bound chromatin structures formed during cell division when an acentric chromosome fragment or an entire chromosome fails to be incorporated into one of the daughter cell nuclei. They are easy to identify in mammalian erythrocytes because of the absence of the main nucleus. An increased frequency of micronucleated immature erythrocytes (MIE) in the bone marrow or blood is indicative of recent exposure to a chromosome-damaging agent.

8.2 History

In a search for a less laborious and less demanding alternative to metaphase chromosome analysis of the bone marrow, Schmid's group at the University of Zurich found that increases in micronuclei and other nuclear anomalies in the bone marrow of Chinese hamsters treated with the cross-linking agent Trenimon correlated with increases in chromosome damage [1]; similar anomalies were found in the bone marrow of other species treated with the drug [2,3]. Nuclear anomalies occur as a result of apoptosis, aberrant chromosome segregation, and aberrant nuclear division [4].

Genotoxic agents were found to cause increases in micronucleated erythrocytes in mice [5–7], particularly in the IE population [8]. The present day mammalian micronucleus test concentrates on MIE to simplify scoring and maximize sensitivity. Because it is less labor-intensive, less technically challenging, detects all agents that cause chromosome breakage as well as nondisjunction (inappropriate or incomplete chromosome segregation at nuclear division) due to spindle damage in the bone marrow, and can be more sensitive, the erythrocyte micronucleus test has generally replaced the bone marrow chromosome aberration test to become the most widely used *in vivo* genotoxicity assay (e.g., [9,10]). Variations including sampling of peripheral blood, specific staining methods, and integration into routine toxicology studies have allowed wider application of the test. Automation of scoring by flow cytometry, image analysis, and laser scanning cytometery has further enhanced the ease of scoring and the potential sensitivity of the method. Standard methodology including acceptable dosing regimens, sampling times, and detection methods for routine regulatory studies is specified by the recently updated and internationally recognized OECD guideline for the mammalian erythrocyte micronucleus test [11], which should be followed for all studies for regulatory submission unless appropriate justification is presented. We strongly recommend referring to that guideline when establishing and performing the test in your laboratory.

8.3 Fundamentals

The standard rodent micronucleus assay involves examination of IEs in bone marrow and sometimes blood. Mammalian erythroblasts undergo maturation in the bone marrow, expelling the nucleus to form IEs but generally retain micronuclei. This cohort of IEs can be identified by various staining methods that depend on their high RNA content or the presence of the CD71 antigen on the cell surface. Over the course of approximately 24 h, the RNA and CD71 marker are lost and the cells are then termed mature erythrocytes (ME). Other terminologies are used (sometimes inappropriately even in this chapter); the correct terms together with the most widely used staining and detection methods are summarized here (Table 8.1).

Table 8.1: Summary of staining methods and terminology

Preparation	Stain	Detection Method	Erythrocyte Stage and Terminology	
			IE	ME
Bone marrow and blood smears	Giemsa[a]	Light microscopy	Polychromatic, PCE	Normochromatic, NCE
Bone marrow and blood smears	Acridine orange[b]	Fluorescence microscopy	Immature	Mature
Supravitally stained blood	Acridine orange	Fluorescence microscopy	Reticulocyte	–
Bone marrow and blood suspensions	CD71 fluorescent antibody	Flow cytometry	CD71-positive	CD71-negative

[a]Other Romanowsky stains can be used in conjunction with or as an alternative to Giemsa, including Wright, Leishman, and May-Grünwald. These stains all rely on polychromatic staining of RNA by the methylene blue component.
[b]Other fluorescent nucleic acid–specific dyes have occasionally been used but do not seem to have any advantage over acridine orange (AO), except for use in automated methods [12]. Nonfluorescent DNA-specific staining methods have been described but are more demanding and do not give such obvious differentiation as does AO (e.g., the modified Feulgen technique [13]).

The test is generally performed in routine laboratory rodent species (i.e., rat and mouse). In the case of the rat, the micronucleated erythrocytes are sticky and rapidly filtered out of the peripheral blood, principally by the spleen. Therefore, when examining rat peripheral blood, analysis should be restricted to the youngest IE population (type I reticulocytes or CD71-positive erythrocytes) to increase sensitivity [14,15]. Even so, the proportion of micronucleated type I reticulocytes in rat blood is relatively low compared with bone marrow [15]; automated methods (principally involving flow cytometry) allow rapid examination of a larger cell population to detect a number of events equivalent to that seen in the bone marrow; therefore, in the case of rat blood at least, automatic scoring has a distinct advantage over manual methods. Either microscopic or validated automated methods are accepted by international regulatory agencies. In mice, when the spleen does not effectively filter out micronucleated cells, the frequency of micronuclei in peripheral blood may be evaluated in ME when the dosing period exceeds the lifespan of the erythrocyte (i.e., approximately 4 weeks in rodents) [16].

Covalent binding, intercalation, or interference with DNA metabolism (replication or repair) can lead to chromosome breakage (clastogenicity), resulting in acentric fragments that subsequently form micronuclei. A second mechanism of formation involves interference with the spindle apparatus by aneugenic agents, resulting in lagging whole chromosomes. Chromosome fragments and lagging chromosomes tend not to be incorporated into one of the daughter nuclei, so they are not usually expelled with the main nucleus when the erythroblast transitions to an IE. Determination of the mechanism of micronucleus formation can be important in establishing a threshold and, therefore, an acceptable safety margin. In the absence of extensive data for individual agents, genotoxins that bind directly to DNA are generally expected to show activity even at low dose levels; therefore, regulatory bodies usually set very low acceptable exposure levels for them. In contrast, indirect agents including aneugens generally show clear thresholds for effects. Treatment with aneugenic agents results in a high proportion of larger micronuclei containing centromeres. Centromere-positive micronuclei can be distinguished using FISH (fluorescence *in situ* hybridization) probes or a fluorescent kinetochore-specific antigen (CREST staining), as described later. The mechanism of induction of MIE is also important in assessing the relevance of other genotoxicity tests.

When samples are scored for the incidence of MIE, the proportion of IEs among the total erythrocyte population [calculated as IE/(IE + ME)] is also assessed. A reduction in this proportion for the test agent–treated group in comparison to the concurrent control group is used as a measure of bone marrow toxicity/suppression, which can sometimes be used as supporting evidence of target organ exposure.

8.4 Test Substance Considerations

If it is known or suspected that the test substance is not systemically distributed and therefore bioavailable in the target organ, then the erythrocyte micronucleus is not appropriate. In certain circumstances, changing the route of exposure may allow higher systemic and target organ exposure levels, that is, e.g., it may be possible to achieve much higher bioavailability of a drug intended for inhalation using intravenous infusion.

Micronucleated erythrocytes can be induced by nongenotoxic mechanisms involving disturbance of erythropoiesis; appropriate precautions should be taken when evaluating materials known or suspected of causing anemia, prolonged hyperthermia or hypothermia, or stimulation of erythropoiesis, as discussed near the end of this chapter (see Section 8.10).

8.5 Study Design

Important aspects of study design, protocol, and reporting requirements are described in ICH, FDA, and OECD guidelines. Various dosing and sampling regimes have been designed to optimize detection of micronucleated cells. The options listed later in this section are generally considered equally acceptable for studies for regulatory submission. Experiments should strictly adhere to national regulations and laws relating to animal experimentation. In addition, the animals should be maintained in a healthy stress-free environment by trained and supervised staff for moral and scientific reasons.

In the case of pharmaceuticals, blood, or plasma analysis ("bioanalytical"), data will usually be available to support the choice of species and route. If the test substance shows reasonable bioavailability, then that information should be summarized in the study report. Otherwise, it may be appropriate to include a bioanalytical component in the micronucleus test itself. In the case of mouse studies, this will usually entail a satellite group with four animals sampled at, for example, three time points near the approximate time when plasma/ blood levels can be expected to be close to be maximum (e.g., 1, 2, and 4 h after oral treatment). In the rat, sampling is facilitated because a larger blood volume can be taken without compromising the animals; therefore, provided that the analytical method is sufficiently sensitive, the same animals can be sampled at each time point. In some cases it may even be possible to sample animals from the main study without interfering with parameters assessed in the test itself. In general, there is no need to produce a detailed toxicokinetic profile; that would necessitate at least twice as many sampling times and an intravenous group to calculate absolute bioavailability. Alternatively, if an appropriately sensitive micro-sampling method is available, then the main group animals can be used to provide toxicokinetic samples provided that all animals are sampled in the same way [17,18]. Whatever the situation, if plasma/blood levels are adequate, then targeting of the organ can reasonably be assumed to occur because the bone marrow is a relatively well-perfused organ.

8.5.1 Animal Source, Housing, Maintenance, and Identification

Animals should be certified as specific pathogen-free and obtained from a reputable accredited supplier (e.g., AAALAC and Class A breeder USDA in the United States). For each experiment, animals should be obtained from a single barrier within a breeding facility. Facility animal care and housing should comply with current guidelines for the country and institution where the work is conducted, but some general guidelines are mentioned here. AAALAC [19] or the Guide for the Care and Use of Laboratory Animals [20] are good sources for information on animal care and housing. On receipt, animals should be checked for age, sex, and general health. Prior to initiating any experimental procedures, rodents should be allowed to acclimate for a minimum of 5 days. Room conditions should be controlled for humidity (40–70%) and temperature (22 ± 3 °C) with a 12-h light/dark cycle, except when interruptions are necessitated by designated activities such as room cleaning. Any animals that show or develop signs of ill health or marked injury on arrival or during the course of acclimation should be removed from the study; if disease is suspected, then the affected animals can be euthanized and subjected to postmortem examination. Animals should be provided food and water *ad libitum* prior to and during experimentation unless appropriately justified.

Individual animals should be identified uniquely (e.g., ear tagging, micro-chipping or biometric). Tail-marking using an indelible marker pen is suitable for temporary identification of individual animals and, if reapplied, is probably the most straightforward method for short-term studies. Animals are normally "randomly" assigned (stratified) to treatment groups based on body weight so that mean and variance in bodyweight are similar for each group. Rodents should be housed in groups of up to five per cage unless this leads to fighting; slightly injured or aggressive animals may be need to be isolated. Each group and sex should be housed separately in cages labeled uniquely with the animal numbers and study identity. All cages should be placed in similar positions in the same room to minimize potential systematic effects; there is no need to randomize cage positions unless that is standard procedure within the laboratory.

8.5.2 Animal Species, Strain, Age, and Sex

The test is usually conducted with young adult rodents (6−10 weeks old at the beginning of treatment); older animals or other species including dog and monkey can be used if the IE population can be identified, the laboratory has adequate historical control data for that species, and appropriate justification is presented in the report. Incidences of micronucleated erythrocytes in various mammalian, bird, and other vertebrate species have been reported [21,22], and many of them could be used for environmental monitoring.

Inbred, hybrid, or outbred animals are acceptable for use if the laboratory has adequate historical negative/vehicle and positive control data. The difference between background rates of micronucleated cells between standard breeds of mice and rats is a matter of debate; in cases in which acridine orange staining has been used, there seems to be a relatively small difference (e.g., [15,23]), whereas other reports indicate high variations between breeds (e.g., [24,25]). To some extent, high variation could be explained by poor or variable technique, especially when using Giemsa-type stains, and background rates in excess of 0.5% should be viewed with suspicion. Most commonly, outbred animals are used for toxicology studies and in the micronucleus test. The reader should be aware of the possibility for a sudden shift in background rates of lesions including MIE if there is a change in the genetics of a particular source of outbred rodents (e.g., if the colony is re-derived consequent to a disease). Although inbred and hybrid strains should be stable and show less variation between individuals, they are substantially more expensive.

Results for male and female animals are usually similar at equi-toxic dose levels [26], in which case the use of only a single sex (usually male) may be justified. However, if sex-related differences such as toxicity, exposure, or metabolism are known or expected, then use of both sexes is recommended. Typically, exposure differences of less than two-fold are not considered significant. For statistical reasons, and because the maximum daily dose level is usually lower, we recommend sampling both sexes when the micronucleus test is integrated into general toxicology studies.

8.5.3 Historical Negative/Vehicle and Positive Control Data

The historical control database should be established during the validation phase of the micronucleus test in a particular laboratory. This validation should confirm that the laboratory obtains MIE values for the positive and, in particular, negative control groups are within the expected range and that the laboratory can detect relatively low doses of clastogenic and aneugenic substances. Laboratories with limited experience should take into account expected values based on published results from reliable sources when establishing their own historical control database. Detailed guidance on developing an adequate database is provided elsewhere [27] and in OECD guideline 474. An adequate negative control database consists of at least 10, and preferably 20, separate experiments. The distribution rather than just the range of individual and group mean values should be taken into account and is expected to be very close to Poisson, with a mean value of approximately 1 MIE per 1000 IE for most breeds of mice and rats.

Outliers in negative control groups are very rare and should be treated with suspicion; values should only be excluded if scientifically justifiable (e.g., animals dosed by routes that cause stress may be considered separately). In general, untreated animals or those treated with the vehicle control by most routes should give very similar MIE values and are included in the distribution. If the staining technique or source of animals changes, then it may be appropriate to reestablish the database.

When establishing the historical control database, it should list all appropriate parameters including individual animal results, date of sampling, vehicle, dose volume and regimen, route of administration, sex, and age to allow in-depth analysis, if needed. In accordance with OECD guideline 474, study reports should show the distribution of group mean results together with range, mean, sample standard deviations and 95% tolerance limits, the time period covered, and the number of data points. The distribution can be useful in interpreting borderline apparent increases in test article—treated groups; in that case, the upper tolerance limit contains 97.5% of mean MIE values obtained from previous experiments. This value can be calculated using the PERCENTILE function in Microsoft Excel, although it can also be approximated using the = NORMINV function once results have been appropriately transformed, for example, $\sqrt{(x + 0.5)}$ can be used if the distribution is close to Poisson.

A similar historical **positive** control MIE database should be established and the distribution should be presented in the report. Historical positive control results tend to show a high degree of variability between animals and experiments and can drift with time, but the concurrent positive control MIE value is expected to be within or close to the distribution of historical control values. Although the distribution should be presented in the report, historical positive control data are not generally of any great importance when interpreting the outcome of a particular study.

Proportions of IEs should also be recorded in the database, but there can be a high variability between animals and, because this proportion decreases with age, any comparisons with historical data are of limited interest; there is normally no requirement or value in presenting historical control results for this parameter in the report.

8.5.4 Number and Size of Treatment Groups

Usually three dose levels of the test substance are used with a minimum of five animals per sex per experimental point being examined. However, if only a single dose of the test substance is administered, only the vehicle control and high-level treatment group need to be sampled at the second time point. If toxic effects that may lead to mortality or early euthanasia are likely, then it may be prudent to add one or two additional animals to the high-level group, particularly when only one sex is being used. If the test substance is not expected to be genotoxic based on *in vitro* results and published information for related compounds, and if the maximum tolerated dose (MTD) is above the standard limit of 2000 mg/kg bodyweight (or 1000 mg/kg/day when the dosing period is ≥ 14), then only a single (high-level) group needs to be dosed with the test substance for comparison with the vehicle control.

Concurrent negative control group(s) should be included in all studies, except in the case of the peripheral blood version of the test, where a pre-dose sample can act as an appropriate negative control. Negative control animals should be treated with an equal volume of the vehicle used to formulate the test substance (or with a similar placebo if the test substance is dosed undiluted). When a laboratory has no previous experience and no published information regarding the use of a particular vehicle, it may be appropriate to screen it for effects in advance of use or to include a concurrent untreated control group. Selection of the solvent/vehicle control is covered in the Formulation chapter of this manual.

Relatively inexperienced laboratories should include a positive control group to help control bias and to demonstrate ability to prepare, stain, and score slides correctly. Typically, this will be a standard chemical administered at only the first time point because multiple administrations will usually greatly reduce the number of IE for examination. The number of animals in the positive control group can justifiably be reduced if a reasonable response is expected. Experienced laboratories with an adequate historical database need only include concurrent positive control groups occasionally (e.g., once every 6 or 18 months). In cases when concurrent positive control animals are not dosed, equivalent samples collected from a previous study should be processed and encoded along with study samples as a procedural control and to minimize potential bias.

The positive control substance at the chosen dose level should cause a consistent moderate increase in micronucleated cells above background levels as established in preliminary experimentation. It is acceptable to dose the positive control group by a standard route (typically oral) that may differ from the test substance. Examples include cyclophosphamide administered at 20 mg/kg to rats, ethyl nitrosourea, and ethyl methanesulfonate. Mitomycin C is a convenient positive control for the mouse micronucleus test because it comes in preweighed 2-mg aliquots in injectable vials. If the test substance is known to be or is suspected of being aneugenic, then it is appropriate to include a second positive control group dosed with a known spindle poison such as colchicine or vinblastine for comparative purposes to facilitate any follow-up examination of samples. Other class-related positive controls may be used when appropriate.

8.5.5 Acute and Repeat-Dose Schedules

The conventional test involves sampling of bone marrow rodents 24 and 48 h after a single dose. Because it is not practical to sample bone marrow from rodents while they are still alive (at least not without contamination with blood), this involves one set of animals for each sampling time with only a high-level group and a vehicle control group needed for the second sampling time. When toxicity is not a factor (i.e., when the standard limit dose is used or the maximum feasible dose is not expected to cause toxicity), then only a single dose level of the test article is needed.

The recently revised OECD guideline prefers approaches that involve sampling only a single set of animals. For example, animals can be sampled 18 to 24 h after the second of two doses administered 24 h apart. Alternatively, mouse peripheral blood can be sampled at two time points between 36 and 72 h after a single dose or a single time point 36−48 h after two doses administered 24 h apart. Comet assay endpoints can be incorporated into the micronucleus test if a third dose is administered 2−6 h prior to euthanasia [28].

If three or more daily administrations of the test substance are given at approximately 24-h intervals, then samples are collected within 24 h (bone marrow) or 40 h (blood) after the last treatment (OECD). This option allows integration of the micronucleus test into repeat-dose general toxicity studies. Both strategies reduce labor costs and the number of animals used in experimentation. In addition, some of the parameters assessed in the routine toxicology studies can be useful in confirming the relevance of micronucleus assessment, including toxicokinetic and erythrocyte parameters. Cytostatic substances can cause a delayed increase in micronucleus production [29]: sampling peripheral blood within the first 2 weeks of an ongoing toxicology study can overcome issues with delay in appearance of micronucleated cells and helps avoid complications arising from bone marrow toxicity following more prolonged administration. Multiple administrations of potent cytotoxic chemicals such as colchicine, dimethylhydrazine, mitomycin C, and monocrotaline results in greatly exaggerated toxic effects, so only low dose levels can be used in longer-term experiments. In such cases, substantial increases in MIE may not be evident [15], although cytotoxic effects (indicative of potential genotoxicity) would presumably be obvious in the bone marrow and/or in other tissues (e.g., on histopathological examination).

Occasional changes to these sampling times may be justifiable based on toxicokinetic/pharmacokinetic information (e.g., if the test substance has a very long biological half-life, then only a single-dose administration may be needed).

8.5.6 Dose Level Selection

The highest dose selected for the micronucleus test is the lowest dose among the following:

1. The limit dose of 2000 mg/kg/day for studies of <14 days or 1000 mg/kg/day for longer studies.
2. The MTD without inducing death, study-limiting toxicity (e.g., body weight loss), bone marrow decrease, or excessive distress or clinical signs necessitating euthanasia. The chosen dose would normally be expected to cause only moderate clinical signs; it should not cause animals to become moribund or cause stressful clinical signs.
3. The maximum feasible/practical based on formulation and route of administration constraints.
4. A dose that induces 50%−80% reduction in the proportion of IE erythrocytes among total erythrocytes in the bone marrow (IE/(IE + ME)) to not less than 20% of negative control levels using conventional staining methods or 5% of control levels when using CD71 staining for flow cytometry [30]. A lower high dose may be justified if the test substance demonstrates saturation toxicokinetics [31].
5. If the test substance is cleared more effectively after multiple administrations, an acute dosing protocol may be justifiable; otherwise, samples should be collected at the earliest compliant time points in a multi-dose study.

When the micronucleus test is integrated into a general toxicology study, the dose levels selected are usually based on appropriate OECD guidance. Under normal circumstances, inclusion of the micronucleated erythrocyte endpoint is considered valid for pharmaceuticals if the top dose selected supports clinical trial purposes. However, if no introductory mammalian cell assay has been performed or if the test is being performed as a follow-up to *in vitro* findings, then dose selection criteria are stricter and the top daily dose should be at least the maximum practical or at least 50% of that which would have been chosen for an acute (standalone) micronucleus test as described [10].

Two lower dose levels in a dedicated micronucleus test are used, except when use of a single dose level is justified in the report as described previously; conventionally, these dose levels are one-half and one-quarter the high dose level, although there are arguments to support the use of only a single high dose when bone marrow suppression is not evident, which is the case for most nongenotoxic chemicals [32,33].

8.5.7 Dose Range-Finding Experiment

If no suitable data exist to support selection of the appropriate dose levels, then a dose range-finding study using a limited number of the same species/breed of animals dosed using the same route and formulation to be used in the actual experiment should be performed. Dose-level selection for integrated studies is covered by ICH and OECD guidelines.

Dose selection for preliminary toxicity testing should take into account any existing toxicity results for that chemical and chemicals with similar structures or biological modes of action. The choice of high level for evaluation will often depend on restrictions applied by the research facility and regulations in force in that country. Two methods of dose range-finding for a dedicated (acute) micronucleus test are described here. In all cases for which little is known about the toxicity of a substance, animals should be observed closely immediately after dosing until clinical signs have abated and at intervals at least until euthanasia at the time planned for final sampling in the main micronucleus test. Animals that show excessive clinical signs or distress should be euthanized immediately and recorded as mortalities.

The up–down approach involves dosing animals sequentially [34], minimizes the number of animals used, and helps avoid animal distress. In this case, a single moderate dose (e.g., 200 mg/kg) is given on day 0 to two animals. In the absence of any severe clinical signs, a second dose is given 24 h later and the animals are maintained at least until the normal sampling time. In the case of severe effects or mortalities, any remaining animals are euthanized immediately. Based on the type, severity of clinical signs (or their absence), and rapidity of onset, a second group of animals is dosed at a corresponding higher or lower dose level on days 1 and 2. This process is repeated until a reasonable approximation of the MTD is obtained (where the MTD is defined as a dose slightly below that expected to cause excessive signs of toxicity, distress, or mortality). For nontoxic test substances, a dose progression might involve a starting dose of 200 mg/kg followed by 625 and 2000 mg/kg, whereas a toxic test substance may start at 200 mg/kg, decrease to 20, and, then, based on absence of clinical signs, should be followed by a dose of 62.5 mg/kg. Test substances of more intermediate toxicity would use the same starting dose but with closer-spaced dose increments of 200, 625, and 1200 mg/kg, for example.

The MTD is not an absolute constant and can vary somewhat between experiments; this could relate to variations in the rate of absorption and bioavailability that, in turn, may depend on various factors, including time of day and, in the case of suspensions, particle size distribution. It is important to control these factors so that unexpected levels of toxicity are not seen in the main test.

8.5.8 Dose Administration

The test substance can be administered by a variety or routes, including oral gavage, subcutaneous injection, or intravenous infusion. Other routes such as inhalation or administration with drinking water or diet may very occasionally be justified; inhalation is technically challenging and will often limit the dose that can be given, whereas it is difficult to control exposure levels using dietary routes. The most appropriate route is the anticipated major route of human exposure (often oral) and/or one that provides maximum expected systemic exposure in terms of AUC (blood levels over time normally expressed as area under the curve). Formulation is simplified if stability in the vehicle/solvent has been demonstrated for the duration of the dosing period. The maximum amount of test substance that can reasonably be administered depends on the recommended maximal dose volume for a particular route and the rate of administration. Animals should be observed for clinical signs of toxicity at least twice daily (usually 0.5 to 1 h and 3 to 4 h after the dose or at Tmax if known); depending on the severity of clinical signs, intermediate checks may be needed. Any animals exhibiting clinical signs of excessive toxicity should be euthanized. In the case of orally dosed animals, it is good practice to perform a postmortem macroscopic examination to check for evidence of misdosing, such as fluid in the lungs or damaged esophagus.

8.5.9 Dose Volume

Outline guidance on the recommended maximum volumes is given in OECD 474; scientists should be aware of more detailed guidance for specific routes of administration given in standard textbooks and peer-reviewed journals (e.g., [35,36]). For oral gavage, the usual maximum volume administered should not exceed 10 mL/kg bodyweight except for aqueous formulations, for which the maximum recommended volume is 20 mL/kg. Dose volume is calculated based on individual animal bodyweight recorded as soon as practical prior to treatment.

8.6 Manual Methods

8.6.1 Equipment and Consumables

Most of the equipment and materials used in the conventional test will be available in a well-equipped laboratory including the following:

1. Bench-top centrifuge
2. Cardboard slide trays
3. Glass or stainless steel slide staining dishes with stainless steel slide racks
4. Disposable centrifuge tubes
5. Microscope slides with frosted end for labeling, coverslips, mounting medium (e.g., Permount or DPX)
6. Blood collection supplies, such as syringes, needles, butterfly needles, and others
7. Depending on blood collection technique, heparin-coated capillary tubes (e.g., Fisher Scientific cat #22-260-950)
8. Fetal calf serum (FCS) or fetal bovine serum (FBS)
9. Methanol
10. Dissecting equipment including scissors and small bone shears/cutters
11. Metered CO_2 source for euthanasia
12. Hanks' balanced salts solution (for rat bone marrow)
13. High quality light or fluorescent microscope with plan objectives

8.6.2 Reagent Preparation

8.6.2.1 Fetal calf serum

The serum does not need to be sterile, but it does need to be free of microbial growth. If frozen, then serum should be thoroughly thawed before aliquoting into amounts of an appropriate size and frozen again before storage. To use, the serum should be thoroughly thawed and then filtered through a 0.22-μm syringe filter to remove particulate. With the exception of horse serum, other types of serum may give acceptable results if heat-inactivated.

8.6.2.2 Acridine orange

Acridine orange ($HCl.H_2O$) is mutagenic and light-sensitive. It can be prepared as an aqueous stock solution at 1 mg/mL, filtered and sterilized into appropriate aliquots, and then stored at 4 °C in the dark for up to 2 months. It can also be purchased as hemi(zinc chloride) salt. Whatever form is used, the final concentration needs to be adjusted empirically and standardized to optimize differential (metachromatic) staining of RNA and DNA.

8.6.2.3 Giemsa stain—Gurr's improved R66

Giemsa powder 3.8 g

Glycerol 250 mL

Methanol 250 mL

Although the original recipe was confidential, the aforementioned recipe produces identical results. Mix the components, stir continuously at 37 °C overnight, and then filter through cotton wool (cotton ball) or use a Buchner funnel with filter paper attached to a vacuum pump. Store the stain solution in tightly sealed amber bottles in a solvent cupboard.

8.6.3 Sample Preparation

Sample preparation and staining is perhaps the most critical aspect of the micronucleus test. You should establish methods to optimize cell density, morphology, differentiation of mature and immature erythrocytes, and good staining of nuclear material before attempting to perform the test; poor preparations are not acceptable. As with all cytogenetic tests, time and effort during setting up the assay will be greatly rewarded later.

8.6.4 Microscopic Methods

Slide racks can be cleaned by soaking in 50% acetic acid and then air-dried before use to remove any stain residue that, in the case of fluorescent stains in particular, can interfere with subsequent staining. Glass microscope slides with a frosted end should be permanently labeled with animal and study identities using an 2H pencil. These slides should be placed in a stainless steel rack, rinsed in methanol, air-dried, and then stored in a dust-free environment until use. In all cases, label and prepare at least three slides/smears for each animal—one is for analysis, the second is a backup, and, in the case of fluorescent staining, the third is for archiving. Additional positive control slides may be made to act as procedural checks for subsequent studies if desired; in this case, the study identity should be omitted.

8.6.4.1 Blood smears

Using a needle and syringe, or a butterfly needle with cannula (shortened by cutting the end off), collect blood from a lateral tail vein directly into K_2EDTA-coated tubes while agitating and place blood on chipped ice. Blood sampling can be facilitated by prewarming the animal using an infrared lamp. Place a 5-μL drop of blood close to the nonfrosted end of microscope slide. Place a second microscope slide in front of the drop at an approximately 45-degree angle and draw it back until a meniscus of blood travels along the slide. While applying slight downward pressure, push the second slide steadily forward so that a thin layer of blood evenly covers most of the slide. Allow the smear to air-dry. Prepare two to three replicate slides for each animal.

8.6.4.2 Mouse bone marrow smears

1. Dispense 2 mL FCS into a disposable centrifuge tube labeled with the animal identity.
2. Euthanize the animals one group at a time.
3. Excise a femur from each animal while removing the proximal epiphysis. This is most easily done by clearing the back of the femur and knee joint of tissue using scissors and then dislocating the knee while pulling on the lower leg. Cut the femur close to the hip using scissors or bone shears. Insert a 21-gage needle fitted to a 2-mL syringe into the cut end of the bone, and then draw the FCS up through the bone before expelling it back through the bone into the tube to create a suspension. Repeat with the second femur using the same serum unless the femur is required for another purpose. Repeat the aspiration to disperse any cell aggregates.
4. Centrifuge the suspensions at 300 g for 5 min.
5. Pour off and discard the supernatant, flick the tube, and resuspend the cells in 30 µL fresh FCS; use a correspondingly smaller amount if only one femur has been used.
6. Place 4 µL of cell suspension on the end of the corresponding labeled microscope slide and prepare a smear as described for blood.

8.6.4.3 Rat bone marrow smears

Rat bone marrow contains a substantial amount of extracellular material and benefits from an additional washing step as described here:

1. Dispense 5 mL fresh or sterile Hanks' balanced salts solution into each disposable centrifuge tube labeled with the animal identity.
2. Euthanize the animals one group at a time.
3. Excise a femur from each animal as described for mice. Insert a 21-gage needle fitted to a 5-mL syringe into the bone and draw the FCS up through the bone before expelling it back through the bone into the tube to create a suspension. Repeat the aspiration to disperse any cell aggregates.
4. Centrifuge the suspensions at 300 g for 5 min.
5. Pour off and discard the supernatant, flick the tube, and resuspend the cells in 2 mL FCS.
6. Centrifuge the suspension at 300 g for 5 min.
7. Pour off and discard the supernatant, flick the tube, and resuspend the cells in 170 µL fresh FCS. If the tibia is used in place of the femur, then the volume of the final addition of FCS should be reduced appropriately.
8. Place 4 µL of cell suspension on the end of the corresponding labeled microscope slide and prepare a smear as described for blood.

8.6.4.4 Smear fixation and staining

Allow the smears to air-dry, place them in a clean stainless steel slide rack, fix in methanol for approximately 10 min, and leave to dry before storing in a dust-free environment. Mouse blood and bone marrow slides can be stained with Giemsa as described; however,

AO staining is preferred because it provides better differentiation between immature and mature erythrocytes (particularly for blood smears), and micronuclei are much easier to spot because they fluoresce intensely. Note that Giemsa (or any of the other Romanowsky dyes including Leishman and Wright) are not suitable for staining rat bone marrow smears because of the presence of mast cell granules, which tend to adhere to erythrocytes and appear similar or identical to micronuclei using these stains [37]. Therefore, DNA-specific stains (usually AO) should always be used in the rat bone marrow test.

8.6.4.5 Giemsa staining

Giemsa is a mix of azure, methylene blue, and eosin. It should be diluted in purified water because the presence of solutes causes the components to form a complex precipitate, resulting in poor and variable staining as well as stain deposit on the slides. The following procedure is similar to that described previously [38] and that described by Gollapudi and Kamra [39]. At least one unstained slide per animal should be held in reserve in case of technical problems or in case subsequent additional analysis (e.g., centromeric staining) is required. Slide staining machines are often used to stain hematology smears, but these give inferior results and are slower than the manual method described here.

1. Prepare fresh 10% stain solution by dilution of 1 volume of Gurr's improved R66 Giemsa stain with 9 volumes of purified water. Mix well and filter through cotton (ball or wool) or a filter paper using a Buchner funnel to remove any small amount of particulate. Note that Giemsa stain solution is available in many different formulations; most give inferior results to R66.
2. Immerse the slides for 5 min in purified water.
3. Transfer the slides to the 10% Giemsa solution and stain for 10 min.
4. Immerse the slides for 5 min in purified water.
5. Immerse the slides for 5 min in fresh purified water. Alternatively differentiate in buffered distilled water (pH 6.8) for 5 min.
6. Drain then a Air-dry.
7. Place the slides in cardboard slide trays.
8. Mount each slide directly with a 24 × 60-mm coverslip (cover glass) using two drops of DPX or Permount in a fume cupboard.
9. Allow the mountant to harden prior to coding of slides. This can be accelerated by using a warm (50°C) oven, but ensure that the slides do not overheat.

Immature/polychromatic erythrocytes stain blue-gray (methylene blue polychromasia), whereas mature/normochromatic erythrocytes are counterstained orange by the eosin component of Giemsa. Nuclei and micronuclei stain red to purple.

8.6.4.6 Acridine orange staining

AO staining for the micronucleus test was originally described many years ago [40–42]. The simplest AO method involves wet-mounting of slides (after coding) directly in aqueous

100 µg AO per mL solution. Dispense two 5-µL aliquots of AO directly onto the smear and immediately lay a 60-mm coverslip on top. Check for an area of the slide with good staining and morphology under a low-power objective before proceeding with analysis.

Alternately, slides can be stained under yellow safelight or subdued lighting:

1. Dip the slides in Gurr's pH 6.8 0.004 M phosphate buffer and then transfer them to 125 µg AO solution for 30 s.
2. Rinse the slides in fresh Gurr buffer and then place them in a second container of fresh Gurr buffer for 10 min.
3. Transfer slides to a third container of fresh Gurr buffer for 15 min. Rinse slides in a fourth container of fresh Gurr buffer.
4. Wipe the back of the slide to remove excess buffer and place a coverslip over the top of the slide.

Smears should be examined soon after mounting using a fluorescence microscope with a blue excitation filter and a yellow barrier filter. IE stain orange, ME stain dull green, and nuclear material including micronuclei stain intense bright yellow/green (Figures 8.1 and 8.2). If the coloration varies from this, then the stain concentration may need to be adjusted: red staining of most material indicates the concentration is too high, and general yellow or green staining without orange/red coloration indicates the concentration is too low. The slides should be scored in a room with subdued lighting, especially if the light source in the microscope is not a high-intensity one. After analysis, the coverslip can be removed after soaking the slide in purified water to allow subsequent checking of slides by a second analyst. AO stain slides fade on examination (it may be helpful to include an antifading agent in the mounting medium) and should be regarded as temporary. They also dry out fairly quickly (unless stored in a wet box); therefore, they should be discarded following confirmation of results by the study supervisor. Unstained back-up slides should be mounted with coverslips using DPX or Permount for protection and archived with the study for potential retrospective investigation.

8.6.4.7 Supravital staining of blood

AO supravital staining can be used with blood from any appropriate species. It is the preferred method of staining for rats because analysis can be restricted to only the youngest population of IEs (type 1 reticulocytes) in which the endoplasmic reticulum (stained orange) occupies most of the cytoplasm [13,14]. In this way, the impact of splenic filtration of MIE from the blood is reduced.

1. Collect four or five drops of blood from each animal as described previously into a 2-mL heparinized tube and agitate.
2. Add an approximately equal volume of FCS to each tube before storing the samples at 4 °C overnight; most of the platelets, which otherwise tend to stain with AO, making analysis more difficult, disappear/fade during this period.

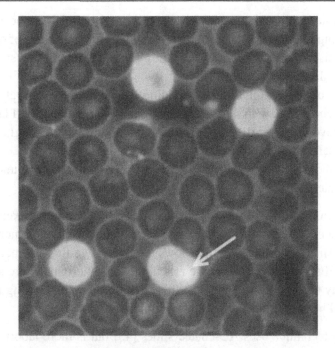

Figure 8.1
Blood smear stained with AO. Arrow points to a micronucleus inside an IE.

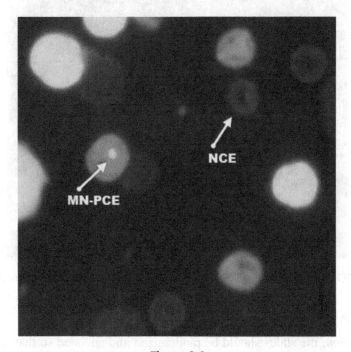

Figure 8.2
Bone marrow smear stained with AO. MN-PCE indicates a micronucleated immature erythrocyte (MIE), whereas NCE indicates a mature erythrocyte (ME).

3. Wipe a prewashed slide with a medical wipe and remove any lint on the central area of the slide by scraping with a second slide, or use a quick squirt from a can of compressed air.
4. Remove and discard most of the supernatant plasma from the blood samples that will have settled following overnight storage.
5. Dispense 1 μL of a 1-mg/mL aqueous acridine orange onto the central area of the cleaned slide and mix it with 4 μL blood using the micropipette tip. Place a clean lint-free 32-mm coverslip over the mixture. This method produces a single-cell layer of immobilized cells showing consistent staining throughout.
6. Examine the slides under oil immersion optics using a fluorescence microscope fitted with appropriate filters for AO.

The staining pattern is similar to that described for fixed preparations, except the morphology of the endoplasmic reticulum is preserved and is stained a more intense orange. In this case, the extracellular background shows a faint orange fluorescence, ME appear dull green/khaki, IEs show a bright orange reticulum, and micronuclei are a very bright green/yellow. Only type I erythrocytes (i.e., those with reticulum covering most of the cytoplasm) should be scored for the presence of micronuclei.

A similar staining technique uses AO-coated slides [43] but is more laborious and tends to lead to patchy staining.

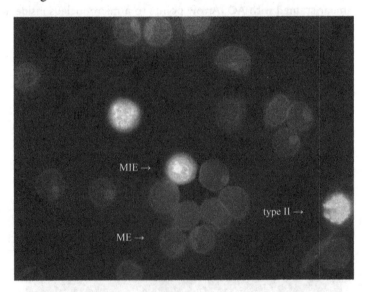

Rat blood AO supravital stain showing a type I reticulocyte with a micronucleus (MIE).

8.6.4.8 Microscopic evaluation

Prior to examination, the slides should be randomized and encoded so that the reader is not aware of the treatment group. This can be done using the random function in a spreadsheet program and printing the slide numbers out on self-adhesive labels that are fixed over the top of the animal ID without obscuring the study number. Saving the slide code electronically facilitates decoding and sorting of results later. If no positive control group was included in the study, then positive control slides from a previous study should be included prior to staining and coding.

The reader should be trained in accordance with the facility's SOPs and their ability should be confirmed using a set of standard slides bearing in mind that not all staff show an aptitude for slide-reading. The study scientist should regularly reevaluate one or two slides from each study together with any slides giving unexpected results. It is useful for the slide reader to make a note of the vernier location of the first nine MIE on each slide to facilitate slide review. In that case, a calibrated vernier stage is needed, the microscope ID should be recorded in the raw data, and the slides should always be oriented in a consistent way (e.g., label on the left). The microscope should have high-quality optics, flat wide field, high resolution, and low chromatic and spherical aberration; for example, high-magnification objectives should be planapo or plan fluor, and for light microscopy the sub-stage condenser should be a suitable match. The slide reader should be trained in cleaning and setting up the microscope correctly (i.e., using Köhler illumination in the case of transmitted light). When reading a slide, the reader should examine ("count") all the relevant cells in a field before moving rapidly to the next field (i.e., not move slowly across the slide while counting). The SOP should define a systematic approach to scanning the slide so that none of the fields examined overlap, although that would be evident using fluorescence microscopy because of the fading. The microscope should be set up on a vibration-proof bench or a homemade stand to dampen vibration. Counts are made using a bench top Denominator tally counter or similar electronic counter on a rubber mat; it is best to use two separate two-channel units to minimize the chance of pressing an inappropriate key when using a multi-channel (blood differential–type) counter: the first counter is used for scoring IE and ME, and the second is used only for recording micronucleated cells.

Bone marrow and blood preparations should be briefly examined under low power to determine an area with good morphology and staining suitable for analysis. The edges and end ("tail") of the smear should be avoided because these tend to contain larger cells and the proportion of IE is not representative. Then, the slide should be examined using an oil-immersion objective—a total magnification of approximately $\times 400$ to $\times 630$ is ideal for routine examination, although higher magnification may be useful during training. For each animal, at least 500 (bone marrow) or 2000 (blood) erythrocytes are scored to determine the proportion of immature erythrocytes, $IE \div (IE + ME)$. At least 4000 IEs per animal should be scored to determine the incidence of micronucleated immature erythrocytes MIE/IE. OECD 474 indicates "If the historical negative control database indicates the mean background MIE frequency is $<0.1\%$ in the testing laboratory, consideration should be given to scoring additional cells." This will likely be the case in rat blood because of the rate of filtration of IE mentioned previously. Although there is no requirement to score MME along with MIE, it can be useful to preclude the presence of micronucleus-like bodies in the preparation [38] and to confirm the absence of a preexisting disease condition that might otherwise lead to a general increase in micronucleated erythrocytes making a particular supply of animals unsuitable (personal observation). MME incidences in control mice are expected to be similar to MIE values (i.e., approximately 0.1% or 1 per 1000); in rats, the value is lower (perhaps 0.01 or 0.02%).

Especially in laboratories with limited experience, it may be useful to stain and code two smears per animal and examine only the better smear. In that case, the slide reader should identify which smear has been examined (e.g., by initialing the label).

8.6.4.9 Identification of micronuclei

Criteria for identification of micronuclei (as well as the distinction between ME and IE) should be defined in the laboratory's SOPs and in the study protocol. Micronuclei are identified by the following criteria:

- Large enough to discern morphological characteristics and coloration but less than one-third the size of a nucleus.
- Should possess a generally rounded shape with a clearly defined outline.
- Should be deeply stained and similar in color to the nuclei of other cells.
- Should lie in the same focal plane as the cell.
- Lack internal structure (i.e., pyknotic).
- There should be no micronucleus-like debris in the area surrounding the cell.

Particular note should be made of misshapen ("cuboidal") and large "micronuclei." The latter can result from aneugenic effects [44], whereas the presence of both would be an indication of disruption of erythropoiesis (e.g., secondary to methemaglobinemia) rather than genotoxicity. Micronucleus-like debris can be caused by stain precipitate, dust, or microbial contamination of the FCS. Other inclusions in erythrocytes result from treatment with chemicals (e.g., Heinz bodies resulting from hemoglobin degradation and Q-bodies resulting from treatment with quinacrines); however, their staining characteristics and irregular morphology are quite distinct from that of micronuclei. Application of the precautions described previously and strict criteria indicated here will help to identify and avoid problems.

8.6.5 Records

Suitable forms should be prepared for recording results as per the example here.

Micronucleus Test Results for Encoded Slides Study number: *ABC123*

Microscope ID: No. 3						
	Proportion		MME	IE	MIE	
Slide Code	ie	me				Performed by/Completion Date
1	278	301	0	2000	2	
2	180	391	0	2000	1	
etc						
Comments: Reviewed by:				Date:		

ie, number of immature erythrocytes noted in proportion ie/(ie + me); me, number of mature erythrocytes noted in proportion; MME, number of micronucleated mature erythrocytes observed; IE, number of immature erythrocytes examined for micronuclei; MIE, number of micronucleated immature erythrocytes observed.

Entries should be made by indelible pen or, when permitted by your facility, by direct data entry. Example entries are shown in italics in this form. The microscope should be identified when vernier locations are being recorded.

8.6.6 Identification of Aneugenic Agents

Agents that disrupt the spindle apparatus resulting in micronucleus formation from lagging chromosomes are considered to be potentially aneugenic rather than mutagenic. Distinguishing this mode of induction is important in establishing potential effects and for risk analysis. In particular, spindle poisons need to reach a threshold level of exposure before effects are seen, which greatly assists in establishing an appropriate safety margin. The testing laboratory will usually be aware of spindle damage potential prior to the study; in which case, a main purpose of the test will be to establish the shape of the dose-response curve and confirm a NOEL (no observable effect level) for micronucleus induction in the bone marrow using an appropriate range of dose levels. The presence of predominantly large micronuclei with a high DNA content is symptomatic of spindle poisons [44]. However, more specific methods of identifying micronuclei formed from whole chromosomes are usually preferred as described here. Whatever the situation, positive control slides from animals treated with a clastogenic (e.g., mitomycin C or cyclophosphamide) and an aneugenic agent (e.g., vincristine, vinblastine, or colchicine) should be included for comparative purposes.

Centromeric staining is generally preferred in the mouse because the FISH-staining probe is specific and less subjective than kinetochore staining using the fluorescence-labeled CREST antibody. However, no universal centromeric probe is available for the rat, so the CREST-staining technique is generally used for identifying micronuclei formed from whole lagging chromosomes in that species, although Takeiri et al. [45] have proposed a mixed satellite pan-centromeric probe for use in the rat.

8.6.7 Centromeric Staining Using FISH

Centromeric labeling provides a method of identifying whether a micronucleus contains a centromere. The presence of a centromere signal in micronuclei is assumed to indicate the presence of a whole chromosome. The FISH technique is used with commercially available probes for the centromeres of mouse chromosomes that have fluorescent labels incorporated; CY3 label is red and FITC label is green when viewed through a fluorescent microscope with the appropriate filters.

8.6.7.1 Materials

- 20 × SSC (saline sodium citrate) stock solution = 3 M NaCl (17.53 g/100 mL) + 0.3 M trisodium citrate dihydrate (8.82 g/100 mL)
- 2 × SSC (1 in 10 dilution of stock)
- 2 × SSC with 0.1% Tween 20 (100 μL Tween 20 in 100 mL 2 × SSC)
- 0.4 × SSC with 0.3% Tween 20 (20 mL 2 × SSC + 80 mL water + 300 μL Tween 20)
- Pan-centromeric Star*FISH© paints (human and mouse) are available from Cambio UK

All solutions are prepared by dilution from stock of 20 × SSC, which is stable for 1 year and stored at room temperature.

8.6.7.2 FISH method using programmable hotplate

The FISH method uses a programmable hotplate such as HYBrite or Thermobrite. Care should be taken at all stages of using the chromosome paints to minimize light exposure because they are photo-degraded. Slides should be aged for at least 24 h at room temperature prior to centromeric labeling to dehydrate. The procedure is the same for both human and mouse probes and is as described here.

The HYBrite programmable hotplate is switched on prior to use to allow the hotplate to reach 42°C (approximately 10 min). The slides to be painted are warmed by placing them on the hotplate surface prior to use (see Note 4).

1. The pan-centromeric paint is taken from the freezer to thaw prior to use (at least 15 min).
2. 15–20 μL of mouse centromeric chromosome paint is added to each slide with a small coverslip. The coverslip is then sealed by adding rubber cement/glue around the edges of the coverslip. When the glue has dried, the slides are placed on the HYBrite hotplate. The program has a denaturation step of 69 °C for 5 min, followed by hybridization at 42 °C for between 16 and 40 h.
3. Prepare 0.4 × SSC with 0.3% Tween 20 in glass Coplin jar and place in the water bath with water covering approximately three-quarters of the height of the Coplin jar.

4. Heat to $73 \pm 1\,°C$ and allow approximately 1 h to get to temperature. Place $2 \times SSC$ 0.1% Tween 20 in a Coplin jar at room temperature.
5. Check the temperature of the water bath (see Note 5).
6. Remove slides from Hybrite. Remove glue and gently slide off the coverslips. Place two slides only at one time (see Note 6) in the Coplin jar in the water bath, agitate for 3−4 s, and leave in Coplin jar for 1 min.
7. Transfer slides to Coplin jar containing $2 \times SSC$ 0.1% Tween 20 for 2 min. Drain the slides (N.B. do not allow to dry) and add antifade containing DAPI counterstain. Add large (22×40 mm or 22×50 mm) coverslip and place in card tray. Store flat and in the dark prior to scoring on a suitable fluorescent microscope.
8. Allow temperature in Coplin jar to return to previous level (approximately 5−10 min) before washing the next two slides.

8.6.7.3 Alterative protocol for FISH

If a HYBriteTM machine is not available, then an alternative method must be used for probe hybridization (as described in StarFISH Catalogue and Protocols; available from Cambio).

1. Initially, slides are dehydrated via serial ethanol washing in 70%, 70%, 90%, 90% (v/v) ethanol for 2 min each, followed by 5 min in 100% ethanol.
2. Then slides are denatured in prewarmed 70% formamide (70 mL formamide + 30 mL $2 \times SSC$ solution) at $65\,°C$ for 1.5−2 min.
3. Slides are then quenched in ice-cold 70% (v/v) ethanol for 4 min, followed by subsequent dehydration (as described).
4. The whole chromosome probe, in hybridization buffer, is then warmed to $37\,°C$ and denatured at $65\,°C$ for 10 min.
5. The pan-centromeric probe in hybridization buffer is denatured at $85\,°C$ for 10 min and then immediately put on ice.
6. Finally, the probes would be combined, applied to the slide, and then allowed to hybridize at $37\,°C$ for approximately 16 h in an air-tight, humidified box.
7. Following hybridization, slides should be washed twice for 5 min in 50% formamide/ $2 \times SSC$ at $37\,°C$ and then twice in $2 \times SSC$ for 5 min.

8.6.7.4 FISH: slide checking

Check slides after counterstain and antifade are added to determine the presence of centromeric signals (either red or green) under the microscope in any nucleated cells (blue from DAPI counterstain) to determine that the hybridization has taken place.

8.6.7.5 FISH: slide scoring

Slides are scored using an appropriate fluorescence microscope with triple band pass filter and individual single filters for CY3 and FITC. Scoring is performed on digital counters. Data are recorded on paper. A total of 100 micronuclei should be assessed per slide. In animals with low incidences of micronuclei induction this may not be possible, so scoring should be limited to 20,000 IEs.

8.6.8 Kinetochore Labeling

Kineotochore labeling uses an antikinetochore antibody to determine whether micronuclei contain a centromere. It is used for rat *in vivo* micronucleus or other species for which centromeric paints are not feasible or commercially available. The presence of a kinetochore signal in the micronuclei is assumed to indicate the presence of a whole chromosome.

8.6.8.1 Materials

- *PBS (Phosphate-buffered saline)*. Supplier: Sigma-Aldrich; Storage Conditions: Room temperature. Dissolve each tablet in 200 mL water
- *Tween 20*. Supplier: Sigma-Aldrich; Storage Conditions: Room temperature
- *Vectashield mounting medium with propidium iodine*. Supplier: Vector Lab Inc; Storage Conditions: 4 °C
- *Primary antibody*. Antikinetochore antibody Supplier: Antibodies Inc.; Storage Conditions: −20 °C; Preparation method: Aliquoted into 200 µL volumes
- *Secondary antibody*. Fluorescein isothiocyanate (FITC)-conjugated goat antihuman IgG; Supplier: Antibodies Inc.; Storage Conditions: −20 °C; Preparation method: Aliquoted into 200 µL volumes

8.6.8.2 Methods

Care should be taken at all stages when using the antihuman IgG antibody with fluorescent FITC labels to minimize light exposure because they are photo-degraded. The procedure is therefore split into two distinct phases. Phase 1 can be conducted in the light; phase 2 must be conducted under minimal light to preserve the fluorescent label.

The indirect immunofluorescent labeling of kinetochore proteins is performed as previously described [46]. To preserve the integrity of the kinetochore proteins, cells are fixed in analytical reagent grade methanol at approximately −20 °C for 15 min and then air-dried at room temperature. As soon as the fixative evaporates, the slides are stored in slide boxes in a −20 °C freezer until analysis to preserve the kinetochore epitope.

Phase 1

The slides required for kinetochore labeling are immediately hydrated with PBS on removal from the freezer. While the slides are in the buffer, antikinetochore antibody is diluted 1:1 with PBS. The slides are removed from the PBS after approximately 10 min, allowing any excess PBS to drain off. Next, 100 µL of the diluted antibody is applied to each slide. A flexible plastic coverslip is then gently placed on each slide, spreading the antibody evenly across the surface of the slide. The slides are then incubated in a humidified chamber at 37 °C for approximately 1 h.

After incubation, unbound antibody is removed from the slides by washing in Coplin jars as detailed in steps 1 to 5 here (care is taken not to disturb the cells):

Step 1. Place in PBS for 1 min.
Step 2. Place in PBS containing 1% Tween 20 for 3 min, with gentle agitation.
Step 3. Rinse in PBS.
Step 4. Rinse in PBS.
Step 5. Place in PBS for 5 min.

Phase 2

While the slides are in the final wash (step 5), 10 µL of fluorescein isothiocyanate (FITC)-conjugated goat antihuman IgG is diluted 1:50 (10 µL in 490 µL of PBS). Once the slides have been removed from their final wash and drained, 120 µL of the fluorescent probe is placed onto each slide and spread evenly with a plastic coverslip as in phase 1. The slides are then incubated in a dark humidified chamber at 37 °C for approximately 1 h. After incubation, the slides are washed in a Coplin jar as detailed in steps 1 to 5. Once the slides have been removed from their final wash and drained, two to three drops of Vectashield mounting medium containing propidium iodide are placed onto each slide via a glass coverslip and then placed in a card slide tray for approximately 20 min to develop prior to scoring.

Slide Checking

Slides are assessed using a fluorescent microscope. The presence of kinetochore signals (green) in nucleated cells (red from counterstain) are checked to determine that the hybridization has taken place.

Slide Coding

The Study Director produces a code sheet using an Excel spreadsheet. All slides are allocated a slide code. The slide codes are written or printed on adhesive labels together with the study number. The code labels are applied to the appropriate slides according to the code sheet. The code sheet must be signed and dated by the individual who has performed the coding procedure, and then the code sheet is placed in a sealed envelope. The envelope is only opened after all analyses are complete for decoding. The code sheet is archived as raw data.

Scoring takes place on the red filter to identify the IEs containing micronuclei, and then the red filter is swapped for the green and triple band pass filters to ascertain whether a kinetochore signal is present.

Analysis of Slides

> Erythrocytes appear orange/red.
> Nucleated cells appear bright red.
> Micronuclei appear red; on the green filter, they have a green signal if a kinetochore is present.

One hundred micronucleated erythrocytes are scored and the number of erythrocytes is recorded. If 20,000 or 30,000 erythrocytes are reached and 100 micronucleated erythrocytes are not seen, then scoring is stopped. The number of total erythrocytes scored (i.e., 20,000 or 30,000) is decided on a study-to-study basis by the Study Director.

Scoring is performed on digital counters and results are recorded on paper.

Assessment of results

For each slide, the total number of micronuclei is calculated as the sum of the kinetochore-positive and kinetochore-negative micronuclei (MN); the numbers will be expressed per 2000 IEs scored.

The number of IEs scored is estimated using the group mean percentage of IEs reported in the relevant bone marrow micronucleus study. The group mean percentage from the bone marrow micronucleus study is multiplied by the total number of erythrocytes scored for the same group in the current kinetochore study to calculate the total number of IEs scored per group.

To estimate the induced frequencies of kinetochore-positive and kinetochore-negative MN, the control frequencies for each are first calculated. These will then be deducted from the actual kinetochore-positive and kinetochore-negative MN frequencies in each treated group to give the induced frequencies. The percentages of total induced micronuclei that are kinetochore-positive and kinetochore-negative are then calculated.

8.7 Automated Analysis and Flow Cytometry

Individual semi-automated and fully automated slide scanning systems have been devised and are in use in a few laboratories [30,47]. However, the most widely used and validated automatic system relies on a three-color fluorescent staining method to detect DNA, platelets, and a surface marker of IEs followed by single-laser flow cytometry [48]. Because this is the only widely used and standardized automatic method, it is described in detail in this section.

Advance preparation of specific reagents and software templates is advised to facilitate efficient sample processing. It is also recommended to label all necessary tubes and vials with sample IDs prior to beginning sample processing.

As indicated, many of the reagents and materials required for flow cytometric scoring of micronucleated reticulocytes are provided with MicroFlow kits available from Litron Laboratories (Rochester, NY). Additional materials and supplies that are required but not supplied with the kits are specifically noted.

8.7.1 Individual Reagents

Anticoagulant solution (In Vivo MicroFlow^{PLUS} kit)
Buffered solution (In Vivo MicroFlow^{PLUS} kit)
Long-term storage solution (LTSS) (In Vivo MicroFlow^{PLUS} kit)
Rat anti-CD71 antibody (In Vivo MicroFlow^{PLUS} kit)
DNA stain (In Vivo MicroFlow^{PLUS} kit)
Platelet antibody (In Vivo MicroFlow^{PLUS} kit)
Biological standards (In Vivo MicroFlow^{PLUS} kit)
    Positive control blood samples (fixed)
    Negative control blood samples (fixed)
    Malaria biostandard blood samples (fixed)

8.7.2 Solution and Material Preparation

The following solutions are made fresh daily under sterile conditions. The volumes provided here are shown as the amounts required for one sample. Determine the number of samples you plan to process in a single day and scale up the volumes accordingly. Be sure to include additional volume of the working reagents for the Malaria Biostandard, CD71 set-up sample, and negative and positive controls.

If you are washing fixed samples (both experimental or the provided biological standards) out of LTSS, then the wash solution should contain 1% FCS (v/v). This solution can also be used for preparing the Ab labeling solutions described here, so be sure to factor this additional volume when determining how much buffer solution and 1% FCS are required for both washing samples and preparing the labeling solutions.

Fixative tubes (must be prepared at least 1 day prior to blood collection)

One 15 mL polypropylene centrifuge tube is required per sample; two are needed if fixing in duplicate. Add 2 mL of fixative to each tube and replace caps. Label each tube with the appropriate information. If labels are used, then ensure they are compatible with ultracold storage. It is also helpful to label the cap of each tube. If not using ultracold freezer-compatible labels, then it is helpful to cover the labels with clear tape to protect them from splashed liquids and to prevent them from falling off in the freezer. Place the rack of tubes overnight (or longer) at $-75\,°C$ to $-85\,°C$ to allow for sufficient chilling of the fixative.

Washing solution for samples in LTSS

Combine 5 mL buffer solution with 50 μL FCS for each sample/biostandard in LTSS. Filter through a 0.2-μm filter and keep on ice. This solution can be used on subsequent days if it is made under sterile conditions, refrigerated during storage, and filtered again on the day of use.

Anticoagulant/diluent vials (prepare prior to blood collection)

One vial is required per blood sample; label vial with appropriate information. Aseptically aliquot 350 μL anticoagulant/diluent into each vial and refrigerate until use.

Labeling solution I

Whole blood: Thaw RNase solution and quickly spin along with rat anti-CD71 Ab and platelet Ab to achieve best recovery of solutions. Based on the number of samples that will be processed and analyzed that day, aseptically combine 100 μL of cold buffer solution with 1 μL of RNase Solution and 1 μL rat anti-CD71 antibody per sample in a sterile vessel. Tap gently to mix. This is labeling solution I. Remove 80 μL of labeling solution I and place into a flow cytometry tube. This will receive 20 μL of malaria biostandard and will be used for calibrating the flow cytometer.

Bone marrow: Thaw RNase solution and quickly spin along with rat anti-CD71 Ab and platelet Ab to achieve best recovery of solutions. Based on the number of samples that will be processed and analyzed that day, aseptically combine 100 μL of cold buffer solution with 1.5 μL of RNase solution and 1.5 μL rat anti-CD71 antibody per sample in a sterile vessel. Tap gently to mix. This is labeling solution I. Remove 80 μL of labeling solution I and place into a flow cytometry tube. This will receive 20 μL of malaria biostandard and will be used for calibrating the flow cytometer

Labeling solution II

Add the 0.5 μL platelet Ab per 100 μL of labeling solution I to the same tube as noted and gently mix. This is now labeling solution II. Aliquot 80 μL of labeling solution II into labeled flow cytometry tubes. Prepare one tube for each experimental sample to be analyzed that day, and also one tube each for the malaria biostandard and CD71 setup sample. Cover all tubes containing labeling solutions with foil and store at 2 °C to 8 °C until needed.

DNA staining solution

Aseptically combine 2 mL buffer solution with 50 μL DNA stain in a sterile container based on the number of samples required. Store the DNA staining solution in the dark at 2 °C to 8 °C (not on ice) until needed.

8.7.3 Flow Cytometry Method

Flow cytometric enumeration of MN is routinely performed in mouse and rat blood and bone marrow. This section specifically describes the protocol for rat peripheral blood and bone marrow [4,49,50]. Information on the mouse-specific procedures and assay components can be obtained from Litron Laboratories (Rochester, NY, USA; www. litronlabs.com). Procedures differ somewhat depending on whether blood or bone marrow is being analyzed; these differences are clearly marked in the following section.

8.7.4 Blood Collection

Collect 60 μL to a maximum of 120 μL of blood from each animal directly into vials containing 350 μL anticoagulant/diluent (Litron) and mix gently. Samples can be stored at room temperature for up to 6 h or refrigerated for up to 24 h before fixing. Alternatively, blood can be collected in K_2EDTA-coated tubes (e.g., BD catalog number 367861), where it is stable at 2 °C to 8 °C for 2 days. In this case, invert to mix, remove 100 μL of sample, and dilute in 350 μL anticoagulant/diluent, and then proceed as described here.

8.7.5 Bone Marrow Collection and Processing

8.7.5.1 Prepare cellulose columns

Fractionation of rat bone marrow through microcrystalline cellulose columns is essential for reliable flow cytometric micronucleus analysis. Procedures are similar to those described by Romagna and Staniforth [51].

1. Prepare approximately 1.0 g of cellulose mix per femur by mixing equal portions (by weight) of α-cellulose and Sigmacell cellulose type 50 into a screw-cap bottle. Seal and mix vigorously by inverting and swirling for approximately 5 min.

2. Cut Fisher lens paper into circles to use as filter discs large enough to cover the bottom of a 20-mL syringe barrel without gaps but small enough to easily fit into the syringe.

3. Remove plungers from the 20-mL syringes and insert the circular filter discs into the bottom. Tare the syringe on a balance and add approximately 1.0 g of matrix mix if one femur is to be fractionated and 1.2 g of matrix mix if two femurs are to be fractionated. Tap the syringe upright to lightly pack the matrix material. Insert a modified syringe plunger (rubber tip removed and plastic shaved for easy fit) to very lightly pat down any remaining loose matrix material. Keep upright and cover with parafilm or foil until use.

4. When ready to use, mount columns over 15-mL centrifuge tubes.

8.7.6 Collect and Fractionate Bone Marrow Samples

1. Aliquot 2−3 mL heat-inactivated, filtered FCS into labeled centrifuge tubes (one for each femur).

2. Remove femur(s). Draw up FCS into a 3-mL syringe, insert needle, and flush bone marrow from one femur into the corresponding centrifuge tube.

3. Finely disperse the bone marrow into the FCS by repeatedly aspirating and discharging gently with the syringe into the centrifuge tube. Cap the tube and process other femurs.

4. Centrifuge at approximately $100 \times g$ to $150 \times g$ for 5 min. Aspirate supernatant, leaving 0.5 mL or less of serum. Resuspend pellet into residual serum. At this point, prepare slides, if necessary.

5. Dilute the concentrated bone marrow with approximately 2 mL of buffer solution.

6. Holding the pipette tip just above the center of the column matrix, add the diluted bone marrow drop-wise to premounted columns.

7. Add 13 mL to 14 mL of buffer solution (drop-wise at first so the column matrix is not disturbed) to elute the erythrocytes from the column and collect in 15 mL polypropylene centrifuge tubes. Note that the addition rate can gradually increase after a meniscus forms above the matrix.

8. Centrifuge the eluted erythrocyte fraction at approximately $200 \times g$ to $250 \times g$ for 10 min. Aspirate the supernatant, leaving 200 μL to 300 μL.

9. Resuspend the cell pellet and fix within 4 h.

8.7.7 Fixation of Blood and Bone Marrow Samples

It is extremely important that the tubes containing fixative remain ultracold ($-75\,°C$ to $-85\,°C$) and do not come in contact with vapors from dry ice. CO_2 vapor causes carbonation and cellular aggregation. Therefore, fixative should not be stored in a freezer containing dry ice. If you are unable to fix blood samples DIRECTLY from the $-75\,°C$ to $-85\,°C$ freezer as described here, follow the alternative fixing procedure found on the Litron Labs website (www.litronlabs.com).

Keep fixative in an ultracold ($-75\,°C$ to $-85\,°C$) freezer (a chest freezer is preferred because it maintains temperature better than upright freezers). Perform the following steps very quickly and work near the freezer. Samples can be fixed in duplicate.

It may be helpful for two individuals to perform this procedure, with one filling the micropipettors with diluted blood samples and the other removing the fixative tubes from the freezer. Otherwise, if a single operator is performing the fixation procedure, remove only one tube of fixative from the ultracold freezer at a time. After adding the diluted blood sample, return this tube to the freezer and retrieve the next fixative tube.

1. Immediately prior to fixing, invert the vial containing the sample to ensure a homogeneous suspension. Using a micropipettor, retrieve 180 μL of the diluted whole blood sample. For bone marrow samples that have undergone column clean-up, retrieve 150 μL of the bone marrow suspension.
2. Remove the corresponding labeled 15 mL tube containing fixative from the freezer, uncap, and position the pipette tip approximately 1 cm above the surface of the ultracold fixative.
3. Make sure that the pipette tip does not touch the side of the tube or the surface of fixative, and forcefully dispense the sample directly into fixative (see the diagram on the next page).
4. Cap the tube of fixed sample VERY tightly and vortex briefly (only 3 to 5 s) and return it to the ultracold freezer ($-75\,°C$ to $-85\,°C$). If a vortexer cannot be placed right next to the freezer, then hold the top of the tube with one hand and use your other hand to sharply strike the bottom of the tube several times before returning it to the freezer. (steps 3 through 5 should take no more than 10 s.)
5. Change the pipette tip and repeat steps 1 through 5 for the remaining diluted samples. There should be enough volume in each vial to fix each sample twice, if necessary.
6. If the freezer temperature begins to warm up significantly (i.e., increases by $5\,°C$), then stop processing samples. Wait until the freezer temperature returns to the required range before completing sample fixation. Again, due to their ability to maintain temperature, chest freezers are recommended.
7. Store the samples at $-75\,°C$ to $-85\,°C$ for at least 3 days before washing to store in LTSS or analyzing on the flow cytometer.

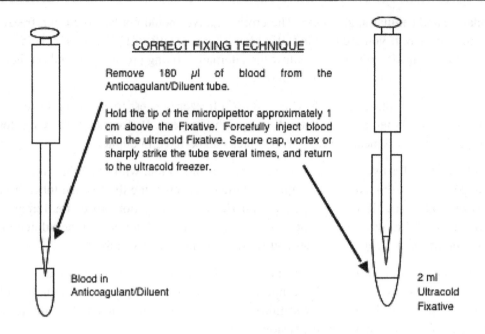

CORRECT FIXING TECHNIQUE

Remove 180 µl of blood from the Anticoagulant/Diluent tube.

Hold the tip of the micropipettor approximately 1 cm above the Fixative. Forcefully inject blood into the ultracold Fixative. Secure cap, vortex or sharply strike the tube several times, and return to the ultracold freezer.

Blood in Anticoagulant/Diluent

2 ml Ultracold Fixative

INCORRECT FIXING TECHNIQUES

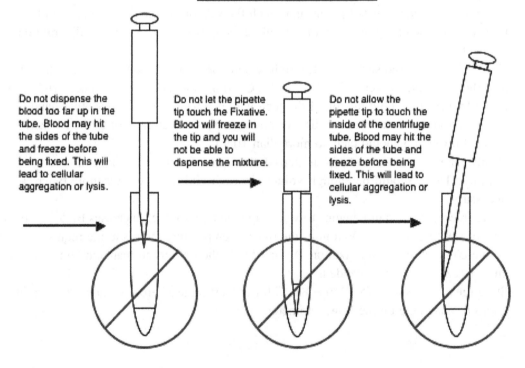

Do not dispense the blood too far up in the tube. Blood may hit the sides of the tube and freeze before being fixed. This will lead to cellular aggregation or lysis.

Do not let the pipette tip touch the Fixative. Blood will freeze in the tip and you will not be able to dispense the mixture.

Do not allow the pipette tip to touch the inside of the centrifuge tube. Blood may hit the sides of the tube and freeze before being fixed. This will lead to cellular aggregation or lysis.

8.7.8 Storage of Fixed Samples

We strongly recommend that methanol fixed samples should be transferred into LTSS as described in Sections 8.6.1–8.6.3. If you have access to a chest-style ultracold freezer that will maintain the fixed samples at the required temperature range consistently, and where the samples can be stored toward the bottom of the freezer, then samples can be maintained in fixative.

If the freezer is not a chest-style freezer, is opened routinely, or the samples cannot be stored away from the freezer door, then samples should be washed out of fixative and transferred into LTSS, as described. Ideally, samples should be transferred into LTSS after they have been in fixative for at least 3 days. It is possible to transfer samples into LTSS many days or even weeks after fixation in fixative, but during this time they are extremely sensitive to temperature fluctuations.

8.7.8.1 Wash samples out of fixative

It may be helpful for two individuals to perform this procedure, with one tapping and opening tubes and the other adding buffer solution. Once two people have become proficient with this procedure, it is possible to remove as many as three tubes from the freezer at a time.

1. Pack buffer solution on ice to achieve an ice-cold, but not freezing, temperature (approximately 45 min).
2. Have a container of ice and a 25 mL pipette ready for aliquoting buffer solution in step d. Perform the following steps as quickly as possible (within approximately 20 s); plan to work at a location adjacent to the freezer.
3. Remove up to three tubes of fixed experimental samples from the ultracold freezer. Quickly place the capped tubes on ice and close the freezer. Tap each tube sharply three or four times (or vortex for 3 to 5 s) to resuspend the cells and loosen the cap on each tube.
4. Immediately add 12 mL of ice-cold buffer solution to each tube. Be careful not to touch the tube with the pipette tip to prevent transfer of sample from one tube to another. Tighten the caps, invert the tubes once to mix the solutions, and immediately replace on ice until all are processed.
5. Repeat steps c and d for additional samples. Note that once buffer solution has been added to the fixed cells, it is important for the tubes to remain on ice or at 2 °C to 8 °C unless otherwise specified.

6. Centrifuge the tubes at approximately $300 \times g$ to $400 \times g$ for 5 min. When centrifugation is complete, quickly remove the tubes and immediately replace them on ice.
7. Aspirate the supernatant from each tube, leaving less than 50 μL of supernatant in which to resuspend cells. Recap the tubes and immediately return to ice.
8. Working with one sample at a time, quickly resuspend the cells in the remaining supernatant by tapping the bottom of the tube or by vortexing. Put the tube back on ice and continue to resuspend the remaining samples.
9. At this point, either transfer cells into LTSS for further storage (Section 11.2) or proceed to labeling (Section 13) and analysis (Section 14).

8.7.9 Transfer Samples to LTSS

After washing out of fixative and resuspending pellets (Section 11.1, steps 1−8), add 1 mL of LTSS to each tube and store at $-75\,°C$ to $-85\,°C$. Samples can also be transferred into cryovials to save freezer space.

8.7.9.1 Wash samples out of LTSS

Ideally, samples and biological standards should be washed on the day they will be analyzed; however, once washed out of LTSS, they are stable for approximately 3 days (stored at 2 °C to 8 °C).

1. Prepare at least 5 mL of buffer solution with 1% FCS for each sample in LTSS and biological standard to be washed. Filter through a 0.2-μm filter and place on ice. (If all of this solution is not used, refrigerate and filter again on day of use or discard and prepare fresh when washing samples on another day.)
    a. If samples are in cryovials, aliquot 5 mL of this buffer solution plus 1% FCS into the appropriate number of labeled 15 mL centrifuge tubes (one tube per sample) and keep on ice.
    b. If samples are in 15 mL tubes, you will add 5 mL of this buffer plus 1% FCS to each tube.
2. Remove the appropriate cells from the ultracold freezer and thaw at ambient temperature.
3. Immediately upon thawing, either aliquot contents into tubes containing 5 mL buffer plus 1% FCS or add 5 mL buffer solution plus 1% FCS to each tube. Invert once to mix, and then place back on ice. Repeat with the remaining samples.

4. Centrifuge the tubes at approximately $300 \times g$ to $400 \times g$ for 10 min. When centrifugation is complete, quickly remove the tubes and immediately replace them on ice.

5. Aspirate the supernatant from each tube, leaving less than 50 μL of supernatant in which to resuspend cells. Recap the tubes and immediately return to ice.

6. Working with one sample at a time, quickly resuspend the cells in the remaining supernatant by tapping the bottom of the tube or by vortexing. Put the tube back on ice and continue to resuspend the remaining samples.

7. After all pellets are resuspended, store the samples at 2 °C to 8 °C or on ice until labeling for flow cytometric analysis.

8.7.10 Label Washed Samples for Flow Analysis

To ensure an accurate reading, it is important that all cells are labeled with the respective Abs and that the cellular RNA is degraded. Therefore, make sure when adding the blood sample to the labeling solution that all of the sample comes into contact with the labeling solution. If a drop of blood is on the side of the tube, then wash it down with the solution already in that tube.

1. With washed samples on ice, tap the tubes to resuspend the cell pellets (if not recently tapped out).

2. Add 20 μL of malaria biostandard to the FCM tube containing labeling solution I. Gently tap to mix.

3. Add 20 μL of malaria biostandard to an FCM tube containing labeling solution II. Add 20 μL of CD71 setup to an FCM tube containing labeling solution II. Gently tap to mix.

4. Add 20 μL of each experimental sample to the appropriately labeled FCM tubes containing labeling solution II. Tap the tubes gently to mix.

5. Return any remaining washed samples to 2 °C to 8 °C for storage.

6. Cover FCM tubes with foil to protect from light and incubate at 2 °C to 8 °C in the refrigerator (preferred) or on ice for 30 min.

7. For peripheral blood samples, after 30 min at 2 °C to 8 °C, tap each tube very gently to resuspend cells and place in new racks (that are not cold). Protect from light and incubate the tubes at room temperature for 30 min to ensure complete degradation of cellular RNA. If room temperature is below 20 °C, then the second 30-min incubation can be modified so that the samples are incubated at approximately 37 °C for 15 min and then at room temperature for 15 min.

8. For bone marrow samples, after 30 min at 2 °C to 8 °C, tap each tube very gently to resuspend cells and place in new racks (that are not cold). Protect from light and incubate the tubes containing the experimental samples at approximately 37 °C for 30 min and the malaria biostandard samples at room temperature for 30 min to ensure complete degradation of cellular RNA.

9. After incubation at room temperature, return the tubes to 2 °C to 8 °C until analysis.

8.7.11 Flow Cytometric Analysis

8.7.11.1 Flow cytometer calibration with biological standards

Please note that the biological standards must first be washed out of LTSS (Section 8.6.3) and labeled (Section 8.7) before being used to calibrate the flow cytometer. The following setup and compensation instructions are specific for CellQuest software, but they should be useful with other software packages. If using FASCDiva software, perform the following steps:

> Open the FACSDiva template (.xml file) for Rat PLUS Blood or Bone Marrow (available for download from the Litron Laboratories website (www.litronlabs.com)). Open the following folders on your computer: My computer >New Volume (D) >BDExport >Templates >Experiment >General.
> Drag the template into the General folder.
> Close this window and start the FASCDiva software.

Click on "Experiment" in the menu bar and create a new folder. Select the new folder and click the "New Experiment" button on the Browser toolbar. The Experiment Template dialog appears. Click the 'General Tab" and select your template.

1. Before analyzing samples, ensure that the flow cytometer is working properly. Follow the manufacturer's instructions for the appropriate setup and quality control procedures. Open the template file.

2. Gently tap the bottom of the tube containing the washed and labeled CD71 setup sample to loosen settled cells. Add 1.5 mL to 2.0 mL of DNA staining solution and place the sample on the flow cytometer. (While this sample is being analyzed, add DNA staining solution to the malaria biostandard samples and place at 2 °C to 8 °C until analysis.) In Plot A, adjust the "Single Cells" region to include the cells of interest and exclude aggregates (see Appendix A).

3. Adjust FL1 PMT voltage so the High CD71-Positive RETs are located just above the lower green demarcation on the Y-axis of Plot E. Adjust FL3 PMT voltage so the NCEs are within the first decade of red fluorescence. The resulting plot should look

similar to the plot shown here. Note: the plot shown is an example of gating used for rat blood; if you are studying mouse blood samples, then refer to the appropriate examples in the mouse-specific manual available at www.litronlabs.com.

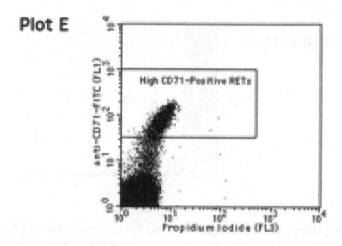

4. Place the malaria biostandard sample in labeling solution I on the flow cytometer. Refrigerate the CD71 Setup sample.
5. Viewing Plot D1, adjust the FL2 PMT voltage until the majority of cells in the lower left area are just to the left of the "Platelets" region. The resulting plot should look similar to the one shown here.

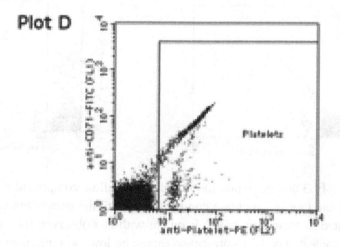

6. Viewing Histogram B, adjust FL3 PMT voltage until the nonparasitized cells approach the first decade of FL3 fluorescence and the first parasite peak is well resolved.

(BD CellQuest users are advised to place the first parasite peak at channel 22 ± 2 on Histogram B.) The location of the nucleated cells should fall in the last half of the last decade of red fluorescence. The resulting plot should look similar to the one here.

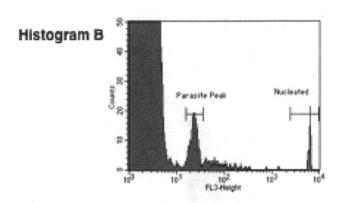

7. Eliminate the yellow (FL2) component of the FITC signal. Adjust FL2-%FL1 compensation to eliminate the yellow component of FITC. Viewing Plot D1, increase compensation until the young FITC-positive cells are positioned directly above the mature FITC-negative cells. Correct compensation is set when cells containing a single parasite are aligned in a vertical plane. See the before and after plots here.

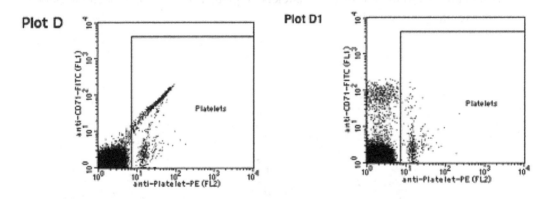

8. Adjust FL2-%FL3 compensation to eliminate the yellow component of propidium iodide. Viewing Plot D2, increase compensation until the parasitized cells show low FL2-associated fluorescence, which is on par with that observed for the NCEs at the origin. The nucleated cells' fluorescence should be low, no more than the first decade of FL2. When compensation is set appropriately, the parasitized cells should not be evident in the "Platelets" region of Plot D1. See the before and after plots of D2 and D1 here.

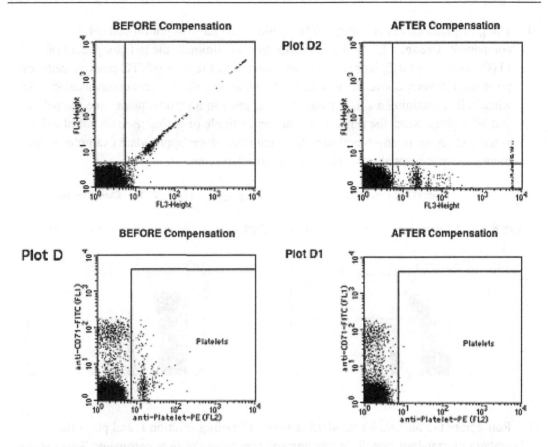

9. Readjust the FL3 PMT voltage, if necessary. (BD CellQuest users are advised to place the first parasite peak at channel 22 ± 2 on Histogram B.) If this is performed, then compensation may need slight adjustments.

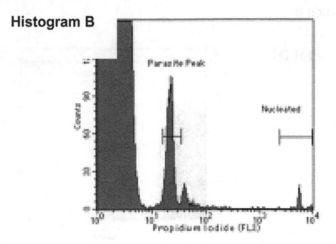

10. The green fluorescent antibody (FITC-conjugated) has a slight far-red (FL3) component. Use the FL3-%FL2 compensation to eliminate the red component of FITC. Viewing Plot E, increase compensation until the young FITC-positive cells are positioned directly above the mature FITC-negative cells. Correct compensation is set when cells containing a single parasite are aligned in a vertical plane. See the before and after plots. Note: the plots shown are an example of gating used for rat blood; if you are studying mouse blood samples, then refer to the appropriate examples in the mouse-specific manual available at www.litronlabs.com.

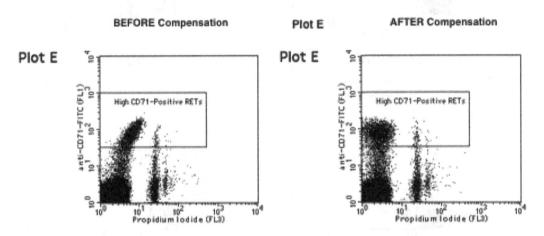

11. Refrigerate the malaria biostandard sample in labeling solution I, and place the malaria biostandard sample in labeling solution II on the flow cytometer. This sample includes the antiplatelet antibody; therefore, it should have FL2-associated fluorescence (PE). Without adjusting voltages or compensation, the resulting plot should look similar to the one here. Refrigerate the malaria biostandard sample in labeling solution II.

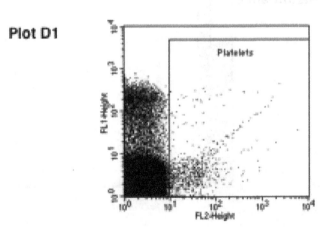

12. Once instrumentation and software settings are configured with the CD71 setup and malaria biostandard samples, continue to monitor the location of the nucleated cell peak of the experimental blood samples throughout the course of an analysis session. This measurement is useful for guarding against instrument drift. If the nucleated cells drift out of position, then use the CD71 setup and malaria biostandard samples stored at 2–8 °C to readjust the instrument as necessary.

13. After calibrating the flow cytometer with the CD71 setup and malaria biostandard samples each day, analyze experimental samples.

8.7.12 Analysis of Experimental Samples

1. It is preferable if the regions and quadrants are not changed between experimental samples. This is why it is worth taking some extra time to carefully consider PMT voltages and compensation settings initially. The region "Single Cells" on Plot A may need to be adjusted between samples (to accurately define the light scatter characteristics of unaggregated cells).

2. If this is your first time using this process, analyze the kit-supplied positive and negative control samples. Otherwise, proceed to the analysis of experimental samples. These samples may also be useful for demonstrating proficiency in the method and providing data regarding so-called scoring controls that may be required for compliance with certain regulatory guidelines. It is up to the user to determine what is necessary to meet such regulatory requirements.

3. It is important to maintain a consistent flow rate; therefore, do not change the flow rate after calibrating your instrument with the biological standard.

4. Analyze experimental samples by adding 1.5 mL to 2.0 mL of DNA staining solution to a sample. Place the sample on the flow cytometer and analyze. It is important not to change the FL3 PMT voltage (malaria biostandard assured this was appropriate), although FL3-%FL2 compensation may need slight adjustment so that RETs sit directly above the NCEs.

5. While one sample is being analyzed, add 1.5 mL to 2.0 mL of DNA staining solution to the next sample and place at 2 °C to 8 °C.

6. To obtain meaningful micronucleus statistics, it is important to use a spreadsheet rather than CellQuest's "% Gated" or "% Total" statistics. A sample spreadsheet is available from the website. Within this spreadsheet, input the number of "Events" observed in the Quadrant Statistics to calculate the following:

% RET = (UL + UR)/(UL + UR + LL + LR)*100

% MN-NCE = (LR)/(LR + LL)*100

% MN-RET = (UR)/(UR + UL)*100

8.7.13 Template Preparation for Flow Cytometric Analyses

Template files have been included with this kit but are specific to CellQuest or FACSDiva software. The next pages show actual screen images of the CellQuest template's graphs and histogram, the gates used for each plot, and how a stop mode of 20,000 reticulocytes was set. Flow cytometry operators who are not using CellQuest software should find these pages valuable for constructing their own data acquisition and analysis template.

It also may be helpful to run single-color compensation controls and use auto-compensation if this is available with the software you are using.

We recommend that if you are using FACSDiva software, you should have parameters of "Height" rather than "Area." When analyzing the single-color control for the DNA stain, adjust PMT voltage so that nucleated cells fall in the last decade of red fluorescence.

Defining Gates:

G1 = R1 = "Single Cells"

G2 = R2 = "Total RBCs"

G3 = R1 and R2 = "Single Cells" AND "Total RBCs"

G4 = R3 = "High CD71-Positive RETs"

G5 = R1 and R2 and R3 = "Single Cells" AND "Total RBCs" AND "High CD71-Positive RETs"

G6 = R1 and R2 and not R4 = "Single Cells" AND "Total RBCs" AND NOT "Platelets"

G7 = R1 and R2 and R3 and not R4 = "Single Cells" AND "Total RBCs" AND "High CD71-Positive RETs" AND NOT "Platelets"

1. Gate for each Plot:

Plot A	No Gate
Plot B	G1
Plot C	G1
Plot D1	G3
Plot D2	G1
Plot E	G3
Plot F	G6

2. Use Gate G7 to set the stop mode. This will allow you to stop data acquisition at a specified number of RETs (typically 20,000). For this gate to work accurately, the lower green demarcation line for region "High CD71-Positive RETs" on Plot E and the horizontal line of the quadrant in Plot F need to be at the exact same Y-value.

3. Save this template file. This template file should be appropriate for all rat blood analyses. To ensure consistency of data, it is preferable for no changes to be made to the location and size of the regions between samples. The exception is the location and size of the Single Cells region on Plot A, which may require minor adjustments.

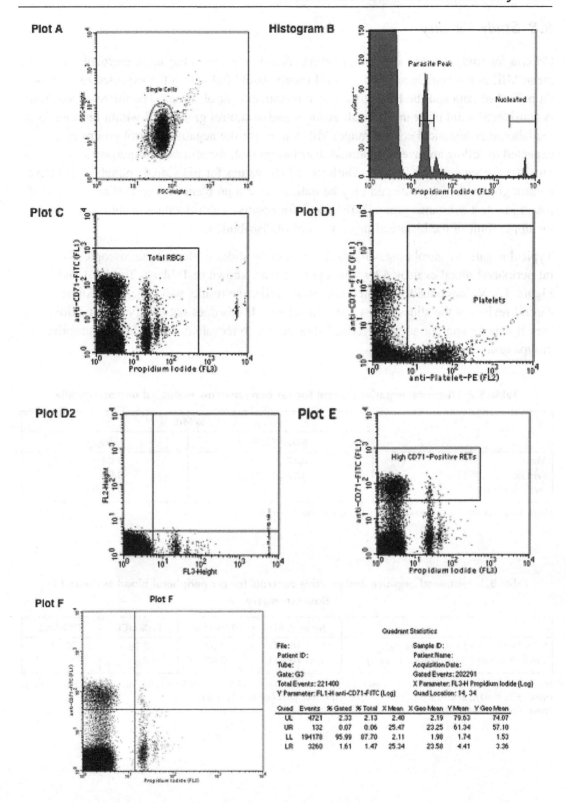

8.8 Study Validity

Criteria for study validity and interpretation should be given in the study protocol. The mean MIE in the vehicle/negative control group should fall within the expected range based on published data and the laboratory's own historical control values. The micronucleus test is considered valid if mean MIE values for negative control groups fall within or close to the laboratory historical control range. MIE values for the negative control groups are expected to follow an inverse binomial distribution that, for all practical purposes, is virtually the same as the Poisson. Outliers in MIE values for individual animals in negative control groups are very rare and may be indicative of a problem or a borderline response if found in a test substance group. MIE values for positive control values should lie beyond the upper limit of the historical negative control distribution.

Typical negative control ranges for rat bone marrow slides evaluated microscopically and rat peripheral blood evaluated by flow cytometry are shown in Tables 8.2 and 8.3 and Figure 8.3. Values outside accepted ranges or borderline results will generally require a careful review of the slides (and vernier locations). If this does not clarify the situation, then it may be appropriate for a second slide-reader to reevaluate slides from appropriate groups under code.

Table 8.2: Historical negative control for rat bone marrow evaluated microscopically

	% MIE	
	Mean (SD)	Range
Male	0.17 (0.04)	0.04–0.36
Female	0.17 (0.04)	0.06–0.47
Individual rats	—	0.0–0.78

Source: Data from 109 studies conducted in 1992–2005 at Bristol-Myers Squibb.

Table 8.3: Historical negative and positive controls for rat peripheral blood evaluated by flow cytometry

	Mean ± SD	95% LCL	95% UCL	99% UCL
VC %MNRET (32 studies, 166 rats)	0.13 (0.03)	0.07	0.18	0.21
CP-10 %MNRET (10 studies, 47 rats)	1.51 (0.53)	0.40	2.6	—

SD, standard deviation; 95% LCL, 95% lower confidence limit (mean − (2 × SD)); 95% UCL, 95% upper confidence limit (mean + (2 × SD)); and 99% UCL = 99% upper confidence limit (mean + (3 × SD)).
Source: Data collected in 2012–2014 at Bristol-Myers Squibb.

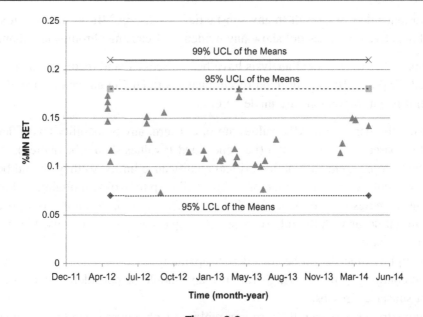

Figure 8.3

Historical vehicle control for rat peripheral blood evaluated by flow cytometry and background frequency of micronucleated reticulocytes (%MNRET) over time. *Source: Data collected from 2012—2014 at Bristol-Myers Squibb.*

8.9 Interpretation of Results and Statistical Analysis

8.9.1 MIE Values

Because male and female animals show qualitatively similar effects in the micronucleus test, when a particular study involves use of both sexes it is generally acceptable to combine the results prior to analysis and interpretation [52]. This maximizes the power of statistical analysis and reduces the likelihood of an inappropriate interpretation. A positive effect (i.e., evidence of chromosome damage) is indicated by a statistically significant increase in the mean MIE value for one or more test substance groups compared to the concurrent control with a mean value and at least one or two individual animal values above the upper tolerance limit (98%) of the historical negative control range. In cases where more than one dose level is available, any such increase is generally expected to be dose-related, although certain mechanisms of activity may result in a plateau or all-or-nothing response (e.g., spindle poisons), or perhaps a downturn at high doses due to cytostatic activity, bearing in mind that the optimal sampling time for detection of effects can be dose- and compound-dependent.

If a test substance does not result in any substantial increase in MIE as defined, it should be considered negative (i.e., does not show any evidence of causing chromosome damage).

Various approaches to statistical analysis have been discussed and recommended (e.g., Lovell [53]) and, bearing in mind recent changes to OECD guidance on study design, some general recommendations are made here.

1. Because only increases in MIE values are of concern, any probability levels determined should be based on the upper tail (i.e., one sided P values should be quoted). Guidelines do not generally define critical significance limits, so they should be defined in the protocol. A critical P value of <0.01 will help to avoid highlighting slight apparent increases that are generally due to chance variation when $P<0.05$ is chosen, which might occur with the relatively small sample sizes commonly used in most standalone studies.
2. Each sampling time should be considered separately.
3. Positive control groups show high variance and should be considered independently of the test substance groups.
4. Nonparametric tests (generally based on ranking) lack power when the group size is limited and should be avoided when only a single sex and/or dose level is being examined.
5. Because MIE values for unaffected animals are expected to approximate to a Poisson distribution, individual values should be subjected to the $\sqrt{(x + 1/2)}$ transformation prior to conventional statistical analysis.
6. MIE results can then be subjected to ANOVA and/or comparison of individual groups using an equivalent t-test, which takes into account the number of comparisons being made (Dunnetts). In general, the response is expected to increase with dose, so an appropriate trend test such as Williams test is arguably more appropriate and powerful [54]. The tests mentioned here are widely used in toxicological and clinical investigations, but more specialized models may be needed under certain circumstances when analyzing results for NOEL or point of departure, in which case you will need the help of a specialist statistician.

8.9.2 Proportion of Immature Erythrocytes

This proportion can be subjected to statistical analysis in a way similar to MIE results, but no transformation is needed prior to analysis. Bone marrow toxicity/depression is indicated by a dose-related (where appropriate) statistically significant reduction in the proportion compared with the concurrent control group. Results for individual studies can be saved in a historical control database for reference purpose, but no comparison needs to be made with previous results. In particular, the proportion of IEs decreases with age, so comparison is only appropriate when animals are of similar ages. Animals treated with a cytotoxic agent such as the positive control are expected to show only a slight or no decrease in the proportion at the first, and usually the only, sampling time for positive controls because of the time taken for the dividing erythroblast population to develop into IEs. In addition, if the positive control samples are derived from an earlier study, then that comparison is inappropriate, especially if the animals are of different ages.

Bone marrow depression in routine testing is unusual and often associated with cytostatic or cytotoxic agents that generally cause increases in MIE in any case. It can also result from indirect effects. It is best not to rely on this as evidence of target organ exposure in routine testing.

8.10 Nongenotoxic Mechanisms of Induction of Micronucleated Erythrocytes

8.10.1 Causes

As discussed previously, foreign bodies and nonnuclear cellular inclusions can be mistaken for micronuclei on occasion. However, the use of good technique coupled with nucleic acid–specific fluorescent staining largely avoids problems with micronucleus-like bodies while providing improved differentiation between immature and mature erythrocytes with fewer borderline cells. Increases in erythrocytes containing micronuclei can occur as a result of irrelevant or nongenotoxic mechanisms, including:

1. Direct stimulation or suppression (followed by rebound) of erythropoiesis, for example, by chemicals with erythropoietic activity including cobalt and erythropoietin itself [55–57]
2. Indirect stimulation of erythropoiesis as a result of anemia, for example, due to excessive internal bleeding or anemia consequent to methemaglobinemia
3. Prolonged departure from normal body temperature
4. A preexisting disease condition in a particular supply of animals

Potential "irrelevant" mechanisms of formation of MIE are described in detail elsewhere [58] and include accelerated erythropoiesis leading to retention of some nuclear fragments during the transition from erythroblast to erythrocyte (i.e., incomplete enucleation) and disruption of the spindle apparatus. In theory, overstimulation of erythropoiesis and hypothermia and hyperthermia could also result in MIE by clastogenicity resulting from disruption of DNA replication and repair processes.

8.10.2 Avoiding and Recognizing Irrelevant Positives

If the test material is likely to disrupt erythropoiesis, then the micronucleus test should be replaced by a conventional bone marrow chromosome aberration test; alternatively, the micronucleus test can be modified to include sampling of bone marrow metaphase cells for potential examination of chromosome damage in the event of an apparent treatment-related increase in MIE, as described for the "cytonucleus test" [59]. For the cytonucleus test, the metaphase arresting agent (usually colchicine) should be given 2 h prior to animal sacrifice because any longer exposure might lead to increases in MIE. In addition, the sampling time for bone marrow should be adjusted to accommodate both the micronucleus and chromosome aberration tests (e.g., 18 and 42 h following a single dose or 18 h after two or more doses).

If the test material is known or suspected of disrupting body temperature, then, in the case of hypothermia, that may be avoidable by supplying supplementary heating or changing to a less susceptible species. In these circumstances and when effects on body temperature are suspected based on clinical signs, it is important to monitor the core temperature of the animals continually.

Increases in MIE as a result of these effects tend to occur at only the second sampling time following a single administration and are generally greatly enhanced by multiple administration. Therefore, a single-dose administration regime is justifiable when a test agent is likely to cause anemia, disruption of erythropoiesis, or prolonged effects on body temperature.

8.11 Limitations of the Rodent Erythrocyte Micronucleus Test

A major limitation of conventional micronucleus tests is that they are only sensitive to genotoxins (or their active metabolites) that are systemically distributed at adequate levels. The micronucleus test has been applied to nonhematopoietic tissues, where it has many of the advantages of the bone marrow test; in particular, the preparation and scoring techniques are relatively simple and the test does not require administration of an arresting agent (so it can be applied to ongoing toxicology studies and human tissues). In this way, it can be used for monitoring male germ cells [60,61] and solid tissues such as liver and GI, where preparation of good metaphase preparations is difficult or impossible [62]. However, fragments from apoptotic cells can appear identical to micronuclei, so results should be interpreted with caution [63]. Apoptosis and micronuclei are jointly termed nuclear anomalies and are particularly obvious in tissues containing dividing cells after treatment with clastogens and spindle poisons [50,64]. Assessment of micronuclei and other nuclear anomalies in tissues other than bone marrow can be useful for screening and quantifying local effects; however, because these assessments are not usually included in routine regulatory submissions, they are not described in detail here.

References

[1] Boller K, Schmid W. Chemische Mutagenese beim Säuger. Das Knochenmark des Chinesischen Hamsters als *in vivo*-Testsystem. Hämatologische Befunde nach Behandlung mit Trenimon. (Chemical mutagenesis in mammals. The bone marrow of Chinese hamsters as an *in vivo* test system. Hematologic evidence after treatment with trenimon). Humangenetik 1970;11(1):35–54.

[2] Matter B, Schmid W. Trenimon-induced chromosomal damage in bone-marrow cells of six mammalian species, evaluated by the micronucleus test. Mutat Res 1971;12:417–25.

[3] Matter BE, Grauwiler J. Micronuclei in mouse bone-marrow cells. A simple *in vivo* model for the evaluation of drug-induced chromosomal aberrations. Mutat Res 1974;23(2):239–49.

[4] Fenech M, Kirsch-Volders M, Natarajan AT, Surralles J, Crott JW, Parry J, et al. Molecular mechanisms of micronucleus, nucleoplasmic bridge and nuclear bud formation in mammalian and human cells. Mutagenesis 2011;26(1):125–32.

[5] Heddle JA, Carrano AV. The DNA content of micronuclei induced in mouse bone marrow by y-irradiation: evidence that micronuclei arise from acentric chromosomal fragments. Mutat Res 1977;44:63–9.

[6] Heddle JA, Hite M, Kirkhart B, Mavournin K, MacGregor JT, Newell GW, et al. The induction of micronuclei as a measure of genotoxicity. A report of the U.S. environmental protection agency gene-tox program. Mutat Res 1983;123(1):61–118.

[7] Heddle JA. A rapid *in vivo* test for chromosomal damage. Mutat Res 1973;18(2):187–90.

[8] von Ledebur M, Schmid W. The micronucleus test. Methodological aspects. Mutat Res 1973;19(1):109–17.

[9] FDA Redbook 2000; Revised July 2007 Toxicological principles for the safety assessment of food ingredients. <http://www.fda.gov/Food/GuidanceRegulation/GuidanceDocumentsRegulatoryInformation/IngredientsAdditivesGRASPackaging/ucm078310.htm>.

[10] International Committee on Harmonisation (ICH). ICH S2(R1) guidance on genotoxicity testing and data interpretation for pharmaceuticals intended for human use. Published in the Federal Register 7 June 2012;77(110):33748–9.

[11] Organization for Economic Co-Operation and Development (OECD). OECD Test Guideline 474: Mammalian Erythrocyte Micronucleus Test. Paris: OECD Publishing; 2014.

[12] Harada A, Matsuzaki K, Takeiri A, Tanaka K, Mishima M. Fluorescent dye-based simple staining for *in vivo* micronucleus test with flow cytometer. Mutat Res 2013;751(2):85–90.

[13] Proudlock RJ, Statham J, Howard W. Evaluation of the rat bone marrow and peripheral blood micronucleus test using monocrotaline. Mutat Res 1997;392:243–9.

[14] CSGMT. Micronucleus test with mouse peripheral blood erythrocytes by acridine orange supravital staining: the summary report of the 5th collaborative study by CSGMT/JEMS.MMS. The Collaborative Study Group for the Micronucleus Test. Mutat Res 1992;278(2–3):83–98.

[15] Hamada S, Sutou S, Morita T, Wakata A, Asanami S, Hosoya S, et al. Evaluation of the rodent micronucleus assay by a 28-day treatment protocol: summary of the 13th Collaborative Study by the Collaborative Study Group for the Micronucleus Test (CSGMT)/Environmental Mutagen Society of Japan (JEMS)-Mammalian Mutagenicity Study Group (MMS). Environ Mol Mutagen 2001;37(2):93–110.

[16] Schlegel R, MacGregor JT. The persistence of micronuclei in peripheral blood erythrocytes: detection of chronic chromosome breakage in mice. Mutat Res 1982;104(6):367–9.

[17] Molloy J, Foster JR, Thomas H, O'Donovan MR, Tweats D, Doherty AT. Does bleeding induce micronuclei via erythropoietin in Han-Wistar rats?. Toxicol Res 2014;3:247–53.

[18] Smith C, Sykes A, Robinson S, Thomas E. Evaluation of blood microsampling techniques and sampling sites for the analysis of drugs by HPLC-MS. Bioanalysis 2011;3(2):145–56.

[19] Association for Assessment and Accreditation of Laboratory Animal Care International. <http://wwwaaalacorg/>; [accessed 16.10.14].

[20] National Research Council (US) Committee for the Update of the Guide for the Care and Use of Laboratory Animals. Guide for the Care and Use of Laboratory Animals. 8th edition ed. Washington (DC): National Academies Press (US); 2011.

[21] Zúñiga-González G, Torres-Bugarín O, Luna-Aguirre J, González-Rodríguez A, Zamora-Perez A, Gómez-Meda BC, et al. Spontaneous micronuclei in peripheral blood erythrocytes from 54 animal species (mammals, reptiles and birds). Mutat Res 2000;467:99−103.

[22] Cristaldi M, Anna Ieradi L, Udroiu I, Zilli R. Comparative evaluation of background micronucleus frequencies in domestic mammals. Mutat Res 2004;559(1−2):1−9.

[23] CSGMT (The Collaborative Study Group for the Micronucleus Test). Strain difference in the micronucleus test. Mutat Res 1988;204(1988):307−16.

[24] Salamone MF, Mavourin KH. Bone marrow micronucleus assay: a review of the mouse stocks used and their published mean spontaneous micronucleus frequencies. Environ Mol Mutagen 1994;23:239−73.

[25] Abrevaya XC, Carballo MA, Mudry MD. The bone marrow micronucleus test and metronidazole genotoxicity in different strains of mice (Mus musculus). Genetics and Molecular Biology 2007;30 (4):1139−43.

[26] Sutou S, Hayashi M, Nishi Y. Sex difference in the micronucleus test. Mutat Res 1986;172(2):151−63.

[27] Hayashi M, Dearfield K, Kasper P, Lovell D, Martus HJ, Thybaud V. Compilation and use of genetic toxicity historical control data. Mutat Res 2011;723(2):87−90.

[28] Pant K, Krsmanovic L, Bruce SW, Kelley T, Arevalo M, Atta-Safoh S, et al. Combination comet/ micronucleus assay validation performed by BioReliance under the JaCVAM initiative. Mutat Res 2015;786-788:87−97.

[29] Maier P, Schmid W. Ten model mutagens evaluated by the micronucleus test. Mutat Res 1976;40 (4):325−37.

[30] Darzynkiewicz Z, Smolewski P, Holden E, Luther E, Henriksen M, François M, et al. Laser scanning cytometry for automation of the micronucleus assay. Mutagenesis 2011;26(1):153−61.

[31] Creton S, Saghir SA, Bartels MJ, Billington R, Bus JS, Davies W, et al. Use of toxicokinetics to support chemical evaluation: informing high dose selection and study interpretation. Regul Toxicol Pharmacol 2012;62(2):241−7.

[32] Hayashi M, Sofuni T. The need for three dose levels to detect genotoxic chemicals in *in vivo* rodent assays. Mutat Res 1995;327:247−51.

[33] Hayashi M, MacGregor JT, Gatehouse DG, Blakey DH, Dertinger SD, Abramsson-Zetterberg L, et al. *In Vivo* Micronucleus Assay Working Group, IWGT. *In vivo* erythrocyte micronucleus assay III. Validation and regulatory acceptance of automated scoring and the use of rat peripheral blood reticulocytes, with discussion of non-hematopoietic target cells and a single dose-level limit test. Mutat Res 2007;627 (1):10−30.

[34] Lipnick RL, Cotruvo JA, Hill RN, Bruce RD, Stitzel KA, Walker AP, et al. Comparison of the Up-and-Down, conventional LD50 and fixed dose acute toxicity procedures. Fd Chem Toxicol 1995;33:223−31.

[35] Diehl KH, Hull R, Morton D, Pfister R, Rabemampianina Y, Smith D, et al. A good practice guide to the administration of substances and removal of blood, including routes and volumes. J Appl Toxicol. 2001;21(1):15−23.

[36] Turner PV, Brabb T, Pekow C, Vasbinder MA. Administration of substances to laboratory animals: routes of administration and factors to consider. J Am Assoc Lab Anim Sci 2011;50(5):600−13.

[37] Miller RC. The micronucleus test as an *in vivo* cytogenetic method. Environ Health Perspect 1973;6:167−70.

[38] Schmid W. The micronucleus test. Mutat Res 1975;31(1):9−15.

[39] Gollapudi B, Kamra OP. Application of a simple Giemsa-staining method in the micronucleus test. Mutat Res 1979;64(1):45−6.

[40]   Hayashi M, MacGregor JT, Gatehouse DG, Adler ID, Blakey DH, Dertinger SD, et al. *In vivo* rodent erythrocyte micronucleus assay. II. Some aspects of protocol design including repeated treatments, integration with toxicity testing, and automated scoring. Environ Mol Mutagen 2000;35(3):234−52.

[41]   Hayashi M, Sofuni T, Ishidate Jr M. An application of acridine orange fluorescent staining to the micronucleus test. Mutat Res 1983;120(4):241−7.

[42]   Hayashi M, Sofuni T, Ishidate Jr M. Kinetics of micronucleus formation in relation to chromosomal aberrations in mouse bone marrow. Mutat Res 1984;127(2):129−37.

[43]   Hayashi M, Morita T, Kodama Y, Sofuni T, Ishidate Jr M. The micronucleus assay with mouse peripheral blood reticulocytes using acridine orange-coated slides. Mutat Res 1990;245(4):245−9.

[44]   Yamamoto K, Kikuchi Y. A comparison of diameters of micronuclei induced by clastogens and by spindle poisons. Mutat Res 1980;71(1):127−31.

[45]   Takeiri A, Motoyama S, Matsuzaki K, Harada A, Taketo J, Katoh C, et al. New DNA probes to detect aneugenicity in rat bone marrow micronucleated cells by a pan-centromeric FISH analysis. Mutat Res 2013;755(1):73−80.

[46]   Ellard S, Mohammed Y, Dogra S, Wölfel C, Doehmer J, Parry JM. The use of genetically engineered V79 Chinese hamster cultures expressing rat liver CYP1A1, 1A2 and 2B1 cDNAs in micronucleus assays. Mutagenesis 1991;6(6):461−70.

[47]   Shibai-Ogata A, Tahara H, Yamamoto Y, Fujita M, Satoh H, Yuasa A, et al. An automated new technique for scoring the *in vivo* micronucleus assay with image analysis. Mutagenesis 2014;29(1):63−71.

[48]   Dertinger SD, Torous DK, Hayashi M, MacGregor JT. Flow cytometric scoring of micronucleated erythrocytes: an efficient platform for assessing *in vivo* cytogenetic damage. Mutagenesis 2011;26 (1):139−45.

[49]   Garriott ML, Piper CE, Kokkino AJ. A simplified protocol for the mouse bone marrow micronucleus assay. J Appl Toxicol 1988;8(2):141−4.

[50]   Goldberg MT, Blakey DH, Bruce WR. Comparison of the effects of 1,2-dimethylhydrazine and cyclophosphamide on micronucleus incidence in bone marrow and colon. Mutat Res 1983;109:91−8.

[51]   Romagna F, Staniforth CD. The automated bone marrow micronucleus test. Mutat Res 1989;213 (1):91−104.

[52]   Tamura RN, Garriott ML, Parton JW. Pooled inference across sexes for the *in vivo* micronucleus assay. Mutat Res 1990;240(2):127−33.

[53]   Lovell DP, Anderson D, Albanese R, Amphlett GE, Clare G, Ferguson R, et al. Statistical Analysis of In Vivo Cytogenetic Assays. In: Kirkland DJ, editor. Statistical Evaluation of Mutagenicity Test Data. UKEMS Sub-Committee on Guidelines for Mutagenicity Testing, Report, Part III. Cambridge: Cambridge University Press; 1989. p. 184−232.

[54]   Bretz F, Hothorn LA. Statistical analysis of monotone or non-monotone dose-response data from *in vitro* toxicological assays. Altern Lab Anim 2003;31(Suppl. 1):81−96.

[55]   Suzuki Y, Nagae Y, Ishikawa T, Watanabe Y, Nagashima T, Matsukubo K, et al. Effect of erythropoietin on the micronucleus test. Environ Mol Mutagen 1989;13(4):314−18.

[56]   Suzuki Y, Nagae Y, Li J, Sakaba H, Mozawa K, Takahashi A, et al. The micronucleus test and erythropoiesis. Effects of erythropoietin and a mutagen on the ratio of polychromatic to normochromatic erythrocytes (P/N ratio). Mutagenesis 1989;4(6):420−4.

[57]   Suzuki Y, Shimizu H, Nagae Y, Fukumoto M, Okonogi H, Kadokura M. Micronucleus test and erythropoiesis: effect of cobalt on the induction of micronuclei by mutagens. Environ Mol Mutagen 1993;22(2):101−6.

[58]   Tweats DJ, Blakey D, Heflich RH, Jacobs A, Jacobsen SD, Morita T, et al. Report of the IWGT working group on strategies and interpretation of regulatory in vivo tests I. Increases in micronucleated bone marrow cells in rodents that do not indicate genotoxic hazards. Mutat Res. 2007;627(1):78−91.

[59]   Albanese R. The cytonucleus test in the rat: a combined metaphase and micronucleus assay. Mutat Res 1987;182:309−21.

[60] Kallio M, Lähdetie J. Analysis of micronuclei induced in mouse early spermatids by mitomycin C, vinblastine sulfate or etoposide using fluorescence in situ hybridization. Mutagenesis 1993;8(6):561–7.

[61] Tates AD. Validation studies with the micronucleus test for early spermatids of rats. A tool for detecting clastogenicity of chemicals in differentiating spermatogonia and spermatocytes. Mutagenesis 1992;7 (6):411–19.

[62] Morita T, MacGregor JT, Hayashi M. Micronucleus assays in rodent tissues other than bone marrow. Mutagenesis 2011;26(1):223–30.

[63] Tolbert PE, Shy CM, Allen JW. Micronuclei and other nuclear anomalies in buccal smears: methods development. Mutat Res 1992;271(1):69–77.

[64] Proudlock RJ, Allen JA. Micronuclei and other nuclear anomalies induced in various organs by diethylnitrosamine and 7 12 dimethylbenz[α]anthracene. Mutat Res 1986;174(2):141–4.

CHAPTER 9

The Rodent Bone Marrow Chromosomal Aberration Test

Ray Proudlock

Boone, North Carolina, USA

Chapter Outline

9.1 Introduction 324
9.2 History 324
9.3 Related Methods 325
9.4 Study Design and Performance 326
    9.4.1 Vehicle/Negative Control and Formulation 326
    9.4.2 Positive Control Group 327
    9.4.3 Sex and Group Size 327
    9.4.4 Number of Groups 327
    9.4.5 Evidence of Target Organ Exposure 328
    9.4.6 Dose Selection 328
    9.4.7 Dose Administration 328
    9.4.8 Treatment Schedule 329
    9.4.9 Animal Observations 329
    9.4.10 Animal Euthanasia 329
9.5 Terminal Procedures 330
    9.5.1 Equipment 330
    9.5.2 Consumables 331
    9.5.3 Advance Preparation 331
    9.5.4 Bone Marrow Collection 332
    9.5.5 Slide Preparation 333
    9.5.6 Slide Staining 333
    9.5.7 Slide Examination 334
    9.5.8 Calculations and Reporting of Results 334
    9.5.9 Acceptability of the Study 335
    9.5.10 Evaluation and Interpretation of Results 335
    9.5.11 Test Report 337
    9.5.12 Integration into Other Studies 339
    9.5.13 Cytonucleus Test 339
Appendix 340
References 341

Genetic Toxicology Testing.
DOI: http://dx.doi.org/10.1016/B978-0-12-800764-8.00009-4
© 2016 Elsevier Inc. All rights reserved.

9.1 Introduction

The rodent bone marrow chromosome aberration test was widely used in the 1970s and 1980s for evaluating the systemic genotoxic potential of chemicals [1–4] but has been largely supplanted by the erythrocyte micronucleus test. Both tests show similar sensitivity to bone marrow clastogens [5,6], but the micronucleus test has perceived advantages in terms of simplicity, ease of automation, adaptability, and speed of scoring. In addition, the micronucleus test can be used to detect aneugens, a class of genotoxic agents that is not consistently identified using the chromosome aberration test [7]. However, the aberration test is useful in cases in which the test material could cause micronuclei by nongenotoxic mechanisms, including prolonged departure from normal body temperature and depression or stimulation of erythropoiesis, either directly or as a consequence of anemia caused by hemolysis or methemoglobinemia. These micronuclei can be large, with unusual shapes, and are probably a result of incomplete enucleation during erythroblast maturation. In such cases, the chromosome aberration test has the advantage that chromosomal defects can be observed directly in the same sensitive target organ. The test uses slide preparations and scoring methodologies that are very similar to those of the *in vitro* chromosome aberration test and, as in that test, the main endpoint measured is chromosome breakage (clastogenicity) in cells arrested at metaphase. DNA damage resulting from covalent binding, intercalation, or interference with DNA replication or repair can all result in chromosome breakage. The bone marrow is an ideal tissue for examination because it contains a large proportion of sensitive dividing cells that are readily harvested and processed as a suspension without the need for any releasing or enzymatic digesting agents. In addition, because the bone marrow is a well-perfused organ, it is expected to receive good exposure to any clastogens or active metabolites that are systemically distributed.

9.2 History

The essential elements of the test include colchicine administration to accumulate cells in metaphase, hypotonic treatment, and then fixation of cells in suspension as described for mice by Ford and Hamerton [8]. Early clinical studies were performed to assess the effect of radiation and cytotoxic drugs on bone marrow chromosomes [9,10], whereas laboratory studies generally used Chinese hamsters (*Cricetulus griseus*) that, with a diploid chromosome count of 22, have relatively few and larger chromosomes, which greatly facilitates chromosome analysis [11–13]. However, group housing and breeding of Chinese hamsters are difficult because females of this species are very aggressive toward other hamsters [14]. Technical improvements in the quality of metaphase preparations mean that the test now generally uses the standard laboratory rodent species, most commonly rat or occasionally mouse [15–18].

The first OECD international guideline for the bone marrow chromosome aberration test (often referred to as the metaphase test) was published in 1984, when the test was widely used for regulatory submissions. This guideline was subsequently revised in 1997 and 2014. Most regulatory agencies, including those of the US, EU, and Japan, defer to OECD guidelines in terms of assay performance and study design, although the US FDA and ICH include some additional guidance and clarification [19,20].

9.3 Related Methods

A guideline for the conduct of the spermatogonial chromosomal aberration test was produced by OECD in 1997, and it was last updated in 2014 [21]. Although the spermatogonial test has the advantage of detecting genotoxicity in the organ most relevant for evaluating heritable chromosome defects, the methods required to prepare good metaphase preparations are more demanding and the test does not seem to have any advantage over the bone marrow test in terms of sensitivity [22,23]. Attempts have been made to assess chromosome damage in tissues that receive more direct exposure to chemicals [24,25]. However mechanical, chemical, and enzymatic methods used to isolate single cells generally result in poor preparations with a large amount of debris; to some extent, the debris in spermatogonial and intestinal tissue preparations can be removed by the hydrolysis step if the Feulgen staining technique is used. However, because of the relative simplicity of the methods and the quality of preparations, the incidence of micronuclei has become an increasingly successful alternative measure of cytogenetic damage in solid tissues [26].

Sampling and culturing blood samples in the presence of a mitogen to stimulate lymphocyte cell division *ex vivo* with subsequent analysis of chromosome preparations have been used to assess accumulated chromosome damage [27]. This technique has been fairly widely used in the biomonitoring of accumulated cytogenetic defects in exposed workers but, even though it could be incorporated into ongoing toxicology studies, it does not seem to have been adopted to any great extent.

Detection of sister chromatid exchanges (SCEs) resulting from induction of homologous recombination repair was at one time considered a promising genetic toxicology screen. In this case, animals are dosed repeatedly or continuously labeled with the base analog bromodeoxyuridine (BUDR), and then colchicine is administered a few hours before bone marrow is harvested; metaphase preparations are made as in the chromosome aberration test. Chromatids are differentially stained light and dark at the second metaphase (after the start of BUDR labeling); using the continuous labeling scheme mentioned here, one chromatid will have one BUDR-substituted DNA strand and both strands in the sister chromatid will contain substituted DNA. Metaphases are then scored for the incidence of reciprocal interchanges evident as symmetrical exchange of light and dark regions between the adjacent regions of the sister chromatids. A substantial increase in SCEs per metaphase is considered indicative of induction of recombination repair resulting from DNA damage [28,29]. Presumably, this test has not been incorporated into regulatory requirements because, like the other tests described in this section, it is technically demanding and does not offer any perceived advantage over other *in vivo* tests for general screening, although it and a related *ex vivo* lymphocyte method are occasionally included in the testing of gasoline additives in the United States [30].

9.4 Study Design and Performance

The following section covers aspects of general study design based on regulatory guidelines ICH S2(R1) and OECD 475. The details of animal housing, feeding, and identification, as well as the details of dose selection, formulation, and administration specified by OECD, for the test are almost identical to those described for the *in vivo* rodent micronucleus test. Usually, young (6–10 weeks old on arrival) rats or mice are used and are assigned to groups (randomized or stratified) based on individual bodyweight so that each group has similar averages and variances in bodyweight. Although rats or mice are commonly used for the test, the OECD guideline indicates that other species, including nonrodents, may be used when scientifically justified.

9.4.1 Vehicle/Negative Control and Formulation

The vehicle should have no toxic or irritant effect at the dose volume used, and it should not be suspected of chemical reaction with the test material. Aqueous vehicles such as water, saline, or aqueous suspending agents are generally preferred because they can be given in larger volumes without causing adverse effects. Although vegetable oils are occasionally used, these are not chemically defined or biologically inert and make chemical analysis of formulations (to support stability and achieved concentration) difficult. They also tend to get on the animals' fur, which complicates clinical observations of signs such as pilo-erection.

Formulations should be homogenous and freshly prepared, except when data are available to support stability, in which case it may be advantageous to formulate ahead of time (e.g., to allow chemical analysis to confirm formulation acceptability prior to dosing). Formulations for intravenous administration should be close to physiological in terms of acidity and tonicity.

Usually, the negative control group is treated with the vehicle used to formulate the test substance. Alternatively, when appropriate, the negative control group can be treated with a placebo that is similar to the (formulated) test material. The negative control group should be treated at approximately the same time and in the same way as the test material groups.

9.4.2 Positive Control Group

A positive control group should be included at the first sampling time at a dose level expected to cause a moderate increase in aberrant metaphases. In cases in which the laboratory has a reasonable historical positive control database, this group can be reduced in size or omitted altogether. In the latter case, scoring controls (unstained slides) from a previous experiment using the same species should be included, stained, and encoded together with those from the current study. Whatever the situation, the positive control does not need to be administered in the same way (e.g., by the same route) as the test article. Convenient positive controls administered orally as aqueous solutions include cyclophosphamide monohydrate at 10 mg/kg for rats and mitomycin C at 6 mg/kg for mice.

9.4.3 Sex and Group Size

Only one sex usually needs to be tested unless substantial differences in systemic toxicity, metabolism, bioavailability, or bone marrow toxicity are expected or seen, such as in preliminary testing. Each group should consist of five animals (five males plus five females if both sexes are used). Particularly when using only one sex, consideration should be given to having additional animals available in case one or two animals from the high dose group need to be replaced, for example, due to unscheduled euthanasia resulting from unacceptably severe clinical signs.

9.4.4 Number of Groups

Except as noted in the next paragraph, normally three dose levels of the test item are evaluated at the first (main) sampling time, and only the high dose needs to be sampled at the second time point. The concurrent negative (vehicle) control group is normally sampled at both time points. A positive control group is normally included at the first sampling time, except as discussed previously. Therefore, a typical standard study consisting of a single sex would involve sampling a minimum of 25 animals at the first time point and 10 animals at the second time point. Any additional animals that have been dosed as potential replacements (e.g., at the high dose level) should also be sampled to maximize the statistical power of the test.

Deviations from the standard study design mentioned should be justified with appropriate supporting information in the report. Intermediate and low doses are not required at either sampling time if the high dose produces no observable toxic effects (particularly cytostatic or cytotoxic effects in the bone marrow) and if there is no indication of genotoxicity from *in vitro* genotoxicity studies or data from structurally related substances, provided there is supporting evidence of target organ exposure. If the laboratory has an adequate and stable historical control database, then a negative control group may be omitted at the second sampling time.

9.4.5 *Evidence of Target Organ Exposure*

Blood or plasma toxicokinetic data using the same species, formulation, and route are appropriate to support target organ exposure because bone marrow is considered a well-perfused organ. If supporting evidence of target organ exposure is available (the OECD guideline indicates that it is expected), then it should be presented in the report. As in other *in vivo* genotoxicity tests, consideration should be given to inclusion of a toxicokinetic element (with blood or plasma analysis) in the study to demonstrate systemic bioavailability if that information is not already available, particularly when the test is used to further evaluate the relevance of *in vitro* findings. A substantial dose-related reduction in the mitotic index may be used as indirect evidence of exposure, however, that is usually only seen with cytotoxic or cytostatic substances that are clastogenic in any case.

9.4.6 *Dose Selection*

The high dose should be the least of the following:

- the maximum tolerable
- the maximum achievable based on formulation, animal welfare, and route of administration
- the standard dose limit of 2000 mg/kg per administration.

Although the test is not normally performed over dosing periods of more than 14 days, in such cases the dose limit is 1000 mg/kg/day. Two lower doses are usually also used in addition to the high dose, with these being 50% and 25% of the high dose, although a dose interval of up to fourfold is acceptable.

9.4.7 *Dose Administration*

As with the micronucleus test, the dosing route should take into account the likely route of maximal human exposure (in terms of bioavailability) while ensuring adequate levels of target organ exposure. Intraperitoneal injection is not generally considered relevant to the human exposure situation and, like the oral route, could result in first-pass elimination; administration in the diet or drinking water is complicated in terms of assessment of exposure levels as well as time and duration of exposure. Oral, subcutaneous, and intravenous infusion routes are generally the most relevant and practical in terms of volumes of material that can be administered. If infusion or intravenous injection is chosen, then solubility of the material in both the formulation and, subsequently, in the blood must be taken into account. For specialist routes like infusion and inhalation, the scientist should collaborate with experts in that field to minimize technical problems and stress to the animals.

9.4.8 Treatment Schedule

Infusion and inhalation routes typically involve exposure over a period of 4−8 h in a single day. Other routes of exposure usually involve a single bolus injection; in some cases, that may be split into two administrations given 2−3 h apart (e.g., if the dose volume is large). Animals are sampled after a period approximately equivalent to 1.5 times the normal average cell-cycle time, which, for rats, mice, and Chinese hamsters, equates to 12−18 h after completion of treatment. For other species, it would be necessary to determine the bone marrow cell-cycle time based on published information or experimentally. The negative control and high-level groups are sampled again 24 h after the first sampling time to allow potentially slow absorption or metabolism of the test material or cell-cycle delay. Changes to these sampling times may be justifiable, for example, if they are based on toxicokinetic data for a compound that has a very long biological half-life.

Animals are treated with an appropriate dose of metaphase-arresting agent soon before euthanasia. Colchicine should be formulated in sterile 0.9% saline at 0.4 mg/mL and then administered by intraperitoneal injection at 10 mL/kg bodyweight 2−5 h (rats) or 3−5 h (mice) prior to euthanasia and sampling.

9.4.9 Animal Observations

Animals should be examined visually at least once during the acclimation period and at least twice daily after treatment. Additional checks should be included at appropriate times based on anticipated and observed effects of treatment. Clinical signs and mortalities should be recorded. Any animals that show signs of morbidity, distress, or excessive clinical signs should be euthanized immediately for humane reasons and recorded as mortalities. If mis-dosing is suspected, then the animals should be subjected to macroscopic postmortem examination (e.g., to check for perforated esophagus or the presence of dose in the lungs). All animals should be individually weighed on arrival, just prior to dosing, at least once per week during repeat dose studies, and at euthanasia. As mentioned, individual bodyweight may be used to allocate animals to groups so that each group is stratified with a similar average and variance in bodyweight.

9.4.10 Animal Euthanasia

Animals should be killed by a humane method at the scheduled time. The method will depend on the species as well as local and national regulations; a simple method suitable for adult rodents involves exposure to a gradually increasing (metered) concentration of carbon dioxide as described by UK Home Office schedule 1 and AMVA (http://www.nc3rs.org.uk/euthanasia/). Using this procedure, animals are initially anesthetized and then die as a result of overdose while unconscious rather than dying as a result of asphyxiation due to oxygen shortage. This method has the advantage that it avoids clotting of the bone marrow (and blood). Death should be confirmed by checking the pinch reflex and ensured by severing the main blood vessels in the leg during excision of the femur. Although bone marrow is usually obtained from both femurs of each animal, only one femur or the tibias may be used if necessary.

9.5 Terminal Procedures

Note that the two critical phases of sample preparation are the initial addition of fixative to the cells and the dropping of the fixed cells onto the slide. In the first case, the procedures described here should be followed exactly. In the second case, the conditions in the laboratory can have a great impact on the spreading of the metaphases. The fixation preserves the morphology of the chromosomes; it contains methanol, which is a dehydrating fixative and causes shrinkage of the cells, as well as acetic acid, which is a hydrating fixative and causes swelling of the cells. In the presence of water at the fixation and slide-dropping steps, the acetic acid causes hydrolysis of the cytoplasm, which allows the metaphases to spread. If hydrolysis is inadequate, then the metaphases will bunch and form a clump, especially if the humidity is too low at the cell-dropping step. It is helpful to monitor humidity; if this is low and metaphases appear bunched during a preliminary trial, then this should be remedied as described in the procedures.

9.5.1 Equipment

Much of the following list is also used for the rodent erythrocyte micronucleus test:

1. Dissecting tools: scissors, plain bone cutting shears (for rats), and forceps.
2. Microscope slides with a frosted end. Plain slides can be used if an automated slide labeling/etching system is available.
3. Stainless steel slide racks, which should be cleaned by washing in 50% acetic acid then dried.
4. Cardboard slide trays.
5. Slide storage system for archiving slides; cardboard systems are most economical and least liable to damage the slides.
6. Centrifuge: bench-top, low speed.
7. Vortex mixer with variable speed.
8. Fume hood/cupboard.
9. Binocular light microscope with high-quality flat-field achromatic optics and parfocal objectives: medium power plan objective ($16\times$ or similar) and high-power oil immersion ($100\times$). The oil immersion lens should be plan apochromat (Planapo), although plan fluorite may be preferred if the microscope will also be used for fluorescence work. Investment in a high-quality microscope is critical to facilitate accurate assessment of chromosome damage and minimize operator fatigue. Most good, modern microscopes use infinity-corrected extra-low-dispersion (ED) glass lenses and

Köhler illumination to optimize image quality. If you have a limited budget, then consider buying a second-hand microscope because a good microscope will last a lifetime if properly cared for; in this case, ensure the lenses are not damaged (scratched or with deterioration of the cement between components of compound lenses). Carl Zeiss Axio Scope, Leica DM, Nikon Labophot II, and Olympus BX all have good reputations and are, arguably, the only makes worth considering.

10. Vibration-proofed bench.
11. Two-channel bench-top tally counter (e.g., Denominator-type).

9.5.2 Consumables

Adhesive labels with code number (code numbers can be generated in Excel using the random function and then printed onto sheets of adhesive labels), you will need four replicate labels per animal (assuming up to four replicate slides may be examined). The slide code should be printed out and a separate sheet and saved electronically to decode results later. The following will also be needed:

1. Polypropylene centrifuge tubes with caps, 15 mL.
2. HBSS: Hank's balanced salt solution buffered with bicarbonate, freshly prepared or sterile to avoid microbial growth.
3. Disposable 5 mL syringes fitted with 20 G needles (rat) or 2 mL syringes with 21 G needles (mice).
4. Hypotonic: 0.075 M potassium chloride (5.6 g KCl per liter in purified water).
5. Fix: a ratio of 3 volumes of methanol to 1 volume of glacial acetic (ethanoic) acid prepared just prior to each use (often incorrectly referred to as Carnoy's fluid).
6. Pasteur pipettes; the polypropylene ones are most convenient.
7. Stain: Giemsa, Gurr's Improved R66 freshly diluted 1 part to 9 parts purified water and then filtered.
8. Purified water.
9. Results sheets/forms.

9.5.3 Advance Preparation

1. Microscope slides with a frosted end should be handled using gloves to avoid transfer of grease from the skin. Slides are labeled with the study and animal identities using an HB pencil. If necessary, they can be cleaned by soaking in methanol overnight before drying (slides sometimes have a residue of detergent from the manufacturing process).
2. Prepare Hypotonic and then warm the solution before use for 15–30 min in a 37°C water bath.
3. Prepare the HBSS. If prepared from powder or concentrate, then an appropriate amount of sodium bicarbonate must be added to achieve a final concentration of 350 mg/mL. Most conveniently, this is achieved by addition of 4.7 mL of 7.5% w/v sodium bicarbonate per

liter. The bicarbonate solution should be fairly fresh and tightly sealed to minimize deterioration. Dispense HBSS aliquots (5 mL for rats, 2 mL for mice) into polypropylene centrifuge tubes (1 per animal); each tube should be labeled uniquely with the animal identity. The rack (and/or) tubes should also be labeled with the study number.

9.5.4 Bone Marrow Collection

1. Just after euthanasia of each animal, process each femur in turn as detailed below. Note that the initial steps prior to addition of the hypotonic solution are identical to those used for the rat micronucleus test.
2. Remove the skin and most of the underlying tissue from the upper part of the back of a rear leg by using scissors and cutting close and parallel to the bone. Then, dislocate the knee joint while pulling the lower leg away from the animal. Clear the femur of any remaining muscle by scraping using the scissors, and cut it as close to the body of the animal as practical using bone shears; scissors may be used for young mice. In this way, most of the femur is excised and open at the proximal end, with the distal epiphysis still intact.
3. Push the needle of the needle–syringe assembly well into the opening of the bone, and then push the bone toward the bottom of the corresponding centrifuge tube so that it is toward the bottom of the HBSS. Using the needle to hold the bone against the inside of the tube, draw the HBSS into the syringe through the top (open end) of the femur and then discharge it back into the tube. Discard the empty femur, and then repeat the process for the second femur before aspirating and discharging the suspension via the syringe once more. In this way, virtually all the cells in both femurs will be in a fine suspension in tube.
4. Centrifuge the tubes at 1000 rpm in a bench top centrifuge for 5 min. Then, decant and discard the supernatant. Bring the cells back into suspension by "knocking" (flicking by hand) the tube or use a vortex mixer.
5. Add hypotonic until the total volume is approximately 10 mL. At this point the red blood cells will lyse; therefore, for mice in particular, the presence of cells in the suspension and subsequent pellets on centrifugation will not necessarily be obvious.
6. Put the tubes in a water bath at approximately 37°C for approximately 10 min; this time is not critical because the cells will swell almost immediately.
7. Gradually add 2 mL of fix to the cell suspension while mixing continuously at low speed using a vortex mixer.
8. Centrifuge the tubes at 1500 rpm for 5 min. Then, decant and discard the supernatant.
9. Resuspend the cells in the residual solution by gentle flicking. Then, add approximately 2 mL of fix while mixing continuously.
10. Add additional fix to the 10 mL mark. Then, leave tubes at room temperature for at least 30 min. Alternatively transfer the tubes to a refrigerator and store overnight.

11. Centrifuge the tubes at 1500 rpm for 5 min. Then, remove most of the supernatant, allowing approximately 1 mL to remain before resuspending the cells as before and making up to 10 mL with fix.
12. Cells should be stored refrigerated at least overnight at this stage, but they can be stored at approximately 4°C for several months provided that the centrifuge tubes are compatible with the fix.

9.5.5 Slide Preparation

1. Centrifuge the tubes at 1500 rpm for 5 min. Then, remove and discard the supernatant. Resuspend the cells in the residual fix.
2. Add fresh fix up to approximately 10 mL.
3. Centrifuge the tubes at 1500 rpm for 5 min. Remove and discard the supernatant. Resuspend the cells in the residual fix.
4. Add sufficient fix to each tube to produce a slightly cloudy suspension.
5. Prepare a single trial slide. Put a drop of cell suspension onto a clean slide using a clean Pasteur pipette. Air-dry, and then check the quality of the preparation using a (phase contrast, if available) microscope. The metaphases should be well spread but intact, with well-defined chromosomes. Note that metaphase spreading and adherence to the slide occur within a few seconds.
6. If the metaphases are bunched, then that indicates the atmosphere is too dry. In that case, the slide should be held close to the surface of a 70°C water bath while the suspension is dropped onto the slide.
7. Prepare four slides from each animal. Then, allow them to completely air-dry in the fume hood.
8. Cap and retain any residual fixed material to produce additional slides later if necessary.

9.5.6 Slide Staining

1. Immerse the slides for 5 min in purified water.
2. Transfer the slides to 10% Giemsa solution and stain for 10 min.
3. Immerse the slides for 5 min in purified water.
4. Immerse the slides for 5 min in fresh purified water.
5. Air-dry.
6. Place the slides in cardboard slide trays.
7. Mount each slide directly with a 24 × 60 mm coverslip (cover glass) using two drops of permanent mountant (e.g., DPX or Permount) in a fume cupboard.
8. Allow the mountant to harden. This can be accelerated by using a warm (50°C) oven, but ensure that the slides do not overheat.
9. Randomize and encode the slides prior to reading, obscuring the animal identification but not the study number.

9.5.7 Slide Examination

Slide examination and scoring are performed as described for the *in vitro* chromosome aberration test. Check the slide by eye to pick an area for examination that contains a reasonable cell density. Using the microscope with a medium power object, count the numbers of nonmitotic and mitotic cells in the field using the tally counter before moving *directly* to an adjacent field. Avoid scanning gradually across fields, which would probably result in "travel sickness." Move to each new field in a systematic manner to avoid scoring the same field twice. Once a total of at least 1000 cells have been evaluated, record the values obtained on the results form. Similarly, scan the slide systematically under medium power for readable metaphases. As each is found, examine it under high power, check that the cell is of readable quality with a normal chromosome complement ($2n \pm 2$ centromeres), examine readable metaphases for aberrations, and record the number and type of aberrations as well as the number of centromeres. When viewed under high power, metaphases that are not well spread with clearly defined chromatids in a single stage of condensation and an appropriate number of centromeres, as well as those with a number of overlapping chromosomes, are considered not readable and no result should be recorded for them. Sometimes chromosomes may be poorly defined with a crinkly appearance due to preparation artifacts; metaphases with this effect are considered unreadable. You should continue until a total of 200 metaphases have been scored for that animal, often it will be necessary to examine more than one slide per animal. If less than 200 readable metaphases are available or if the slide quality is not considered adequate, then additional slides should be prepared from fixed material and examined.

It may be desirable to record the vernier location for aberrant metaphases to allow retrospective review. In that case, slides should always be orientated in the same way on the microscope stage (e.g., label to the left) and the replicate slide (a, b, c, or d) should be indicated on the form.

9.5.8 Calculations and Reporting of Results

The mitotic index, the number of metaphase cells scored, the number of aberrations per metaphase cell, and the percentage of cells with structural chromosomal aberration(s) should be calculated for each animal. Different types of structural chromosomal aberrations should be listed with their numbers and frequencies. Gaps, polyploidy, and cells with endoreduplicated chromosomes should be recorded separately; these will be reported but are not included in the calculation of the structural aberrant cell frequency. If there is no evidence for a difference in response between the sexes in terms of structural aberrations, then the results may be combined to maximize the power of statistical analysis. Details of toxicokinetic and preliminary investigations (if performed), mortalities and clinical signs, and any other assessments of toxicity made should be reported and, when appropriate, presented in tabular form in the study report.

9.5.9 Acceptability of the Study

Acceptability criteria should be stated in the study protocol and followed in the report. A study is considered acceptable provided that:

1. The quality of the slides is good (i.e., adequate to allow detailed examination for aberrant metaphases).
2. Adequate numbers of dose levels, animals, and cells from each animal have been analyzed.
3. The concurrent negative/vehicle group shows results (% aberrant cells) within the expected range based on published data and the distribution of laboratory historical control results.
4. The positive control group shows a substantial increase in the incidence of aberrant cells compared with the negative/vehicle group, with mean values close to or within the laboratory historical control range.

The potential impact of any deviation from these criteria (e.g., slight reduction in group size at the high dose due to mortality) should be addressed in the report provided that the study as a whole is considered valid. If only a part of a study is considered invalid (e.g., due to excessive mortalities in the high-dose group), then it may be possible to perform a supplementary study with appropriate controls to avoid repeating the whole study.

9.5.10 Evaluation and Interpretation of Results

Evaluation criteria together with details of the proposed statistical analysis should be presented in the study protocol and followed in the report. There has been much debate over choice of appropriate statistical methods for interpretation of *in vivo* genotoxicity tests; in general, the same methods can be used for analysis of *in vivo* chromosome aberration and micronucleus results [31]. Provided the study is well designed with an adequate group size, the outcome of the statistical analysis should reflect an experienced scientist's own interpretation [32]. In accordance with OECD, provided all acceptability criteria are fulfilled, a test material is considered clearly negative if:

1. None of the treatment groups exhibits a statistically significant increase in the frequency of cells with structural chromosomal aberrations (excluding gaps) compared with the concurrent negative control,
2. There is no dose-related increase when evaluated by an appropriate trend test (using three dose groups plus the vehicle/negative control) or an intergroup comparison (single dose group versus the concurrent vehicle negative),

3. Mean values for the test article groups are inside the distribution of the historical negative control data (e.g., Poisson-based 95% control limits), and

4. Bone marrow exposure to the test substance(s) occurred.

Evidence of exposure of the bone marrow to a test substance may include a decrease of the mitotic index or measurement of the plasma or blood levels of the test substance(s). In the case of intravenous administration, bone marrow exposure can normally be assumed. Alternatively, ADME data obtained in an independent study using the same route and same species can be used to demonstrate systemic exposure. Negative results indicate that, under the test conditions, the test chemical does not induce structural chromosomal aberrations in the bone marrow of the species tested.

A test chemical is considered clearly positive if all three of the following criteria are met at one of the sampling times:

1. At least one of the treatment groups exhibits a statistically significant increase in the frequency of cells with structural chromosomal aberrations (excluding gaps) compared with the concurrent negative control.

2. The group mean frequency of aberrant cells is beyond the upper limit of the historical negative control data (e.g., Poisson-based 95% control limits).

3. The increase is dose-related when evaluated with an appropriate trend test.

If only a single (high) dose is examined at a particular sampling time, then a test material is considered clearly positive provided that the first two criteria are met. Statistical tests should use the animal as the experimental unit and, in the case of aberrant cells, be one-tailed because only increases are of interest. In cases in which more than one dose level is examined, the most powerful statistical tests are those that look for overall trend, which is appropriate provided that there is no indication of severe cytostatic activity at the high dose. Aberrant cells are rare and discrete events, so the expected distribution should be approximately Poisson; therefore, a transformation (e.g., $\sqrt{(x + 0.5)}$ where x is the number of aberrant cells found per 200 cells examined) should be applied to approximately normalize the results if the statistical method assumes a Gaussian (normal) distribution. Nonparametric methods based on permutation do not require transformation of results but lack statistical power and are inappropriate when the group size is small (e.g., when performing intergroup comparisons of only a single sex). However, nonparametric trend tests such as Jonckheere's are perhaps the simplest approach to assessing the overall effect of a test material and are less prone to false-positive calls than intergroup comparisons. Whatever the situation, as in all genotoxicity tests, the positive control group (if subjected to statistical analysis) should be analyzed independently of the test material groups.

Any critical probability levels identified in the protocol should be sufficiently conservative to avoid false-positive calls taking into account multiple comparisons (between groups and for each of the two sampling times). For example, reports showing critical values of $P < 0.05$ will often contain * in Tables, implying statistical significance with an associated phrase indicating that the increase is not thought to be "biologically significant"; consider instead adopting a critical P value of 0.01. Before adopting any statistical method or evaluation criteria, the scientist should explore the performance of the test using typical results arranged into borderline cases (i.e., real increases and chance variation) to evaluate the limitations of the methods and set appropriate probability levels for defining "negative" and "positive" results. Unfortunately, statistical analysis involving relatively small group sizes does not necessarily take into account the strength of any apparent response. A step-wise approach that does take this into account would involve not performing any statistical analysis unless any of the treated groups show aberrant cell values substantially above concurrent or expected values based on the historical control range.

Positive results in the chromosomal aberration test indicate that a test chemical induces structural chromosomal aberrations in the bone marrow of the species tested.

In cases where a weak or borderline apparent increase in aberrant cells has been obtained, analyzing more cells or reanalysis of the slides by a second reader may allow a definitive conclusion. If results are still considered borderline, then performance of supplementary testing may be appropriate.

The frequencies of polyploid and endoreduplicated metaphases should be recorded and considered separately from chromosome aberration values. An increase in the number of polyploid/endoreduplicated cells may indicate that the test material has the potential to inhibit mitotic processes or cell-cycle progression. Although often seen in *in vitro* studies, increases in numerical aberrations including polyploidy are rarely, if ever, seen in routine *in vivo* studies. Apparent increases in numerical aberrations and other effects on chromosome structure (such as chromatid separation as a result of centromeric disruption) should be reported as incidental observations. If seen, then they may be of biological importance and worthy of further investigation, but they should not be considered as indicators of genotoxic activity.

9.5.11 Test Report

The test report should include the information listed in OECD guideline 475 including criteria for:

1. supporting evidence of systemic or target organ exposure
2. classification of aberrations
3. considering a study valid/acceptable
4. judgment as positive, negative, or inconclusive.

Table 9.1: Cytogenetic examination and statistical analysis

Treatment	Dose mg/kg	MI	RMI[a]	No Cells Examined Male (♂)	No Cells Examined Female (♀)	No Cells Examined ♂ and ♀	% Aberrant Cells[a] ♂	% Aberrant Cells[a] ♀	% Aberrant Cells[a] ♂ and ♀	
First (16-h) Sampling Time										
Vehicle	0	5.0	100	1000	1000	2000	0.2	0.8	0.5	ns
Test item	500	4.5[ns]	90	1000	1000	2000	0.6	0.0	0.3	
Test item	1000	3.7*	84	1000	1000	2000	1.0	0.4	0.7	
Test item	2000	3.0**	60	800	1000	1800	0.8	0.6	0.7	
Cyclophosphamide	10	5.8[ns]	116	600	600	1200	7.3	11.3	9.3	**
Second (40-h) Sampling Time										
Vehicle	0	5.1	100	1000	1000	2000	0.2	0.8	0.5	
Test item	2000	5.7[ns]	111	1000	1000	2000	0.8	0.6	0.7	ns

MI, Mitotic Index; RMI, Relative Mitotic Index (vehicle = 100%).
Results of statistical analysis using exact permutation for intergroup comparisons (vehicle/negative vs positive control) or linear-by-linear test for trend in Cytel StatXact (test item plus vehicle control groups):
**$P \leq 0.001$ (highly significant).
*$P \leq 0.01$ (significant).
[ns]$P > 0.01$ (not significant).
[a]Occasional apparent errors of 1% in RMI or 0.1% in % aberrant cells may occur due to rounding of values for presentation in the table.

Results should be presented in detail for individual animals (as shown in Appendix Table A.1) and, together with the outcome of statistical analysis, presented in a summary table. An example summary table is presented (Table 9.1).

In this largely fictitious example, the test material did not cause any significant increase in the incidence of cells with chromosome aberrations at either sampling time. There was some evidence of mitotic inhibition as indicated by a dose-related reduction in mitotic index at the first sampling time, although the bone marrow seemed to have recovered by the second sampling time.

The OECD guideline indicates that laboratory historical negative and positive control data with ranges, means, standard deviations, and 95% control limits/percentiles for the distribution as well as the time period covered and number of observations should be presented [33]. Ideally, the laboratory should generate results for at least 10 experiments (i.e., 20 control groups) before embarking on regulatory studies [33]. Most or all of these results can be generated during the internal development and validation of the test, particularly if both an untreated and a vehicle group are included in each phase of the validation. Although the control database should include all appropriate parameters (e.g., vehicle, dose volume), these results can be considered jointly (i.e., as a single distribution) unless any has a clear effect on the incidence of aberrant cells. The historical negative control results are doubly important because they show whether the current control values are within normal limits and whether incidences for the test material are above the expected range for that laboratory. The distribution of group mean results can be generated as a simple chart in Excel or similar spreadsheet program, which can also be used to calculate 95% tolerance limits, with these being the 2.5 and 97.5 percentiles of the distribution of transformed group total results. These limits should approximately coincide with observed limits once the size of the database is adequate.

9.5.12 Integration into Other Studies

The chromosome aberration test is not usually integrated into other studies because metaphase arresting agents might interfere with some of the parameters assessed in those studies. In addition, chromosome aberrations in the rapidly dividing cells of the bone marrow become evident at the first metaphase after their induction. Most visible chromosome aberration are lethal to the cell and are lost, so no accumulation of aberrant cells would be expected after multiple treatments. Multiple administrations of genotoxic agents might also reduce the sensitive cell population and, therefore, the sensitivity of the test. If a multidose treatment regime is used for the chromosome aberration test, then bone marrow should be sampled at a single time point (12−18 h after the last treatment).

9.5.13 Cytonucleus Test

In certain cases, such as when it is suspected that the test material might increase micronucleated erythrocytes by a nongenotoxic mechanism [34], it may be desirable to combine the chromosome aberration and micronucleus endpoints in a single study [35,36,37]. In this case the study design, the dosing regimen, and the sampling times are adjusted to comply with both tests. For example, rats should be treated with the test substance twice at 24 h intervals and then euthanized; bone marrow should be harvested 18 h after the second dose and 3 h after administration of colchicine. Note that the animals should not be treated with colchicine any earlier than this to avoid the potential induction of micronuclei by the arresting agent itself [38]. The bone marrow suspension should be divided into two fractions, with 10% being used for smear production and 90% processed and fixed for potential metaphase preparation. The bone marrow smears should be processed and examined for micronucleated erythrocytes as described in this volume. Metaphase preparations only need to be prepared and examined if there is an apparent treatment-related increase in micronucleated erythrocytes. In this case, it would be advisable to consider inclusion or additional investigations (e.g., blood reticulocyte counts or body temperature measurements) to support a nongenotoxic mode of micronucleus induction mechanism.

Appendix

Table A.1: Individual animal results at the first (16-h) sampling time

Treatment	Dose (mg/kg)	Animal ID		MI	No. of Cells Examined	No. of Aberrant Cells	No. of Aberrations[a]					Incidental Observations			
							b	e	B	E	O	g	G	P	C
Vehicle	0	M	101	3.7	200	2	2	0	0	0	0	0	2	0	0
		M	102	3.3	200	0	0	0	0	0	0	2	0	0	3
		M	103	6.7	200	0	0	0	0	0	0	1	0	0	0
		M	104	5.0	200	0	0	0	0	0	0	0	0	0	3
		F	105	7.2	200	3	3	0	0	0	0	0	0	0	0
		F	106	4.4	200	1	1	0	0	0	0	0	0	0	2
		F	107	3.7	200	2	2	0	1	0	0	0	0	0	4
		F	108	6.8	200	0	0	0	0	0	0	0	0	0	0
		F	109	3.6	200	2	1	0	1	0	0	0	0	0	2
Test item	500	M	110	5.3	200	1	1	0	0	0	0	0	0	0	2
		M	111	3.8	200	1	2	0	0	0	0	0	0	0	0
		M	112	3.4	200	2	1	0	0	0	1	0	0	0	2
		M	113	5.3	200	0	0	0	0	0	0	0	0	0	1
		M	114	3.8	200	1	1	0	0	0	0	0	0	0	0
		F	115	4.6	200	0	0	0	0	0	0	0	0	0	1
		F	116	4.8	200	0	0	0	0	0	0	0	0	0	1
		F	117	8.0	200	0	0	0	0	0	0	0	0	0	1
		F	118	3.9	200	0	0	0	0	0	0	0	0	0	2
		F	119	4.8	200	0	0	0	0	0	0	0	0	0	0
Test item	1000	M	120	3.0	200	2	1	0	0	0	1	0	0	0	3
		M	121	3.1	200	1	1	0	0	0	0	0	0	0	0
		M	122	3.1	200	2	0	1	1	0	0	0	0	0	13
		M	123	5.0	200	1	1	0	0	1	0	0	0	0	2
		M	124	4.4	200	4	3	1	0	0	0	0	0	0	2
		F	125	3.8	200	1	1	0	0	0	0	0	0	0	8
		F	126	4.9	200	1	0	0	1	0	0	0	0	0	4
		F	127	4.9	200	0	0	0	0	0	0	0	0	0	0
		F	128	5.1	200	2	2	0	0	0	0	0	0	0	1
		F	129	3.3	200	0	0	0	0	0	0	0	0	0	2
Test item	2000	M	130	4.3	200	0	0	0	0	0	0	1	0	0	11
		M	131	—	—	Dead									
		M	132	2.2	200	0	0	0	0	0	0	0	0	0	4
		M	133	3.0	200	5	4	0	0	0	1	0	0	0	16
		M	134	2.9	200	1	1	0	0	0	0	0	0	0	7
		F	135	4.0	200	0	0	0	0	0	0	0	0	0	5
		F	136	2.2	200	3	1	0	2	0	0	0	0	0	15
		F	137	2.0	200	1	0	1	0	0	0	0	0	0	2
		F	138	3.0	200	1	0	0	0	0	0	0	0	0	2
		F	139	2.8	200	1	0	0	1	0	0	0	0	0	10

(Continued)

Table A.1: (Continued)

Treatment	Dose (mg/kg)	Animal ID		MI	No. of Cells Examined	No. of Aberrant Cells	No. of Aberrations[a]					Incidental Observations			
							b	e	B	E	O	g	G	P	C
CP	10	M	140	3.1	200	11	9	0	4	0	0	0	0	0	5
		M	141	6.5	200	21	17	3	6	0	0	0	0	0	4
		M	142	2.0	200	12	10	1	6	0	0	1	0	0	0
		F	145	7.2	200	23	14	3	8	0	0	0	0	0	4
		F	146	6.5	200	31	19	7	14	0	0	0	0	0	5
		F	147	6.7	200	14	10	4	5	1	0	0	0	0	0

Chromatid aberrations: b, e, and g indicate break, exchange, and gap, respectively. Chromosome aberrations: B, E, G, and O indicate break, exchange, gap, and other, respectively (includes pulverized chromosomes and cells with >8 aberrations). Numerical aberrations: P, C, and CP indicate polyploidy and endoreduplication, centromeric disruption, cyclophosphamide monohydrate, respectively.
[a]g, G, P, and CD are excluded from the calculation of % aberrant cells.

References

[1] Preston RJ, Au W, Bender MA, Brewen JG, Carrano AV, Heddle JA, et al. Mammalian *in vivo* and *in vitro* cytogenetic assays: a report of the U.S. EPA's gene-tox program. Mutat Res 1981;87(2):143—88.

[2] Preston RJ, Dean BJ, Galloway S, Holden H, McFee AF, Shelby M. Mammalian *in vivo* cytogenetic assays. Analysis of chromosome aberrations in bone marrow cells. Mutat Res 1987;189(2):157—65.

[3] Richold M, et al. *In vivo* cytogenetics assays. In: Kirkland DJ, editor. Basic mutagenicity tests, UKEMS recommended procedures. UKEMS subcommittee on guidelines for mutagenicity testing. Report. part I revised. Cambridge: Cambridge University Press; 1990. p. 115—41.

[4] Tice RR, Hayashi M, MacGregor JT, Anderson D, Blakey DH, Holden HE, et al. Report from the working group on the *in vivo* mammalian bone marrow chromosomal aberration test. Mutat Res 1994;312(3):305—12.

[5] Kliesch U, Danford N, Adler ID. Micronucleus test and bone-marrow chromosome analysis: a comparison of 2 methods *in vivo* for evaluating chemically induced chromosomal alterations. Mutat Res 1981;80(2):321—32.

[6] Shelby MD, Witt KL. Comparison of results from mouse bone marrow chromosome aberration and micronucleus tests. Environ Mol Mutagen 1995;25(4):302—13.

[7] Marrazzini A, Betti C, Bernacchi F, Barrai I, Barale R. Micronucleus test and metaphase analyses in mice exposed to known and suspected spindle poisons. Mutagenesis 1994;9(6):505—15.

[8] Ford CE, Hamerton JL. A colchicine, hypotonic citrate, squash sequence for mammalian chromosomes. Stain Technol 1956;31(6):247—51.

[9] Pedersen B. Chromosome aberrations in blood, bone marrow, and skin from a patient with acute leukaemia treated with 6-mercaptopurine. Acta Pathol Microbiol Scand 1964;61:261—7.

[10] Bell WR, Whang JJ, Carbone PP, Brecher G, Block JB. Cytogenetic and morphologic abnormalities in human bone marrow cells during cytosine arabinoside therapy. Blood 1966;27(6):771—81.

[11] Schmid W, Staiger GR. Chromosome studies on bone marrow from Chinese hamsters treated with benzodiazepine tranquillizers and cyclophosphamide. Mutat Res 1969;7(1):99—108.

[12] Schmid W, Arakaki DT, Breslau NA, Culbertson JC. Chemical mutagenesis. The Chinese hamster bone marrow as an *in vivo* test system. I. Cytogenetic results on basic aspects of the methodology, obtained with alkylating agents. Humangenetik 1971;11(2):103—18.

[13] Arakaki DT, Schmid W. Chemical mutagenesis the Chinese hamster bone marrow as an *in vivo* test system. Hum Genet 1971;11(2):119—31.

[14] Porter G, Lacey A. Breeding the Chinese hamster (*Cricetulus griseus*) in monogamous pairs. Lab Anim 1969;3:65–8.

[15] Adler ID. Cytogenetic tests in mammals. In: Venitt S, Parry JM, editors. Mutagenicity testing: a practical approach. Washington (DC): IRL Press; 1984. p. 275–306.

[16] Kurita Y, Sugiyama T, Nishizuka Y. Chromosome aberrations induced in rat bone marrow cells by 7, 12-dimethylbenz[a]-anthracene. J Natl Cancer Inst 1969;43(3):635–41.

[17] Rees ED, Majumdar SK, Shuck A. Changes in chromosomes of bone marrow after intravenous injections of 7,12-dimethylbenz(a)anthracene and related compounds. Proc Natl Acad Sci USA 1970;66(4):1228–35.

[18] Datta PK, Schleiermacher E. The effects of cytoxan on the chromosomes of mouse bone marrow. Mutat Res 1969;8(3):623–8.

[19] ICH (International Committee on Harmonisation). ICH S2(R1) Guidance on genotoxicity testing and data interpretation for pharmaceuticals intended for human use. Published in the Federal Register, 7 June 2012, vol. 77, no 110, p. 33748–9.

[20] US FDA. Redbook 2000 toxicological principles for the safety assessment of food ingredients, short-term tests for genetic toxicity. <http://www.fda.gov/Food/GuidanceRegulation/GuidanceDocumentsRegulatory Information/IngredientsAdditivesGRASPackaging/ucm2006826.htm>; 2007.

[21] OECD. Guideline for the testing of chemicals, genetic toxicology no. 475: mammalian bone marrow chromosomal aberration test, organisation for economic development and co-operation, Paris, France; 26 September 2014.

[22] Adler ID, Ashby J. The present lack of evidence for unique rodent germ-cell mutagens. Mutat Res 1989;212(1):55–66.

[23] Tates AD, Natarajan AT, De Vogel N, Meijers M. A correlative study of the genetic damage induced by chemical mutagens in bone marrow and spermatogonia of mice. III. 1,3-Bis (2-chloroethyl)-3-nitrosourea (BCNU). Mutat Res 1977;44(1):87–95.

[24] Renner HW, Wever J. Comparison of the mutagenic response in small intestine epithelium and in bone marrow of Chinese hamsters by chemical mutagens. Chemosphere 1988;17(9):1885–90.

[25] Blakey DH. Sister chromatid exchange analysis in the colonic and small intestinal epithelium of the mouse. Cancer Lett 1985;28(3):299–305.

[26] Uno Y, Morita T, Luijten M, Beevers C, Hamada S, Itoh S, et al. Micronucleus test in rodent tissues other than liver or erythrocytes: report of the IWGT working group. Mutat Res 2015;783:19–22.

[27] Doherty AT, Baumgartner A, Anderson D. Cytogenetic in vivo assays in somatic cells. Methods Mol Biol 2012;817:271–304.

[28] Perry PE, Thomson EJ. The methodology of sister chromatid exchanges. In: Kilbey BJ, Legator M, Nichols W, Ramel C, editors. Handbook of mutagenicity testing procedures. 2nd ed. Elsevier Science Publishers BV; 1984. p. 495–529.

[29] Allen JW, Shuler CF, Mendes RW, Latt SA. A simplified technique for *in vivo* analysis of sister-chromatid exchanges using 5-bromodeoxyuridine tablets. Cytogenet Cell Genet 1977;18(4):231–7.

[30] US EPA. Code of Federal Regulations, Title 40, Chapter I, Subchapter C, Part 79 Registration of fuels and fuel additives. *In vivo* sister chromatid exchange assay. <http://www.ecfr.gov/cgi-bin/text-idx?SID=cddec 58988fe4c834d387144fc08bd7a&mc=true&node=se40.17.79_165&rgn=div8>; 1998.

[31] Lovell DP, Anderson D, Albanese R, Amphlett GE, Clare G, Ferguson R, et al. Statistical analysis of in vivo cytogenetic assays. In: Kirkland DJ, editor. Statistical evaluation of mutagenicity test data. Cambridge: Cambridge University Press; 1989. p. 184–232.

[32] Festing MF, Lovell DP. The need for statistical analysis of rodent micronucleus test data. Comment on the paper by Ashby and Tinwell. Mutat Res 1995;329(2):221–4.

[33] Hayashi M, Dearfield K, Kasper P, Lovell D, Martus HJ, Thybaud V. Compilation and use of genetic toxicity historical control data. Mutat Res 2011;723(2):87–90.

[34] Tweats DJ, Blakey D, Heflich RH, Jacobs A, Jacobsen SD, Morita T, et al. Report of the IWGT working group on strategies and interpretation of regulatory *in vivo* tests I. Increases in micronucleated bone marrow cells in rodents that do not indicate genotoxic hazards. Mutat Res 2007;627:78–91.

[35] Albanese R. The cytonucleus test in the rat: a combined metaphase and micronucleus assay. Mutat Res 1987;182(6):309−21.

[36] Krishna G, Kropko ML, Ciaravino V, Theiss JC. Simultaneous micronucleus and chromosome aberration assessment in the rat. Mutat Res 1991;264(1):29−35.

[37] Krishna G, Theiss JC. Concurrent analysis of cytogenetic damage *in vivo*: a multiple endpoint-multiple tissue approach. Environ Mol Mutagen 1995;25(4):314−20.

[38] Miller RC. The micronucleus test as an *in vivo* cytogenetic method. Environ Health Perspect 1973;6:167−70.

CHAPTER 10

The In Vivo *Comet Assay Test*

Marie Z. Vasquez[1] and Roland Frötschl[2]

[1]*Helix3 Inc, Morrisville, NC, USA* [2]*Genetic and Reproductive Toxicology, Federal Institute for Drugs and Medical Devices (BfArM), Bonn, Germany*

Chapter Outline

10.1 Introduction 346
10.2 The *In Vivo* Comet Assay in Regulatory Safety Testing 348
    10.2.1 Follow-Up of Positive *In Vitro* Standard Battery Tests 350
    10.2.2 Follow-Up of Negative *In Vitro* Standard Battery Tests 351
10.3 Fundamentals 351
10.4 Equipment and Nondisposable Supplies 352
10.5 Consumables 354
10.6 Reagents and Solutions 354
    10.6.1 Reagents 354
    10.6.2 Solutions 355
        10.6.2.1 *Mincing Buffer (500 mL final volume)* 355
        10.6.2.2 *1% Normal Melting Agarose (200 mL final volume)* 355
        10.6.2.3 *0.5% Low Melting Point Agarose (200 mL final volume)* 355
        10.6.2.4 *Lysing stock solution (900 mL final volume)* 355
        10.6.2.5 *Working lysing solution (40 mL final volume in Coplin jars)* 356
        10.6.2.6 *10 M NaOH stock (500 mL final volume)* 356
        10.6.2.7 *200 mM EDTA stock, pH 10 (200 mL final volume)* 356
        10.6.2.8 *Alkaline electrophoresis buffer (1 L final volume)* 356
        10.6.2.9 *0.4 M Tris Buffer (1 L final volume)* 356
10.7 Test System 356
10.8 Study Design Considerations 357
    10.8.1 Test Article 357
    10.8.2 Vehicle Selection 357
    10.8.3 Positive Control 359
    10.8.4 Number of Animals 359
    10.8.5 Route of Exposure 359
    10.8.6 Treatment Schedule/Sample Time 360
    10.8.7 Dose Selection and Cytotoxicity 361
    10.8.8 Tissue Selection 361
10.9 Standard Test Procedures 362
    10.9.1 Preliminary Procedures 362
    10.9.2 Sample Collection 363
    10.9.3 Comet Slide Preparation 364

10.9.4 Alkaline Electrophoresis 365
10.9.5 Slide Staining 367
10.9.6 Image Analysis Scoring 367
10.10 Data and Reporting 369
10.10.1 Statistical Analysis 369
10.10.1.1 Normality Test 370
10.10.1.2 Pairwise comparisons 371
10.10.1.3 Trend tests 371
10.10.2 Validity of a Test 372
10.10.3 Positive Response Criteria 372
10.10.4 Cytotoxicity 373
10.10.5 Reporting results 376
10.11 Evaluating Unclear Results 378
10.11.1 Equivocal Results 379
10.11.2 Positive Results 379
10.11.3 Negative Results 380
Acknowledgments 381
References 381

10.1 Introduction

The *in vivo* comet assay is often called the alkaline *in vivo* comet assay, referring to the use of slide electrophoresis buffer with a pH >13. Other versions using electrophoresis buffers with a different (e.g., neutral or 12.1) pH may also be used but, because the alkaline version is considered the most sensitive and therefore the only one regularly included in regulatory submissions, it is the only version discussed in this chapter and hereafter is referred to merely as the *in vivo* comet assay. Under alkaline conditions, some forms of DNA damage (e.g., strand breaks, alkali labile sites, adducts) may be expressed by fragmentation of the nuclear DNA that increases in DNA migration during electrophoresis. Other forms of damage (e.g., cross-links) bind the nuclear DNA decreasing DNA migration (Figures 10.1 and 10.2). DNA strand breaks can be directly induced by ionizing radiation, radiomimetic/ highly cytotoxic chemicals (e.g., chlorambucil), radical-forming chemicals (e.g., hydrogen peroxide) or by substances that physically interact with DNA (e.g., asbestos). Alkali-labile sites (e.g., apurinic/apyrimidinic sites) can be induced by agents (e.g., EMS) making alkyl substitutions in the DNA that are easily susceptible to hydrolysis. Adducts are induced by chemicals that covalently bind to the DNA. Some chemicals bind to just one strand of DNA, whereas other chemicals (e.g., cisplatin) can covalently bind to both strands of DNA, ultimately forming interstrand cross-links.

The alkaline version of the comet assay was first published by Singh et al. in 1988, and one of the first *in vivo* applications of the assay was published in 1993 [1]. In March 1999, at the International Workshop on Genotoxicity Testing (IWGT), an expert panel met to

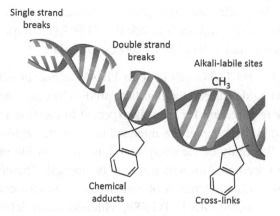

Figure 10.1
Types of DNA damage detectable by the comet assay.

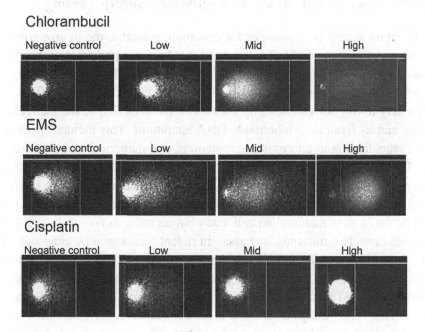

Figure 10.2
The expression of DNA damage in comet where strand breakers and alkylating agents such as chlorambucil and EMS increase DNA migration, but where cross-linkers such as cisplatin decrease DNA migration.

develop the first guidelines for using the *in vitro* and *in vivo* comet assay in genotoxicity testing [2]. Over the next 13 years, the number of *in vivo* comet assay publications more than quadrupled as protocol modifications and improvements were evaluated and recommended. The methodology recommended in 2000 by Tice et al. remains largely unchanged to this day. But validation attempts for the assay that began in 2003 made it clear that technical consistency, attention to detail, and practical experience with the assay were critical factors that would determine its success or failure.

With the adoption of the OECD TG 489 (The *In Vivo* Mammalian Alkaline Comet Assay), the need for a practical guide for conducting these studies has become more significant because the regulatory requirement for them is expected to increase [3]. The recommendations cited in this chapter are intended as a general guide for performing these studies. However, the flexibility of the assay prohibits the inclusion of all the possible protocol components or scenarios for which it may be applied. Therefore, this chapter is limited to describing the critical elements of conducting an *in vivo* comet assay test as outlined by the recently adopted OECD TG 489, with additional details and recommendations by the chapter authors.

10.2 The In Vivo Comet Assay in Regulatory Safety Testing

In regulatory safety testing of substances for genotoxic potential, the *in vivo* comet assay is the most used and recommended follow-up test for substances positive in the *in vitro* mammalian cell tests [3–8]. It is also part of the option 2 standard testing battery for genotoxic potential of pharmaceuticals in the ICH S2(R1) guidance (FDA 2012). Regulatory safety testing for genotoxicity focuses on the detection of the main classes of DNA damage and its fixation in inheritable DNA alterations. This includes gene mutations, clastogenic events leading to chromosome mutations, and numerical chromosome alterations. The two options of standard batteries offered in ICH S2R1 guidelines start with an AMES assay; option 1 includes an *in vitro* mammalian cell assay and an *in vivo* test for chromosomal damage in rodent hematopoietic cells (usually a micronucleus assay), whereas option 2 omits the *in vitro* mammalian cell assay but includes *in vivo* testing in two different tissues, usually a micronucleus assay in rodent hematopoietic cells and an assay in a different tissue with an endpoint different from micronuclei. The test recommended as the second *in vivo* test is a DNA strand breakage assay in liver (Figure 10.3), unless otherwise justified. Subsequent to finalization of OECD TG 489, the most widely used strand break assay is the *in vivo* comet assay. Both options are considered equally suitable for testing the genotoxic potential of any substance. However, substance-specific knowledge may indicate that one option may be preferable. Option 2 with a second *in vivo* test in the liver may, for example, be preferable when the occurrence of short-lived metabolites in liver is expected. An example for such a scenario might be the CB1 antagonist rimonabant where reactive metabolites and protein adducts of the metabolite are generated in liver microsomes [9] and may also be expected to occur *in vivo* in liver. When option 2 is preferred, a combined *in vivo* micronucleus and comet assay should be used when possible to minimize the number of animals used for testing. Adequate exposure in the comet assay can be demonstrated by assessing toxicity in the tissue used by histopathological evaluation, blood

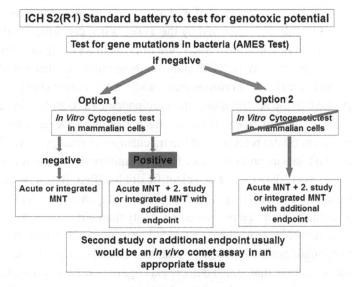

Figure 10.3
Schematic outline of standard battery of genotoxicity tests for pharmaceuticals based on ICH S2 (R1). In the chart, the comet assay is shown as the most generally appropriate complementary *in vivo* assay, although ICH does not indicate which strand break assay should be used. Subsequent to publication of the ICH guidance, the comet assay guideline became the only strand break assay described by a finalized OECD test guideline.

biochemistry toxicity indicators, or other scientifically accepted parameters to prove toxicity in the tissue used or by measuring exposure of drug-related material in the target tissue. The liver is usually expected to be exposed when systemic exposure is demonstrated.

The comet assay and the transgenic mutation assay in rodents (TGR) are also recommended as *in vivo* genotoxicity assays for follow-up of positives in the *in vitro* gene mutation tests. The assays address different genotoxicity endpoints with different impacts on risk assessment. The TGR directly measures gene mutations *in vivo* in any tissue regardless of the genotoxic mode of action of the test compound, whereas the *in vivo* comet assay primarily measures DNA strand breaks. A positive comet result shows exposure to genotoxic compounds inducing DNA strand breaks but not necessarily causing gene mutations. Conversely, compounds causing gene mutations without inducing DNA strand breaks in the process may not be detected by comet but should be positive in the TGR. Therefore, the *in vivo* comet assay as a follow-up for AMES-positive impurities in regulatory testing according to ICH M7 should be used only if convincing evidence is provided that the test compound also induces DNA strand breaks. Such evidence may often be difficult to provide. However, this approach is not founded on convincing experimental evidence, and data directly comparing the *in vivo* comet assay and TGR test for substances inducing gene mutations but not causing DNA strand breaks are lacking. Kirkland and Speit [10] compared the follow-up testing of *in vitro* positive tests with positive carcinogenicity data but negative *in vivo* micronucleus tests in rodents. These data showed that the *in vivo* comet assay detected 90% of the *in vivo* micronucleus negative rodent carcinogens compared to only 50% detected by the TGR. When confirmed mutagens were tested in both the TGR and *in vivo* comet assay, the *in vivo* comet assay detected 100% of the mutagens that tested positive in the TGR and also three mutagens that tested negative in the TGR. These were acrylonitrile, 1,2-dibromoethane, and 1,2-dichloroethane [11–13]. All three substances were positive in the AMES assay and carcinogenic in rodents. This appears to indicate that the TGR is less sensitive than the *in vivo* comet assay for detecting mutagens and not necessarily dependent on the relevance of the mechanism of mutagenicity. Therefore, accepting negative TGR data as proof of lack of *in vivo* mutagenic potential but rejecting negative *in vivo* comet assay data cannot be scientifically justified. Based on the available data at this time, the sensitivity for detecting AMES-positive mutagens and potentially positive rodent carcinogens is higher with the *in vivo* comet assay than with the TGR. However, to further support this conclusion, more data are needed on compounds tested in both assays. With respect to compounds positive in *in vitro* mammalian cell cytogenetic tests, the *in vivo* comet assay has the advantage that it also detects clastogens that are not detectable in the TGR. In addition to these mechanistic considerations, the *in vivo* comet assay has clear economic advantages compared to the TGR. Usually, the comet assay involves only short-term dosing (2–3 doses over 2 days), whereas the TGR normally requires at least 28 daily doses. TGR also requires substantial laboratory resources for extraction of DNA and expression of mutants and much more test substances, animal housing, and laboratory space in dedicated containment areas for handling transgenic organisms. In summary, TGR is more complicated and requires the use of patented rodent strains from limited sources and at a substantial cost. However, the comet assay is easily implemented, takes only 2–3 weeks to conduct from start to finish, and costs between 5- and 10-times less than the TGR. For these reasons, there is more widespread use of the comet assay with more published comet data available compared to the TGR.

10.2.1 Follow-Up of Positive In Vitro *Standard Battery Tests*

According to ICH S2(R1), in cases when a positive result occurs in one of the *in vitro* mammalian cell assays with insufficient weight of evidence for being irrelevant *in vivo*, clearly negative results in two well-conducted *in vivo* assays in appropriate tissues and with demonstrated adequate exposure are considered sufficient evidence for lack of genotoxic potential *in vivo*. In ICH M7—Assessment and control of DNA reactive (mutagenic) impurities in pharmaceuticals to limit potential carcinogenic risk—the *in vivo* comet assay is one option to follow-up an AMES-positive impurity. However, the use of the comet assay instead of a gene mutation assay should be adequately justified. A scientific rational is required when formation of DNA strand breaks or alkali labile sites are formed as premutagenic lesions. This may be deducible from knowledge about the specific mode of genotoxic action of the chemical class the substance belongs to, for example, topoisomerase inhibitors or some alkylators and adduct-forming compounds where strand breaks or alkali labile sites are known to be formed as premutagenic lesions.

10.2.2 Follow-Up of Negative In Vitro Standard Battery Tests

In some cases, tissue-specific follow-up testing may be required even for compounds negative in the standard battery genotoxicity tests. This can happen when such a compound produces positive results in any one of the two standard 2-year carcinogenicity studies in rodents with no plausible mechanistic explanation. In such cases, a genotoxic mode of action may need to be ruled out. An example would be the occurrence of carcinomas in the bladder in a rodent bioassay and no genotoxic effects of the compound in the standard battery genotoxicity tests. This type of tumor is not a common in rodents, and quite a number of bladder-specific genotoxic carcinogens are well known [14]. If there is no convincing evidence that this is driven by a nongenotoxic mechanism, then it may be suspected to be caused by potentially genotoxic activity related to the compound or a metabolite but could not be detected in the genotoxic standard battery tests. Further efforts to identify all relevant metabolites and an *in vivo* follow-up test with investigating effects in the target cells in the bladder may be necessary. The *in vivo* comet assay is one option for investigating genotoxicity in the target tissue. It may be considered suitable, especially when there will be potential metabolites causing DNA damage detectable in the comet assay. Another example would be a substance also with a negative standard battery for genotoxicity but causing a dose-dependent increase in hyperplasia and adenomas and/or carcinomas in intestinal mucosa in rodent bioassays. If there is no clear evidence that this increase is triggered by a nongenotoxic mechanism such as chronic inflammation—induced cell migration and repair proliferation due to local irritation, then a test for DNA damage in the target tissues might be recommended to exclude or verify a genotoxic mechanism. In such a case, the *in vivo* comet assay may be considered a suitable option to measure DNA-damaging activity in intestinal mucosa cells. A negative test result would provide further evidence for nongenotoxic mode of action and exclusion of DNA damaging activity as a potential mechanism. A positive test result, however, would, in general, need additional follow-up whether the DNA damage is caused by DNA-reactive or non-DNA-reactive (indirect) mechanisms.

10.3 Fundamentals

Under alkaline (pH > 13) electrophoresis conditions, some forms of DNA damage (e.g., direct strand breaks, alkali labile sites, DNA adducts) can be expressed as an increase in DNA migration, whereas other forms of DNA damage (e.g., cross-links) can be expressed as a decrease in DNA migration. But nongenotoxic or pre-necrotic/apoptotic mechanisms (e.g., inflammation, excision repair, and oxidative stress excision repair) can also increase DNA migration, whereas post-nectrotic/apoptotic stages (e.g., cell loss, fibrosis) can actually decrease DNA migration [15–16]. So, to avoid making confusing or potentially misleading statements about comet assay measurements and results, the endpoint should be referred to as "DNA migration" rather than "DNA damage" unless additional data supporting the exclusion of nongenotoxic effects can be provided.

Therefore, this chapter only refers to DNA migration. DNA migration is most often defined or described as the density of the migrated DNA (%tail DNA; total pixel intensity of the comet minus the pixel intensity of the head), the distance that the DNA migrated (TL; tail length measured in microns from either the estimated leading or trailing edge of the head), the tail moment (TM; measured in microns as the %tail multiplied by the distance migrated), and/or the Olive tail moment (OTM; measured in microns as the distance between the tail DNA distribution and the Head DNA distribution multiplied by the %tail DNA).

10.4 Equipment and Nondisposable Supplies

The following is a list of the minimal equipment necessary for performing the *in vivo* comet assay tests on a routine basis:

- Animal housing system
- Dosing apparatus
- Electrophoresis gel box, horizontal and recirculating
- Electrophoresis power supply with adjustable regulated voltage (V) and current (mA) settings.
- Forceps
- Freezer ($-20\,°C$)
- Heat block or water bath ($37\,°C$)
- Ice flaking machine
- Image analysis system including microscope with camera mount, CCD camera, PC, and software

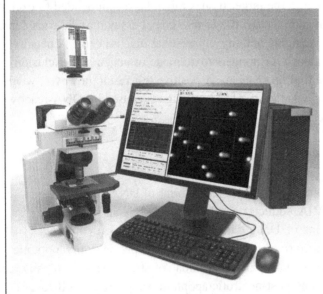

Image courtesy of Andor Technology, an Oxford Instruments Company
- Micropipettes, adjustable (e.g., 20, 200, and 1000 µL)
- Microwave
- Mincing scissors

(Continued)

(Continued)

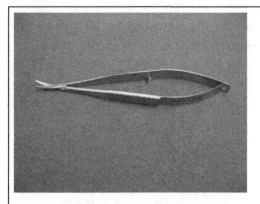

Image courtesy of Global Surgical Instruments
• Opaque plastic Coplin jars

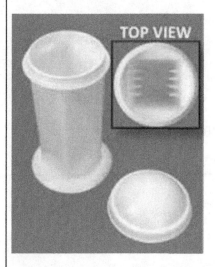

Image courtesy of Newcomer Supply
• pH meter with Tris-compatible electrode
• Pipettor
• Pyrex bottles and beakers
• Refrigerator (4 °C)
• Slide boxes
• Slide warmer (37 °C)
• Stir plate
• Surgical scissors
• Ultra-low freezer (−70 °C)

NOTE: Depending on the location and environment within the facility where slides will be prepared and stored, a dehumidifier may also be necessary to maintain a constant relative humidity (RH) of 60% or less.

10.5 Consumables

Detailed descriptions of the reagents and solutions used in routine testing are provided in the Reagents and Solutions section. The following is a list of common consumables typically used for testing with comet:

- Coverslips, glass, 24 × 50 mm
- Dosing needles
- Dosing vials
- Glass disposal boxes
- Microcentrifuge tubes
- Microscope slides, glass 25 × 75 mm or 3 × 1 inch
- Pipette tips
- Pipettes (5, 10, 25, and 50 mL)
- Utility or medical wipes

10.6 Reagents and Solutions

10.6.1 Reagents

Ca^{2+} and Mg^{2+} free Hanks' balanced salt solution (HBSS)

Ca^{2+} and Mg^{2+} free phosphate-buffered saline (PBS)

Dimethylsulfoxide (DMSO)

HCl (to pH solutions)

Low melting (37 °C) point agarose (LMP)

Na_2 EDTA

NaCl

NaOH

Normal melting agarose (NMA)

Nucleic acid stain (e.g., SYBR™ Gold, ethidium bromide)

Triton X-100

Trizma base

10.6.2 Solutions

10.6.2.1 Mincing Buffer (500 mL final volume)

To 400 mL Ca^{++} and Mg^{++} free Hank's balanced salt solution, add Na_2EDTA to a final concentration of 20 mM and DMSO to a final concentration of 10% v/v. Adjust pH to 7.4–7.7. Store at room temperature for up to 3 months.

NOTE: DMSO will crystallize and come out of solution at temperatures <20°C. Do not store the mincing buffer under refrigerated or cold temperatures. It is important to ensure that the pH of the mincing buffer is 7.4–7.7 before use to avoid degradation of samples. Verification and adjustment (as necessary) of the mincing buffer pH is recommended between uses.

10.6.2.2 1% Normal Melting Agarose (200 mL final volume)

Add 2 g normal melting agarose (NMA) to 200 mL PBS. Using a microwave, bring mixture to a boil and mix thoroughly to ensure it is completely dissolved and homogenous. Prepare fresh for each use, reboiling and remixing as necessary to ensure that it remains hot and homogenous throughout use. Discard any unused portions.

10.6.2.3 0.5% Low Melting Point Agarose (200 mL final volume)

Add 1 g low melting point agarose (LMP) to 200 mL PBS. Using a microwave, bring mixture to a boil and mix thoroughly to ensure it is completely dissolved and homogenous. Prepare fresh and equilibrate to $37 \pm 3°C$ in a heat block or water bath before use. Freshly prepared LMP may be aliquoted to smaller vials and stored refrigerated for up to 6 months. To use LMP that has been aliquoted and stored, use a microwave to reheat the aliquots and bring them to a boil. Mix and equilibrate to $37 \pm 3°C$ before use.

NOTE: Stored aliquots may only be used once because repeated heating will change the concentration. After use, any unused portion remaining in the vial should be discarded.

10.6.2.4 Lysing stock solution (900 mL final volume)

Add 146.1 g NaCl, 37.2 g Na_2EDTA, 1.2 g Trizma base, and 7–9 g NaOH to 700 mL dH_2O and stir until dissolved. Adjust the pH to 10 and adjust the final volume to 900 mL with dH_2O. Verify a final pH of 10 and adjust as necessary. Store at room temperature for up to 6 months.

10.6.2.5 Working lysing solution (40 mL final volume in Coplin jars)

Mix 36 mL of lysing stock solution with 0.4 mL Triton X-100 and 4 mL DMSO. Maintain on ice or refrigerated until use.

NOTE: The working lysing solution should be cold when comet slides are first submerged. But DMSO will crystallize and come out of solution at temperatures less than 20°C, so the working lysing solution should be placed under cold conditions within 8 h or less of use.

10.6.2.6 10 M NaOH stock (500 mL final volume)

Slowly add 200 g of NaOH to 300 mL dH$_2$O. Use care because heat will be generated. Dissolve and make final volume to 500 mL with dH$_2$O. Store at room temperature for up to 2 weeks.

10.6.2.7 200 mM EDTA stock, pH 10 (200 mL final volume)

Add 14.9 g Na$_2$EDTA to 150 mL dH$_2$O. While stirring, adjust pH to 9–11 to facilitate dissolution of the Na$_2$EDTA. Once in solution, adjust the pH to 10 and adjust the final volume to 200 mL with dH$_2$O. Adjust final pH to 10 as necessary. Store at room temperature for up to 2 weeks.

10.6.2.8 Alkaline electrophoresis buffer (1 L final volume)

Add 30 mL of 10 M NaOH stock and 5 mL 200 mM EDTA stock to 965 mL dH$_2$O and mix. Prepare fresh immediately before use. Discard any unused solution.

10.6.2.9 0.4 M Tris Buffer (1 L final volume)

Add 48.5 g Trizma base to 900 mL dH$_2$O and mix. Adjust pH to 7.5 and adjust the final volume to 1 L with dH$_2$O. Store at room temperature for up to 6 months.

10.7 Test System

All animal procedures should be in compliance with the applicable Animal Welfare and government regulations and reviewed by the institutional animal care and use committee (IACUC) or equivalent. Although common laboratory strains of rats and mice (rodents) are typically used for *in vivo* comet assay studies, the comet assay can be applied to any species and/or strain. Only healthy young adult animals (e.g., 6- to 10-week-old rodents at the start of treatment) should be used unless scientifically and ethically justified. Depending on the specific species, animals should be maintained under the appropriate environmental conditions and provided the absorbent bedding with an unlimited supply of feed and water. Although fasting animals before dosing is common for toxicity studies, this is contraindicated for comet assay studies because fasting can perturb homeostasis in multiple tissues and potentially confound comet. Animals should be housed in a manner that minimizes stress, and they should be sufficiently acclimated to the laboratory conditions before use. Each animal should be uniquely identified and randomly assigned to dose groups. To minimize interanimal variability, weight variation of animals at the start of dosing should be minimal, not exceeding $\pm 20\%$ of the mean weight of each sex. And each animal should be dosed based on its individual body weight immediately prior to dosing.

10.8 Study Design Considerations

The study design for the routine testing of chemicals is outlined in OECD TG 489. Studies for regulatory submission should generally follow this guidance and be performed under GLP guidelines. However, the flexibility of the comet assay and the OECD guidelines allow for significant variations in the application of the assay and the manner in which it is applied. The details of every study design should be carefully considered to ensure that they are scientifically justified and appropriate for each test article. This section will cover specific considerations and/or additional information related to the recommendations in OECD TG 489.

10.8.1 Test Article

The comet assay can be used to evaluate the genotoxicity of many test articles including, but not limited to, industrial chemicals, pharmaceuticals, nanoparticles, consumer products, medical devices, environmental contaminants, complex mixtures, and impurities. To ensure that the study design selected is appropriate for each test article, species, and tissue evaluated, the intended/expected route of human exposure, ADME (absorption, distribution, metabolism, and excretion), structural alerts, and toxicity data for each test article should be determined in advance and addressed appropriately in the study design. As a strand break assay, the standard alkaline comet assay cannot detect aneuploidy directly. However, comet can be used to detect DNA–DNA cross-links that may be a useful very early predictor of at least one mechanism of aneuploidy induction even at cytostatic or cytotoxic doses [17–18] that would otherwise make detection of aneuploidy very difficult using cytogenetic methods. The OECD TG 489 states that the standard alkaline comet assay protocol has not been optimized for detecting cross-links *in vivo*. However, evidence exists in the literature suggesting that the standard protocol can detect cross-links *in vivo* when the baseline levels of DNA migration are high enough to detect a decrease in migration as a result of cross-linking [16–19]. So, regardless of the OECD disclaimer, regulators are likely to critically evaluate decreases in DNA migration as potentially indicative of cross-link induction.

10.8.2 Vehicle Selection

Depending on the intended route of administration and the solubility of the test article, almost any standard vehicle for preparing dosing solutions or homogenous suspensions may be used. This can include, but is not limited to, water, saline, or different types of methylcellulose. But the effect of the vehicle on the initial site of contact tissue (e.g., forestomach, stomach, and duodenum for oral administrations) should be evaluated before it is used to ensure that it does not induce low levels of irritation/inflammation that can increase the baseline levels of DNA migration in multiple tissues, both locally and peripherally [20]. This is of particular concern for viscous vehicles and/or mixtures with detergents that may be used for less soluble compounds or impurities because high background levels of DNA migration decrease the sensitivity of the assay and can potentially invalidate a study (Figure 10.4).

If the effect of the vehicle on the tissues selected for evaluation is unknown, and/or if the use of an irritant vehicle is unavoidable, then the number of daily administrations should

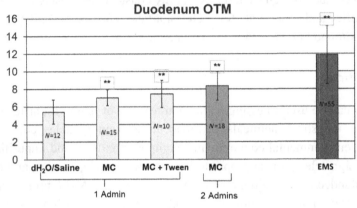

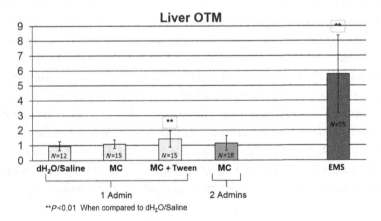

Figure 10.4

Background DNA migration levels induced by dH_2O/saline, methylcellulose (MC), or methylcellulose and Tween in the duodenum and liver following a single daily administration or two daily administrations. N = the number of experiments with identical study designs using the same viscosity and brand name of components.

be three or fewer to minimize the potential confounding effects of vehicle-induced inflammation that can enhance or even indirectly induce a genotoxic response unrelated to the test article exposure [16,21,22].

10.8.3 Positive Control

A concurrent positive control dose group should be included in every study design because it will be necessary to defend the validity of the study and the methods used. This should be carefully considered when integrating the comet assay in a repeat dose toxicity study that does not usually include a positive control dose group. The positive control and the concentration at which it will be administered should induce DNA strand breaks in all of the tissues that will be evaluated with comet. Ethyl methanesulfonate (EMS; CAS No. 62-50-0) is the most common positive control of choice because it produces DNA strand breaks in all the tissues that have been studied [23]. Other positive controls (e.g., methyl methanesulfonate, ethyl nitrosourea) may be used as long as the laboratory can reliably achieve a positive response in the tissues intended for evaluation. When a test article is suspected to induce a specific type of damage (e.g., cross-links), one may be tempted to incorporate a positive control compound to induce that specific type of damage. Special caution should be taken when attempting this because the positive control compound may not necessarily induce the specified damage in the tissue(s) intended for evaluation. For example, the DNA–protein cross-linker formaldehyde induces damage in the nasal mucosa (site of first contact) of rats following inhalation exposure with no evidence of systemic exposure or DNA damage in the blood or any other tissues [24–26]. So, in a study intended to evaluate the induction of cross-links in the liver following oral exposure, formaldehyde is not likely be an appropriate positive control for inducing DNA–protein cross-links in the liver.

10.8.4 Number of Animals

OECD TG 489 recommends the inclusion of at least three test article dose groups, one concurrent vehicle control group, and one concurrent positive control dose group with at least five analyzable animals per dose group per sex evaluated. The dose range should include the maximum dose (MTD, maximum feasible dose, maximum exposure or limit dose) and at least one nontoxic dose. Depending on the toxicity of the test article, dosing more than five animals per dose/sex and/or more than three test article dose groups in a study may minimize the risk of having to conduct additional studies in cases where the toxicity is determined to be too high. It is important to note here that toxicity refers to local tissue toxicity rather than animal mortality.

10.8.5 Route of Exposure

The route of exposure for the comet assay should be based on the intended or expected route of human exposure. This is particularly important when oral ingestion of some drugs (e.g., ophthalmic tetrahydrozoline hydrochloride) is specifically contraindicated due to toxicity, metabolic, and/or absorption issues. There are currently no data attesting to the sensitivity of the comet assay to detect damage induced by administrations in the feed or drinking water. So, a method for using feed or the drinking water as the route of exposure in comet assay regulatory submissions cannot be described or recommended at this time.

10.8.6 Treatment Schedule/Sample Time

OECD TG 489 guideline recommends that animals receive two or more daily treatments with samples collected once at 2–6 h or at the Tmax after the last treatment. A single treatment with multiple sample times may be used in cases where the test article induces excessive toxicity following repeat administrations. Although the guidelines allow for the incorporation of comet into repeat dose studies, doing so has logistical limitations and, as noted by the guidelines, repeat administrations can induce excessive toxicity. Low levels of inflammation immediately after chemical injury can indirectly increase DNA damage in tissues [16,20,22]. Meanwhile, the postinjury cell proliferation and remodeling phases that occur in every tissue after 3 days or more (Figure 10.5) can reduce detectable DNA damage back to baseline levels as cells repair the damage or die and are replaced by undamaged/fibrotic tissue. For this reason, and because comet can detect damage after less than 24 h of exposure, conducting *in vivo* comet studies as acute studies with three or fewer daily administrations is recommended. Where possible, dosing intervals and sample times should be selected based on the intended human exposure conditions and the ADME of the test compound. Animal dosing should be scheduled in a manner that minimizes timing variations between individual animals and dose groups. The time between each

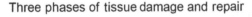

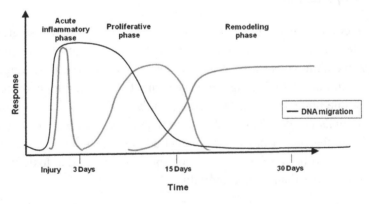

Figure 10.5

Tissue repair timeline showing why acute (≤3 daily) dose administrations may be more appropriate for the comet assay [23].

animal dosing should be consistent and sufficient enough to allow for all of the required sample collection and processing for each animal to be completed at the specified sample time (e.g., 4 h after dosing).

10.8.7 Dose Selection and Cytotoxicity

As stated in Section 10.8.4 and in the OECD TG 489 guidelines, the dose range evaluated should include the MTD and at least two additional dose levels including at least one noncytotoxic dose. Tissue toxicity can increase DNA migration [16,23,27], making it impossible to distinguish between genotoxic and cytotoxic increases in DNA migration. Therefore, special care should be taken to ensure that the dose range evaluated with comet includes doses that are noncytotoxic in each of the tissues evaluated. Some tissues will be more sensitive than others depending on the test compound and study design. So, the lowest dose at which cytotoxicity is induced in any evaluated tissue should be considered the MTD for a comet study. The best measurements of cytotoxicity for the comet assay should detect at the cellular level the pre-necrotic/apoptotic changes associated with homeostasis perturbation (inflammation, caspase activation, glycogen depletion, etc.) because these are most likely to induce and/or coincide with an increase in DNA strand breaks. Membrane permeability assays (e.g., trypan blue exclusion) and necrosis detection methods do not contribute much to the interpretation of DNA migration increases because membrane-compromised/dead cells and their DNA are quickly dispersed and lost during the cell lysis and electrophoresis steps. As a consequence, the detection of membrane-compromised/dead cells in a tissue is more likely to explain the absence of an increase in DNA migration due to excessive cytotoxicity and the subsequent loss of damaged cells.

10.8.8 Tissue Selection

The organ of choice for the comet assay will often be the liver as the main metabolizing and usually well-exposed organ. However, there may be cases where the best choice of target organ for the *in vivo* comet assay may be different from liver. As much as possible, the ADME data, the toxicity, and any available carcinogenicity data should be considered. When there are distribution data showing highest exposure in an organ other than liver and negligible metabolism in liver, the organ with highest exposure may be the organ of choice for the tissue investigated in the comet assay. For example, regarding orally administered drugs, with limited absorption, no relevant metabolites, and highest exposure in the intestinal mucosa, the *in vivo* comet assay in intestinal mucosa cells may be preferential to a liver comet assay. Drug metabolites may also have severe effects in extrahepatic target organs due to transport to the organ or organ-specific metabolism [28]. This is important especially when reactive metabolites are generated predominantly in extrahepatic tissues. In cases where data from metabolic studies and data on organ toxicity from repeated dose toxicology studies provide evidence that relevant reactive metabolites may occur and cause genotoxic effects in extrahepatic tissues, those data should be taken into account when choosing the most relevant tissue for the second *in vivo* assay. For substances with high toxicity in organs others than liver, the follow-up *in vivo* test should also include the tissues where the most significant substance toxicity occurs. This can be the tissue of the site of contact, for example, intestinal mucosa. This frequently happens when orally applied substances cause irritations in stomach or intestinal mucosa. For substances with positive results in carcinogenicity studies, the affected tissue should also be considered as a potential tissue for testing. When, for example, precarcinogenic or carcinogenic lesions are seen in the bladder, the bladder may be considered a relevant tissue.

Additional examples that, on a case-by-case basis, may justify the evaluation of tissues other than the liver are provided here:

ADME examples: Compounds that concentrate in the lung or any other tissue may be evaluated in that tissue. One that demonstrates minimal absorption and/or that is completely excreted/degraded after a short (<6 h) time period may be evaluated in the primary site of excretion (e.g., colon, bladder).

Toxicity examples: Compounds that induce nephrotoxicity without a clear nongenotoxic mechanism should be evaluated in the kidney. A compound that induces sterility may need to be evaluated in the reproductive tract.

Carcinogenicity examples: A compound that induces mammary tumors may be evaluated in the mammary gland if there is no clear rational for a nongenotoxic mechanism. Hormone-regulating tissues (e.g., ovary, adrenal glands) may be considered if there is mechanistic or pathological evidence for such tissues as a potential secondary drug target because damage induced in tissues of the endocrine system may induce the upregulation of uncontrolled cell division in undamaged peripheral tissues such as the mammaries.

10.9 Standard Test Procedures

10.9.1 Preliminary Procedures

Before any samples can be collected and comet slides prepared or processed, the following preliminary procedures must be performed:

1. At least 24 h before dipping the microscope slides in agarose, label the frosted end using a histology marker (e.g., Fisher Secureline™ marker II) specifically resistant to ethanol, NaOH, Triton X-100, and DMSO. Each slide should be labeled with the necessary identifiers (e.g., Study ID, sample ID, etc.) (Figure 10.6). Allow the markings to completely dry.
    NOTE: Most standard permanent markers (e.g., Sharpies), pencil markings, insufficiently dried markings, and printed labels will bleed or come off as comet slides

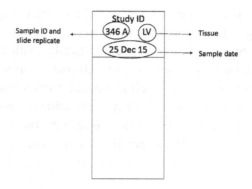

Figure 10.6
Example labeling for comet slides.

are subjected to lysis and electrophoresis. Markers that bleed during lysis can also induce DNA damage in the gel-embedded cells.

2. Dip the prelabeled microscope slides up to the frosted end in freshly prepared boiling hot 1% NMA.
3. Quickly remove the slide from the agarose, wipe the back of the slide to remove the excess agarose, and place the slide horizontally on a flat surface to dry. Slides may be air-dried at room temperature at a RH of 60% or less or placed on a warming unit.
4. Once dried, slides should be stored at room temperature and at a RH of 60% or less.
   NOTE: Dipped slides that are dried and/or maintained at a RH more than 60% are the most common cause of the cell layer of gel falling off the slide during or immediately after electrophoresis.
5. At least 30 min before use, prepare and mix thoroughly the working lysing solution and store cold.
6. At least 30 min before use, prepare the 0.5% LMP and allow it to equilibrate to $37 \pm 3°C$.

10.9.2 Sample Collection

1. With the exception of the blood that can be collected before necropsy, all comet tissue samples should be collected immediately after the animal is euthanized.
2. As soon as possible after collection, all comet samples should be immediately placed in mincing solution and maintained on ice to minimize endogenous DNA degradation that can increase variability.
3. Samples may be rinsed with additional mincing solution as necessary to remove excess blood and/or debris.
4. To prepare a cell suspension for slide preparation, tissues should be quickly minced or aspirated in the mincing buffer and maintained cold.

NOTE: Other methods such as epithelial scraping and enzymatic digestion have been successfully used for preparing cell suspensions. However, the extended time and/or 37°C incubations required for these procedures can be logistically challenging at necropsy and contribute to higher background DNA migration levels and/or variability in comet samples. Further, the DNA damage in one specific cell population from a tissue comprising a heterogeneous mixture of cells is an unreliable representation of damage (i.e., mutations) that can result from cell signaling and interactions within the tissue microenvironment [11]. Therefore, the fastest and simplest method possible for collecting and preparing cell suspensions from tissues is recommended over more extensive or cell-specific isolation methods.

10.9.3 Comet Slide Preparation

CRITICAL NOTE: Predipped slides and comet slides with cells should only be prepared and stored under low (≤60%) humidity conditions to maintain slide integrity and minimize variability that can be caused by agarose absorbing moisture from the environment. High humidity during slide preparation is the primary cause of variability and of gels falling off the slide during/after electrophoresis.

1. For each sample, at least two replicate comet slides should be prepared. If the low-molecular-weight (LMW) DNA diffusion assay (see Section 10.9 for details) will also be performed, then prepare at least three replicate slides.
2. For each comet slide prepared, a 5−10-μL aliquot of cell suspension should be mixed with 75 μL equilibrated 0.5% LMP and layered on top of a predipped and dried 1% NMA slide (Figure 10.7).

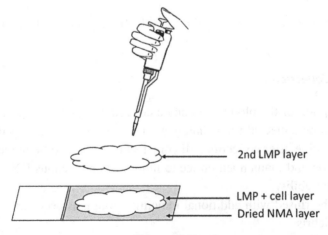

2nd LMP layer

LMP + cell layer

Dried NMA layer

Figure 10.7
Agarose layers for comet slide preparation.

3. Immediately cover the cell/LMP mixture with a coverslip and place the slide horizontally on a cold flat surface to allow the agarose to solidify.
4. Gently remove the coverslip and add a second layer of 75 μL 0.5% LMP to the slide. Replace the coverslip, place the slide horizontally on a cold flat surface, and keep the slide cold until it can be placed in the working lysis buffer.
5. Remove the coverslip and slowly lower the slide into cold, freshly prepared working lysing solution in an opaque Coplin jar or other light-protected container.
6. Lyse the cells in cold working lysing solution for at least 1 h. Slides may be maintained cold in lysing solution for up to 4 weeks before electrophoresis. However, it is recommended to electrophorese all slides within 72 h of preparation to minimize variability and potential loss of sensitivity because samples tend to diffuse over time.

NOTE: There is no evidence that exposure to fluorescent lighting during slide preparation contributes to background levels of DNA migration in comet samples. Therefore, filtered, incandescent, and/or yellow (gold) lights should be used during comet sample processing and slide preparations.

10.9.4 Alkaline Electrophoresis

1. Prepare fresh electrophoresis buffer and verify that the pH is higher than 13.
2. Remove slides from lysis and rinse with neutral pH buffer (e.g., 0.4 M Tris) to remove any residual lysing solution detergents.
3. Place slides lengthwise on the raised surface between the anode and cathode of a horizontal gel box, making sure to place them as close together as possible.
4. Fill the buffer reservoirs on either end of the gel box with the electrophoresis buffer until the liquid level covers the slides.
5. Maintain the slides submerged in the alkaline buffer at 4°C for 5–60 min to allow the DNA to unwind/denature.
   NOTE: Options for maintaining the 4°C temperature are illustrated here (Figure 10.8). The use of a cold room is also an option. However, care should be taken to avoid storing the power supplies and gel boxes in the cold room or refrigerator where moisture can corrode electrical components and connectors.
6. After unwinding, electrophorese the slides at 4°C and at a constant voltage (approximately 0.7 V/cm measured as the distance between the anode and cathode) with the current (mA) and wattage set to vary during the run.
7. Immediately after starting electrophoresis, adjust the current (mA) to the desired range by slowly raising or lowering the level of buffer.
   NOTE: The current of 300 mA that is frequently reported in the literature is just an arbitrary set point initially selected to ensure that the buffer volume at the start of electrophoresis is sufficient to cover the slides and is consistent across multiple

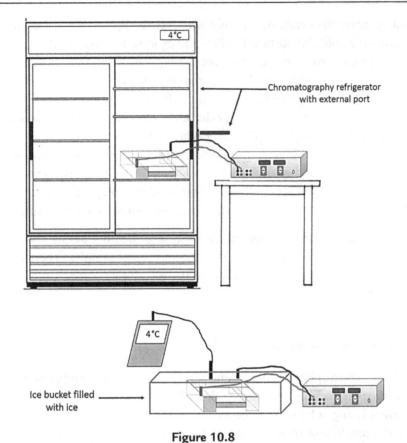

Figure 10.8
Example methods for maintaining 4°C temperature during electrophoresis by the use of a chromatography refrigerator or packing the gel box in ice.

electrophoresis runs. The actual mA reading selected by each laboratory should be based on these criteria using their specific gel boxes and slide thicknesses. It is normal for the current to fluctuate slightly during electrophoresis because resistance changes over time. In cases where the current changes dramatically due to a system failure, the power supply will be unable to compensate and will typically shut off due to standard UL required safety features.

8. Electrophorese slides for 5–40 min.

NOTE: The optimal duration for unwinding and electrophoresis is dependent on the tissue, experimental conditions, laboratory environment/equipment, and the type of damage (cross-links vs. strand breaks) that are being evaluated. Each laboratory will need to determine the best times for these steps based on their own criteria (e.g., achieved sensitivity) and adjust as necessary as experimental conditions/objectives change.

9. After electrophoresis is complete, gently remove the slides from the gel box and rinse them in 0.4 M Tris buffer (pH 7.5) to neutralize them.

10. Slides may now be immediately stained and scored, or they may be immersed in alcohol, air-dried, and stored at room temperature until they can be scored at a later time.

NOTE: Slides that are immersed in alcohol before drying should be allowed to air-dry for at least 12 h before attempting to stain. Any alcohol residue remaining on the slide can inhibit some stains.

10.9.5 Slide Staining

Slides may be stained with any nucleic acid stain (e.g., SYBR™ gold, ethidium bromide, silver stain). The type of stain(s) used by each laboratory will depend on the stain availability and the type of microscope (fluorescent vs. bright field), filter(s), and/or CCD camera/imaging system that will be used. For simplicity, the description is only based on the most common SYBR™ and Ethidium bromide stains.

1. Freshly prepare the desired stain according to manufacturer recommendations.
2. Add at least 200 μL stain to each 25×75-mm slide to saturate and rehydrate the gel and coverslip.
3. Keep the stained slide protected from light as you allow the gel to absorb the stain for at least 10 min.
4. Immediately before scoring, drain any excess stain from the slide.

10.9.6 Image Analysis Scoring

Although comet assay slides may be scored manually, the use of image analysis is recommended in the OECD guidelines for regulated studies. Image analysis systems typically include a computer with image analysis software, a microscope, and a CCD camera. For simplicity, the description here is based on an image analysis system with the Andor Technology Komet™ software installed on a PC and connected to a CCD camera mounted on a fluorescent microscope. However, other image analysis software (e.g., Comet IV, OpenComet) may be used. And when comets are stained with a nonfluorescent stain (e.g., silver), a light microscope may be used.

NOTE: The quality and consistency of images acquired by image analysis systems are highly dependent on the maintenance, quality, and settings of the components. For regulated studies, image analysis systems must be validated and maintained according to user specifications that include, but are not limited to, the GLP requirements for recordkeeping and the use of electronic data and signatures (FDA 21 CFR Part 11).

Microscope

- Microscope objectives should be of the appropriate (e.g., $20 \times$) magnification, clean, and free of oils.
- Filters appropriate for the selected stain should be installed.

- The light source should have sufficient remaining hours to ensure consistent illumination throughout scoring.
- The light source should be centered and focused appropriately to ensure that there is uniform illumination throughout the field of view.

CCD Camera

- The camera settings (e.g., brightness and contrast) should be adjusted to ensure that images of both heavily damaged and minimally damaged cells can be captured as accurately as possible without frequent setting changes.

Software

- The image analysis software should be calibrated with the microscope, light source, and camera that will be used for scoring.
- Measurements should be calibrated and set to the desired units (e.g., microns).
- The software should minimally include the ability to measure the comet TL, %tail, and OTM or tail moment, as well as components required by FDA 21 CFR Part 11 for electronic data (e.g., electronic signatures, audit trails).
- The formula used to calculate the OTM or tail moment should be provided by the software vendor so that it can be reported and measurements can be appropriately compared to data that may be generated by other image analysis systems.
- Validation of the software with the connected components (PC, microscope, camera) including any data capture mechanism should be completed before the system is used to collect or analyze comet study data.

For simplicity, the description here is only based on the real-time analysis of live images captured from a comet slide mounted on a microscope stage.

1. Slides should be coded so that the scorer does not know the treatment group of the sample scored.
2. Position the objective over a central region of the slide, avoiding the edges of the slide/gel.
3. With a live image on the computer screen, capture an image of a comet cell, making sure that the region of interest (ROI) includes only one entire comet without any obvious debris in the ROI or background field (Figure 10.9).
4. When collecting measurements, the image analysis system should accurately identify the head and tail regions of the comet. Some manual adjustments to the ROI and/or the position of the cell in the ROI may be necessary to ensure that images are captured correctly (see Figure 10.10). However, frequent manual adjustments by an inexperienced scorer attempting to perfect each and every measurement are often highly variable and therefore less reliable than the automated measurements of most image analysis systems with the appropriate settings.

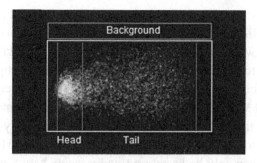

Figure 10.9
Proper comet/ROI position.

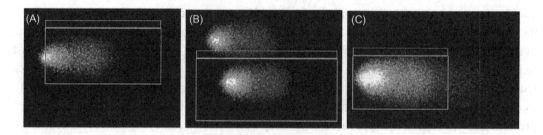

Figure 10.10
Examples where manual adjustments of ROI may be necessary: (A) head region cut off; (B) other comet/debris in background region; and (C) tail region cut off.

5. To ensure that sufficient statistical strength is achieved, OECD TG 489 recommends scoring from two to three slides per sample at least 150 cells per tissue per animal with at least five animals per dose group.
6. At least the %tail, TL, and the OTM or TM measurements should be collected by image analysis for each sample.

NOTE: OECD TG 489 recommends visual scoring of "hedgehogs" defined as comets without a clearly defined head because they are not readily detected by image analysis. Because the guidelines exclude image analysis of these comets, they are not addressed in this section.

10.10 Data and Reporting

10.10.1 Statistical Analysis

Statistical analysis should be conducted using the individual animal data as the experimental unit of exposure. OECD 489 allows the use of the %tail, tail moment, or TL endpoint for evaluation of comet assay data, but it recommends the use of % tail and does not specify which statistical methods should be used. The endpoint and statistical methods selected should be specified in the protocol before the study start and should be consistent for all tissues evaluated within a study. When considering which statistical methods to use, it is critically important to note that all of the endpoints measured by image analysis, including the %tail, are continuous measurements rather than discrete or count-based measurements such as %MN. This means that unlike count-based measurements, the %tail can be any value within the intensity range of the image analysis system with an infinite range of values with up to 10 significant digits (i.e., quantitative). However, the discrete or count-based %MN data can only be based on fixed integers between 0 and 100 (i.e., qualitative). Based on the experience of Moller and Loft [24] and our significant experience evaluating multiple sets of real comet study data from compounds that were later confirmed as genotoxic/nongenotoxic, comet data appear to be sufficiently robust, requiring only simple statistical methods that can be run using the most basic statistical software. And these methods can effectively use individual animal means (vs. medians) calculated as the overall mean of the total cells scored per animal. Using these values, standard pairwise tests (e.g., Dunnett's, Student's t-tests) and trend tests (e.g., linear regression, Kendall rank test) with minor adjustments for distribution and variance homogeneity can be effectively used to determine positive responses as required by OECD TG 489. Recommendations are presented for two different approaches that may be used. In each case, individual animal means should be used and each test should be run as a two-tailed test with a 95% confidence level evaluating for either an increase or decrease in DNA migration. Because experience has proven that statistical analysis with log-transformed data yields results similar to analysis with nontransformed data [16,29], we recommend performing the following procedures on nontransformed data:

10.10.1.1 Normality Test

With the vehicle or negative control dose group data, perform a Shapiro–Wilk test to determine the normality of the distribution for the untreated cell population. If the data are normally distributed ($P \geq 0.05$), then use the parametric tests described here. If the data are not normally distributed ($P < 0.05$), then use the nonparametric tests described.

NOTE: The distribution of comet data in different exposure groups is most often skewed and the parametric tests we recommend are robust even when used to compare groups that are not both normally distributed. But in some tissues (e.g., GI tract), the distribution of the background DNA migration in the untreated cell population can be unusually skewed by technical error, an inflammatory response to the vehicle control, or even normal but high cell turnover at the time of sampling. This can significantly affect group comparisons, increasing the risk of false-positive results. Therefore, we recommend using parametric or nonparametric tests based on the distribution normality of the vehicle control dose group.

10.10.1.2 Pairwise comparisons

Parametric tests

Option 1: Perform a Dunnett multiple comparison test comparing each dose group to the vehicle control group.

NOTE: Multiple comparison tests limit type I (false positive) errors by pooling variances across all dose groups. But they are less sensitive than option 2 and therefore may be more prone to type II (false negative) errors, as indicated by multiple tests run with real comet data from confirmed genotoxic compounds tested under regulatory requirements.

Option 2: Perform independent tests to compare each dose group to the vehicle control group. First, perform an F-test to determine the equality of variances between each of the compared groups. For comparisons of groups with equal variances, perform independent or Student t-tests. For comparisons of groups with unequal variances, perform independent t-tests with the Welch approximation for unequal variances (Welch t-test).

NOTE: Independent t-tests limit type II (false negative) errors by taking into account individual variances for each comparison and are therefore more sensitive than option 1. It is well known that indiscriminately performing multiple post hoc independent t-tests comparing all groups to each other in search of any difference significantly increases the risk of type I errors. But our experience with real comet data from confirmed genotoxic and nongenotoxic compounds indicates that using independent pairwise tests as described for a small and predetermined set of comparisons (e.g., 3–5) is more sensitive and specific than using multiple comparison tests.

Nonparametric tests

Option 1: Perform a Steel multiple comparison test comparing each dose group to the vehicle control group.

Option 2: Perform independent Mann-Whitney tests comparing each dose group to the vehicle control group.

10.10.1.3 Trend tests

Parametric test

Linear regression test.

Nonparametric test

Kendall rank correlation test.

NOTE: Although many dose-response curves are nonmonotonic or nonlinear (Figure 10.11), most include linear elements at different points or doses along the response curve.

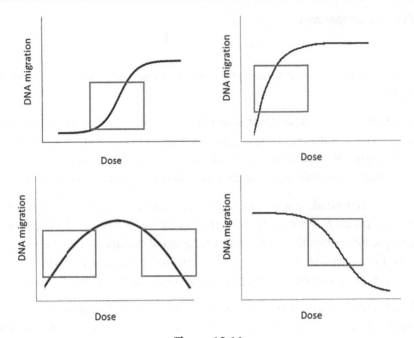

Figure 10.11
Dose-response curves with linear elements that can be detected by standard trend tests.

Therefore, such trend tests can be effective for detecting even nonmonotonic dose responses, especially when more than three exposure groups are included and more than one test with concurrent doses along the dose-response curve are conducted.

10.10.2 Validity of a Test

A valid test must include the following:

a. The administration of the maximum tolerated or maximum feasible dose and at least two additional appropriately spaced doses.
b. Successful analysis of an adequate number of cells (100–150 per sample) and animals (5 per dose). When low cell densities result in less than 100 scorable cells, cytotoxicity and/or technical issues with sample processing should be considered and the validity of the test should be evaluated.
c. For negative studies, the concurrent positive control must induce in each tissue evaluated a statistically significant ($P < 0.05$) increase in DNA migration when compared to the concurrent vehicle control.
d. An appropriate highest dose is used.

10.10.3 Positive Response Criteria

Although OECD TG 489 states that the detection of cross-linking agents is not the primary purpose of the assay as described in the guidelines, it does not exclude their detection as a possibility. Published evidence exists that such agents have been detected *in vivo* as a decrease in DNA migration in some tissues [16,19], so regulators may question whether cross-links have been induced if a decrease in DNA migration is detected. The recommendations in this section are intended to address this possibility as well as the more standard criteria for a positive response as cited in OECD TG 489.

A test article should be classified as positive if the following criteria are met in any tissue evaluated:

a. In the absence of cytotoxicity, at least one dose group exhibits a statistically significant increase (indicative of strand breaks or alkali labile sites) or decrease (indicative of cross-links) in DNA migration when compared to the concurrent vehicle control.
b. A statistically significant dose-related response is detected.

If none of the criteria for a positive response is met, then a test article may be classified as negative as long as the test is valid and there is evidence of target organ exposure or toxicity. OECD TG 489 references the use of historical control data distribution ranges to determine a positive or negative classification. However, the flexibility of the comet assay could limit the amount of historical control data available for every species, vehicle, route, tissue, and number of administrations as required for direct comparisons. In such cases, primary consideration for determining a positive response should be given to criteria a and b. If one but not all of the criteria for a positive response are met, then the test article may be classified as equivocal and additional data or a repeat test with optimized experimental conditions may be necessary. If increases in DNA migration and markers for cytotoxicity are both detected at every dose evaluated, then the result should be considered inconclusive until a repeat study at lower noncytotoxic doses can be conducted.

10.10.4 Cytotoxicity

It has been repeatedly recognized in multiple publications that low levels of toxicity at the cellular level (i.e., cytotoxicity) can increase DNA migration through prenecrotic/apoptotic changes such as inflammation and endonuclease DNA digestion that induce DNA strand breaks before the cell membrane is compromised [16,20]. For this reason, it can be difficult to differentiate between a genotoxic and cytotoxic response with the comet assay. But chronic cytotoxicity that causes tissue necrosis/apoptosis or fibrosis can result in baseline levels of DNA migration due to the loss of damaged cells and their replacement by normal or fibrous tissue [16]. Meanwhile, extreme cytotoxicity or physical damage that can be caused by acute exposure to corrosive or distention-inducing substances that remove, fuse, or blunt the epithelial layer of cells (Figure 10.12) can result in a DNA migration decrease when nonepithelial cells of the test compound-exposed tissue may be compared to the actively dividing epithelial cells from the vehicle control tissue. Therefore, special care should be taken to avoid highly toxic doses and to evaluate for homeostasis perturbations and/or low levels of cytotoxicity using sensitive biomarkers (e.g., cytokine levels, glycogen

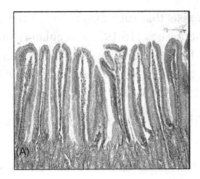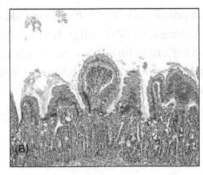

Figure 10.12

(A) Normal duodenal villi in a vehicle control animal. (B) Blunting and fusion of duodenal villi in test compound-exposed animal. Affected epithelium is approximately half the height of the normal epithelium in the vehicle control animal and may show a comparative decrease in DNA migration.

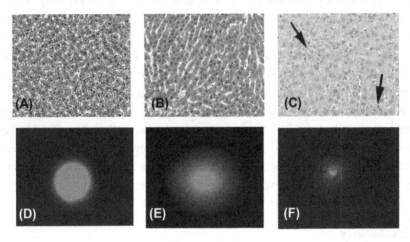

Figure 10.13

H&E-stained liver sections (A–C) and SYBR® Gold–stained LMW DNA diffusion liver samples (D–F) showing effects that can be concordant with DNA migration increases: (A) normal liver from vehicle control; (B) glycogen depletion; (C) minimal inflammation; (D) normal cell with no diffusion; (E) diffused cell with 50–700 kbp LMW DNA fragments; and (F) extremely diffused cell with 180–200 bp LMW DNA fragments.

depletion, LMW DNA diffusion) to aid in the interpretation of comet data. The LMW DNA diffusion assay detects in individual cells the prelethal endonuclease DNA digestion in a replicate set of comet slides that has not undergone electrophoresis and has been successfully applied to detect low levels of cytotoxicity [15,16,30]. However, because this method has proven difficult for some laboratories to master, alternatives such as the histological detection of glycogen depletion (Figure 10.13), minimal to mild levels of inflammation or cytokine biomarkers have shown some promise and appear to be concordant with the LMW DNA diffusion assay and most relevant to comet [16, 20].

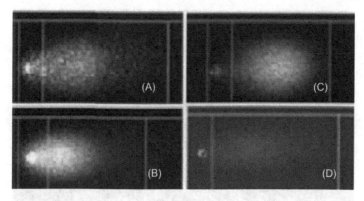

Figure 10.14

Comets that may have been classified "hedgehogs" but that are easily detected and analyzed by the Komet © Image Analysis System. Despite claims that they are indicative of cytotoxicity, these comets are exclusively due to genotoxicity as detected by the acellular comet assay that exposes nuclear DNA-rather than live cells-to test compounds [16].

OECD TG 489 states that "hedgehog" comets that cannot be readily detected by image analysis should be noted and reported separately from the image analysis results. Any relevant increase thought to be due to action of the test chemical should be investigated and interpreted with care. It has been acknowledged in several publications including OECD TG 489 that the etiology of hedgehogs or ghost cells exhibiting extreme DNA damage without a clearly defined head cannot be defined as purely genotoxic or cytotoxic. Therefore, the percentage of hedgehogs should not be reported or interpreted as an indicator of cytotoxicity without additional supporting data. It is also important to note that the definition of a "hedgehog" varies widely from laboratory to laboratory and person to person. Between individuals and even within the guidelines, the definition changes from (a) cells consisting of a small or nonexistent head and diffuse tail to (b) cells without a clearly defined head that cannot be readily detected by image analysis. As evidenced by Figure 10.14, cells with small heads and diffuse tails that may be considered "hedgehogs" by visual assessment can be readily detectable and scorable with image analysis depending on the software, hardware, and system sensitivity and settings (e.g., camera brightness). Figure 10.15 includes an image of what may be considered a "ghost" cell that may not be readily detected or scorable by image analysis. Laboratories should clearly define in advance their classification of "hedgehogs" to ensure consistency between scorers and the interpretation of the data. Because it may be too subjective for a scorer to assess through microscope eyepieces whether a comet is readily detectable by an image analysis system using a digital camera, it may be best and most consistent for scorers to determine the number of what can be considered "hedgehog" or "ghost" comets by counting the number of extremely damaged comets that cannot be accurately scored by image analysis.

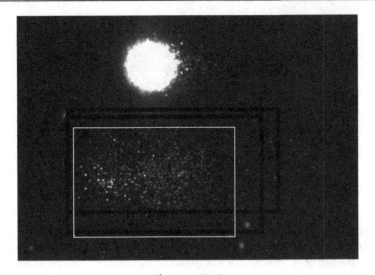

Figure 10.15
Comet that may have been classified as "ghost" that cannot be readily detected or analyzed by image analysis. Image captured with a highly sensitive Andor Technology CCD camera.

10.10.5 Reporting results

Comet data should be reported by tissue and sample time (if multiple sample times are evaluated) in tables that include both individual animal data and dose group means (Example Tables 10.1–10.3). OECD TG 489 recommends calculating the animal mean data as the mean of the two to three replicate slide medians. But historically, many laboratories have been calculating the animal mean as the mean of the total cells scored per animal without taking into account the number of individual replicate slides. The mean of slide medians is a much smaller number than the mean of the total cells analyzed. Therefore, it is critical to clearly report how the animal mean data was calculated and to ensure that the method is consistent with the method used for any historical control data reported to avoid any inappropriate comparisons.

The source and nature of any historical data that may be reported should be controlled and clearly stated in the report to ensure that it is appropriately utilized. If historical control data are used to assist with the interpretation of the study results, then special care should be taken to limit the historical data to studies with the same experimental design (i.e., dose administration route and frequency, sample time), test system (e.g., female Sprague Dawley rats), and vehicle control. But if historical data are merely used to provide proof of proficiency with the tissues evaluated, then an indiscriminate collection of pooled historical control data for each tissue may be reported.

Table 10.1: Liver comet and %LMW: Summary data

Dose (mg/kg)	TL Mean ± SD	OTM Mean ± SD	%Tail Mean ± SD	%LMW Mean ± SD
Positive	45.4 ± 2.24	4.7 ± 0.54	19.7 ± 2.26**	13.8 ± 5.74**
Vehicle	10.9 ± 2.17	0.7 ± 0.19	5.4 ± 0.72	5.2 ± 1.94
25	16.9 ± 2.11	1.1 ± 0.28	7.4 ± 0.90**	6.7 ± 3.67
50	24.1 ± 3.14	1.3 ± 0.12	9.5 ± 0.44**	5.5 ± 2.74
100	33.6 ± 4.08	2.5 ± 0.43	13.1 ± 1.04**	16.2 ± 19.62
	Trend Test P-Value[a]		+ < 0.001**	+0.0221

SD, standard deviation
Data based on 150 cells scored per animal; 5 animals per dose group.
*P < 0.05; **P < 0.01
[a]Dose response increase (+) or decrease (−).

Table 10.2: Liver comet individual animal data

Dose (mg/kg)	Animal No.	TL Mean	TL SEM	OTM Mean	OTM SEM	%Tail Mean	%Tail SEM
Positive 300	384	43.0	1.53	4.6	0.27	19.8	1.08
	385	43.3	1.69	4.6	0.37	18.6	1.14
	355	47.1	1.32	4.6	0.35	18.4	1.12
	364	43.8	1.87	3.8	0.42	16.6	1.27
	381	47.7	1.37	4.8	0.25	21.8	1.07
	375	47.5	1.89	5.5	0.53	22.7	1.40
	Mean ± SD	45.4 ± 2.24		4.7 ± 0.54		19.7 ± 2.26	
Vehicle 0	360	9.7	0.98	0.5	0.07	4.6	0.56
	370	8.5	0.94	0.5	0.11	4.9	0.61
	373	9.4	1.35	0.6	0.16	4.8	0.64
	358	12.7	1.35	0.7	0.16	5.8	0.86
	386	14.2	1.61	0.9	0.16	6.2	0.73
	379	10.7	1.29	1.0	0.32	6.1	0.95
	Mean ± SD	10.9 ± 2.17		0.7 ± 0.19		5.4 ± 0.72	
25	369	20.3	1.86	1.3	0.24	8.3	1.10
	361	17.1	1.80	1.4	0.48	7.8	1.16
	363	17.8	1.81	0.9	0.15	7.0	0.82
	368	15.0	1.04	0.7	0.12	6.5	0.90
	374	14.4	1.52	1.3	0.51	8.5	1.17
	371	16.7	1.47	0.9	0.14	6.4	0.82
	Mean ± SD	16.9 ± 2.11		1.1 ± 0.28		7.4 ± 0.90	
50	362	26.0	1.44	1.4	0.18	10.0	1.00
	376	23.2	1.10	1.3	0.14	9.4	0.85
	377	19.3	0.93	1.1	0.12	9.3	0.96
	382	28.7	1.09	1.3	0.11	9.6	0.81
	357	24.1	1.33	1.2	0.11	10.0	1.01
	365	23.3	1.42	1.4	0.24	8.9	1.03
	Mean ± SD	24.1 ± 3.14		1.3 ± 0.12		9.5 ± 0.44	
100	366	31.2	1.02	2.1	0.31	12.0	1.11
	356	33.5	1.07	2.0	0.23	11.9	0.98
	380	30.8	1.01	2.2	0.27	12.9	1.20
	367	34.9	1.26	3.1	0.56	14.3	1.49
	383	41.1	1.60	2.7	0.30	13.8	0.99
	378	30.3	1.63	2.7	0.52	14.0	1.26
	Mean ± SD	33.6 ± 4.08		2.5 ± 0.43		13.1 ± 1.04	

SEM, standard error of the mean; SD, standard deviation.
Data based on 150 cells scored per animal; Animal means calculated as the mean of total cells scored.

Table 10.3: Liver %LMW individual animal data

Dose (mg/kg)	Animal No.	Diffusion		Total Cells	%LMW
		I	II		
Positive 200	384	84	16	100	16.0
	385	90	10	100	10.0
	355	86	14	100	14.0
	364	92	8	100	8.0
	381	89	11	100	11.0
	375	76	24	100	24.0
				Mean ± SD	*13.8 ± 5.74*
Vehicle 0	360	96	4	100	4.0
	370	95	5	100	5.0
	373	97	3	100	3.0
	358	93	7	100	7.0
	386	92	8	100	8.0
	379	96	4	100	4.0
				Mean ± SD	*5.2 ± 1.94*
25	369	95	5	100	5.0
	361	88	12	100	12.0
	363	98	2	100	2.0
	368	92	8	100	8.0
	374	96	4	100	4.0
	371	91	9	100	9.0
				Mean ± SD	*6.7 ± 3.67*
50	362	98	2	100	2.0
	376	97	3	100	3.0
	377	92	8	100	8.0
	382	91	9	100	9.0
	357	95	5	100	5.0
	365	94	6	100	6.0
				Mean ± SD	*5.5 ± 2.74*
100	366	96	4	100	4.0
	356	93	7	100	7.0
	380	45	55	100	55.0
	367	87	13	100	13.0
	383	97	3	100	3.0
	378	85	15	100	15.0
				Mean ± SD	*16.2 ± 19.62*

Diffusion Classifications: I, condensed DNA; II, diffused DNA; SD, standard deviation.
Data based on 100 cells scored per animal.

10.11 Evaluating Unclear Results

Additional follow-up to a comet study result may be necessary to definitively classify a statistically equivocal result as positive or negative, to discount a statistically positive response as an artifact or cytotoxicity-related, or to defend the reliability of a negative result. The decision to follow-up must be determined on a case-by-case basis for each test compound and should take into account all of the available data and information. Because every scenario cannot be addressed and all approaches may not be applicable in every situation, this section is limited to discussing only a few cases where additional data may be useful and provide recommendations for these approaches. It is important to stress that in keeping with the premise that the comet assay is not a one-size-fits-all test, neither are the follow-up approaches cited in this section.

10.11.1 Equivocal Results

Equivocal results can occur, and then a statistically significant increase or decrease (response) in DNA migration is detected at one or more dose concentrations, but the response is not statistically dose-related (i.e., linear). This can be caused by a biphasic or nonmonotonic dose response influenced by cytotoxicity at the higher doses [15], or it may be an artifact of tissue-specific variability unrelated to the genotoxicity of a test compound. When a hormetic response is suspected, additional statistical analysis excluding the cytotoxic dose(s) may be conducted to determine the presence of a linear dose response in the absence of cytotoxicity. This could provide the confidence required to make a more definitive positive or negative classification. However, it is important to note that any such exclusion should be justified based on documented cytotoxicity data and the results of both analyses with and without any excluded dose group(s) should be reported. When an equivocal result is suspected to be an artifact, the confounding effects of physiological events (e.g., cell turnover, stress, inflammation) that can be a normal function of the cell type (e.g., epithelial) or caused by the dosing procedure or vehicle should be evaluated. This is of particular concern in apoptotic-prone epithelial tissues (e.g., GI tract), in which these physiological events may be exacerbated by the physical characteristics (e.g., viscosity) of the dose formulation and/or the dose frequency [16,31]. A repeat study may be conducted to determine the reproducibility of any significant DNA migration response that does not appear to be dose-related and/or is a suspected artifact. A nonreproducible and nondose-related effect detected at a single dose concentration is most likely an artifact and could allow for a negative classification if all other genotoxicity, pharmacological, and structural data support this conclusion. However, a reproducible but not dose-related change in DNA migration may be indicative of a steep dose response and could be classified as positive.

10.11.2 Positive Results

False-positive results may be caused by the homeostasis perturbations (e.g., incomplete excision repair, cell cycle arrest, inflammation) that can occur before cell membranes are compromised and necrosis/apoptosis is detectable by histopathology. Depending on the dose concentration and the administration frequency, these effects can increase DNA migration at the site of contact as well as peripherally in other tissues as the tissue responds to cellular injury and the systemic inflammatory response progresses. But because cytotoxicity-related increases in DNA migration are most likely to be detected by comet during the early or prelethal stages of cell injury, samples should be evaluated for these potentially confounding effects after 3 days or less of dosing and assessments should specifically evaluate for the presence of minimal to moderate levels of inflammation and/or single-cell necrosis/apoptosis. If the MTD used for the study was based on whole animal (vs. tissue) toxicity, or if tissues were sampled after more than 3 days of dosing, then a repeat study with lower and/or less frequent dose administrations to minimize the potentially confounding effects of cytotoxicity may be the best method for identifying the true nature of a detected positive response. If a positive response is not detected at the noncytotoxic doses, then the test compound may be classified as negative if all other genotoxicity, pharmacological, and structural data support this conclusion. However, it is important to note that genotoxicity and cytotoxicity are often parts of the same continuum [16]. Genotoxic and cytotoxic events frequently overlap with and induce the other. So, the absence of a comet response at noncytotoxic doses alone is not likely sufficient to defend a negative classification in the absence of additional supporting data.

10.11.3 Negative Results

False-negative results may be caused by any variety of issues and/or combination of issues including but not limited to: (1) poor sensitivity due to inadequate technical execution; (2) the evaluation of the incorrect target organ(s)/sample time(s) for a specific compound; and (3) the loss and replacement of damaged cells due to the postlethal stages of extreme or chronic cytotoxicity. For example, the inability to analyze at least 100 cells per sample with at least 50 cells per replicate slide may be indicative of poor sample preparation processes that may require adjustments before results could be considered reliable. A potent clastogen, gemifloxacine mesylate has been reported in the literature as testing negative in the liver of rats after 28 days of dosing [32]. But the Withdrawal Assessment Form published by the EMEA in 2009 [33] reported a positive response in the liver after only 24 h with no evidence of systemic accumulation from repeat dosing. It also reported that the kidney is the target organ of toxicity for gemifloxacine mesylate in the rat, with the compound mostly excreted unmetabolized after 24 h. The negative comet result in the liver after 28 days of dosing may therefore be due to the inappropriate dose frequency/sample time used for this study. Although a positive response was detected in the liver after 24 h, the kidney may have also been appropriate to evaluate, considering that it is the target organ for this compound and the compound is not metabolized. As stated in previous sections of this chapter and as clearly evidenced in the literature [32,33], sampling after more than three daily doses may be inappropriate and/or too cytotoxic to detect the genotoxicity of some compounds with comet. A negative result in the liver should be assessed with caution when a compound is unmetabolized and/or when there is evidence that it targets other organs. The study design and execution of all studies should be critically evaluated to ensure that the study was applied appropriately. When the design or execution are suspect, a repeat study correcting for any such deficiencies should be conducted.

Acknowledgments

Disclaimer
Opinions and recommendations expressed in this publication are those of the authors and do not necessarily reflect those of the institution with which he/she may be affiliated.

References

[1] Pool-Zobel BL, Guigas C, Klein R, Neudecker C, Renner HW, Schmezer P. Assessment of genotoxic effects by lindane. Food Chem Toxicol 1993;4:271–83.

[2] Tice RR, Agurell E, Anderson D, Burlinson B, Hartmann A, Kobayashi H, et al. Single cell gel/comet assay: guidelines for *in vitro* and *in vivo* genetic toxicology testing. Environ Mol Mutagen 2000;35:206–21.

[3] Frötschl R. Experiences with the *in vivo* and *in vitro* comet assay in regulatory testing. Mutagenesis 2015;30(1):51–7.

[4] Committee on Mutagenicity of Chemicals in Food, Consumer Products, and the Environment (COM). Guidance on Strategy for Genotoxicity Testing of Chemicals for Mutagenicity; 2011.

[5] U.S. Food and Drug Administration. Guidance for Industry and Review Staff: Recommended Approaches to Integration of Genetic Toxicology Study Results; 2006.

[6] International Conference on Harmonization of Technical Requirements for Registration of Pharmaceuticals Intended for Human Use (ICH) Guidance on Genotoxicity Testing and Data Interpretation for Pharmaceuticals Intended for Human Use S2(R1); 2011.

[7] European Food Safety Agency (EFSA). Minimum Criteria for the acceptance of *in vivo* alkaline comet assay reports. EFSA J 2012;10(11):2977.

[8] ICH Guidance. S2(R1) on genotoxicity testing and data interpretation for pharmaceuticals intended for human use; availability. Fed Regist 2012;77(110):33748–9.

[9] Thorsell A, et al. Use of electrochemical oxidation and model peptides to study nucleophilic biological targets of reactive metabolites: the case of rimonabant. Chem Res Toxicol 2014;27(10):1808–20.

[10] Kirkland D, Speit G. Evaluation of the ability of a battery of three *in vitro* genotoxicity tests to discriminate rodent carcinogens and non-carcinogens III. Appropriate follow-up testing *in vivo*. Mutat Res 2008;654:114–32.

[11] Sasaki YF, Saga A, Akasaka M, Ishibashi S, Yoshida K, Su YQ, et al. Detection of *in vivo* genotoxicity of haloalkanes and haloalkenes carcinogenic to rodents by the alkaline single cell gel electrophoresis (comet) assay in multiple mouse organs. Mutat Res 1998;419:13–20.

[12] Lambert LB, Singer TM, Boucher SE, Douglas GR. Detailed review of transgenic rodent mutation assays. Mutat Res 2005;590:1–280.

[13] Sekihashi K, Yamamoto A, Matsumura Y, Ueno S, Watanabe-Akanuma M, Kassie F, et al. Comparative investigation of multiple organs of mice and rats in the comet assay. Mutat Res 2002;517:53–75.

[14] Cohen SM. Urinary bladder carcinogenesis. Toxicol Pathol 1998;26(1):121–7.

[15] Vasquez MZ. Combining the *in vivo* comet and micronucleus assays: a practical approach to genotoxicity testing and data interpretation. Mutagenesis 2010;25(2):187–99.

[16] Vasquez MZ. Recommendations for safety testing with the *in vivo* comet assay. Mutat Res 2012;747:142−56.

[17] Wynne P, Newton C, Ledermann J, Olaitan A, Mould T, Harley J. Enhanced repair of DNA interstrand crosslinking in ovarian cancer cells from patients following treatment with platinum-based chemotherapy. Br J Cancer 2007;97(7):927−33.

[18] Murray D, Jenkins W, Meyn R. Kinetics of DNA cross-linking in normal and neoplastic mouse tissues following treatment with cis-diamminedichloroplatinum(II) *in vivo*. Cancer Res 1985;45:6446−52.

[19] Struwe M, Geulick K-O, Junker U, Christian J, Zimmer D, Suter W, et al. Detection of photogenotoxicity in skin and eye in rat with the photo comet assay. Photochem Photobiol Sci 2008;7(2):240−9.

[20] Downs T, Crosby M, Hu T, Kumar S, Sullivan A, Sarlo K, et al. Silica nanoparticles administered at the maximum tolerated dose induce genotoxic effects through an inflammatory reaction while gold nanoparticle do not. Mutat Res 2012;745:38−50.

[21] Roth R, Luyendyk J, Maddox J, Ganey P. Inflammation and drug idiosyncrasy—is there a connection? J Pharmacol Exp Ther 2003;307(1):1−8.

[22] Westbrook A, Wei B, Braun J, Schiestl R. Intestinal mucosal inflammation leads to systemic genotoxicity in mice. Cancer Res 2009;69(11):4827−34.

[23] OECD TG 489. OECD Guidelines for the Testing of Chemicals: *in vivo* Mammalian Alkaline Comet Assay; 2014.

[24] Swenberg J, Moeller B, Lu K, Rager J, Fry R, Starr T. Formaldehyde carcinogenicity research: 30 years and counting for mode of action, epidemiology, and cancer risk assessment. Toxicol Pathol 2013;41 (2):181−9.

[25] Speit G, Schütz P, Weber I, Ma-Hock L, Kaufmann W, Gelbke H-P, et al. Analysis of micronuclei, histopathological changes and cell proliferation in nasal epithelium cells of rats after exposure to formaldehyde by inhalation. Mutat Res-Genet Toxicol Environ Mutagen 2011;721(2):127−35.

[26] Neuss S, Moepps B, Speit G. Exposure of human nasal epithelial cells to formaldehyde does not lead to DNA damage in lymphocytes after co-cultivation. Mutagenesis 2010;25(4):359−64.

[27] Burlinson B, Tice R, Speit G, Agurell E, Brendler-Schwaab S, Collins A, et al. Fourth international workgroup on genotoxicity testing: results of the *in vivo* comet assay workgroup. Mutat Res 2007;627(1):31−5.

[28] Orhan H. Extrahepatic targets and cellular reactivity of drug metabolites. Curr Med Chem 2015;22(4):408−37.

[29] Moller P, Loft S. Statistical analysis of comet assay results. Front Genet 2014;5(292):1−4.

[30] Speit G, Vesely A, Schutz P, Linsenmeyer R, Bausinger J. The low molecular weight DNA diffusion assay as an indicator of cytotoxicity for the in vitro comet assay. Mutagenesis 2014;29(4):267−77.

[31] Damsch S, Eichenbaum G, Tonelli A, Lammens L, Van den Bulck K, Feyen B, et al. Gavage-related reflux in rats: identification, pathogenesis, and toxicological implications (review). Toxicol Pathol 2011;39:348−60.

[32] Rothfuss A, O'Donovan M, De Boeck M, Brault D, Czich A, Custer L, et al. Collaborative study on fifteen compounds in the rat-liver Comet assay integrated into 2- and 4-week repeat-dose studies. Mutat Res 2010;702(1):40−69.

[33] European Medicines Agency Pre-Authorisation Evaluation of Medicines for Human Use: Withdrawal Assessment Report for Factive. Procedures No. EMEA/H/C/995; 2009.

CHAPTER 11

The Pig-a Endogenous Gene Mutation Assay

Jeffrey C. Bemis, Svetlana L. Avlasevich and Stephen D. Dertinger

Litron Laboratories, Rochester, NY, USA

Chapter Outline

11.1 Introduction 384
11.2 History 384
11.3 Fundamentals 385
11.4 Study Design 389
    11.4.1 Animal Species/Strain/Sex/Age 389
    11.4.2 Number of Animals Per Experimental Group 390
    11.4.3 Group Selection/Identification 390
    11.4.4 Negative and Positive Controls 390
    11.4.5 Acute or Integrated Repeat-Dose Studies 390
        11.4.5.1 Dose-range finding 391
        11.4.5.2 Top dose and dose spacing 391
        11.4.5.3 Timing of sample collection 391
        11.4.5.4 Assay configurations 391
11.5 Equipment 392
11.6 Consumables 393
11.7 Reagents and Recipes 393
    11.7.1 Solution and Materials Preparation 393
        11.7.1.1 Buffered salt solution plus 2% FBS 394
        11.7.1.2 Working nucleic acid dye plus counting beads solution 394
        11.7.1.3 Working antibody solution 394
        11.7.1.4 Working anti-PE MicroBead suspension 394
        11.7.1.5 Aliquot anticoagulant solution and Lympholyte®-Mammal 394
11.8 Method Overview 395
11.9 Blood Collection 396
11.10 Leukodepletion and Platelet Removal 397
11.11 Sample Labeling 397
11.12 Column Separation and Sample Staining 400
11.13 Flow Cytometric Analysis: 96-Well Plate-Based
     Protocol 403
11.14 Tabulating and Summarizing Results 409

Genetic Toxicology Testing.
DOI: http://dx.doi.org/10.1016/B978-0-12-800764-8.00011-2

383

11.15 Evaluation and Interpretation of Results   410
 11.15.1 Statistics 410
 11.15.2 Criteria for a Valid Assay 411
 11.15.3 Comparison to Historical Controls 411
 11.15.4 Biological Relevance 411
11.16 Flow Cytometric Template Preparation   412
11.17 Example Plots   414
11.18 Storage and Shipment of Blood Samples   414
11.19 Aspiration of Postcolumn Samples   416
References   416

11.1 Introduction

Endogenous mutation assays based on inactivation of the phosphatidylinositol glycan complement class A (*Pig-a*) gene are well described in the literature [1,2]. These methods are based on loss of *Pig-a* gene function leading to the elimination of cell surface expression of specific proteins associated with glycosylphosphatidylinositol (GPI) anchors. The method described here covers analysis of mutant phenotype cells in blood samples obtained from laboratory rodents. This method is compatible with acute as well as more protracted (e.g., 28 days) exposure schedules. Given the kinetics of formation and manifestation of genotoxicant-induced mutant phenotype cells, a general rule of thumb is that approximately 2 weeks must elapse since the initiation of treatment before one would expect to see a significant response. Upon blood collection, red blood cells are isolated by centrifugation, labeled with antibodies, and depleted of nonmutant cells via immunomagnetic column separation. For each sample, a precolumn and a postcolumn fraction are analyzed via flow cytometry, and the mutation frequencies in the mature and immature erythrocyte populations are determined.

11.2 History

Assessment of mutation in rodent models has historically focused on alterations in specific gene loci (e.g., *HPRT, GPA*) [3,4]. Even the more recent development of transgenic rodent models (Big Blue®, Muta™ Mouse, *gpt*-delta) for the detection of mutation relies on mutagen-induced alteration of an inserted transgene [5]. This fundamental approach of detecting mutation via examination of specific reporter genes is also the basis for the so-called *Pig-a* gene mutation assay. In this system, inactivation of the *Pig-a* gene leads to an inability of the cell to produce functional GPI anchors that are used to target specific proteins to the cell surface. This altered cell surface phenotype is readily assessed via antibody-based labeling coupled with flow cytometric analyses. The presence of the

Pig-a gene and its associated pathways in mammalian systems suggests that it can be applied to numerous laboratory models, and data to date establish the application of the method in both rat and mouse [6,7].

In addition to the extensive body of work surrounding rodent-based *Pig-a* assays found in the literature, there is also a wealth of information on the human disease associated with *Pig-a* inactivation. Paroxysmal nocturnal hemoglobinurea (PNH) is a hematological disorder that arises following loss of *PIG-A* gene function in hematopoietic stem cells. Sufficient accumulation of "mutant offspring" from affected progenitor cells leads to intravascular lysis of red blood cells (RBC) in peripheral circulation, and eventually the mutation results in bone marrow failure. Modern clinical methods for diagnosis of PNH commonly use flow cytometry [8]; however, a large percentage of the peripheral red blood cell population must be affected by the mutation to result in clinical manifestation of PNH. Thus, even the "high-sensitivity" methods that exist in the clinic are only designed to report on mutant frequency as low as 0.01% and are not optimized for very rare event analysis such as one would experience in a laboratory rodent-based model of mutagenesis (e.g., baseline mutant frequency of one per million in RBC).

With regard to the types of mutations that have been associated with PNH, Nishimura et al. [9] demonstrated the presence of insertions, deletions, and base substitutions in affected subjects. In addition to the large body of work that exists to establish the biology and diagnostic parameters surrounding human *PIG-A* mutation, it is within the context of PNH research that Araten first described the potential for the *PIG-A* gene locus to serve as an *in vivo* mutation assay [10,11]. Subsequently, other groups have investigated *Pig-a* mutation to examine mutator phenotype in cancer [12], spontaneous somatic mutation rates [13], and development of a methodology for identification of mutagenic genotoxicants for regulatory safety purposes [1].

11.3 Fundamentals

Whether one is describing human or rodent, as explained here, the inactivation of *Pig-a* gene function is the basis for this assay. One key advantage of this particular gene locus for a mutation assay is that the *Pig-a* gene is located on the X chromosome. This means that in both sexes there is only one functional copy of the gene. In males this is due to their XY status of the sex chromosomes, and in females one of the two X chromosomes is inactivated via gene silencing [14]. Any mutation that then leads to loss of function of the single active copy of the *Pig-a* gene eliminates the formation of a protein that is essential for the first step in the synthesis of GPI anchors (Figure 11.1). These anchors are utilized by the cell to attach specific proteins to the external surface of the plasma membrane, and it is these proteins that provide convenient target(s) for labeling with fluorescent antibodies. Although there are reagents that can bind directly to GPI anchors (e.g., FLAER), several

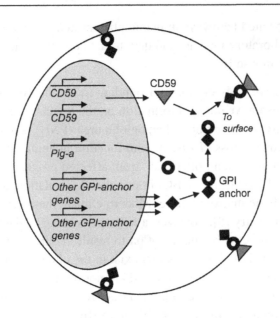

Acquisition of cell surface CD59-negative phenotype via gene mutation

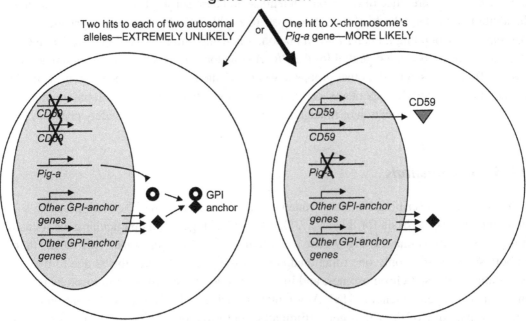

Figure 11.1
Schematic of GPI anchor formation and impact of *Pig-a* mutation.

Pig-a assays, including the one described here, use antibodies raised against the proteins attached to the cell surface via the GPI anchor.

Wild-type (WT) cells express the normal cell-surface phenotype associated with cells possessing an intact *Pig-a* gene (e.g., CD59 expression on the surface of rat red blood cells), but mutant cells lack this phenotype. This is the basis by which the assay classifies cells as either mutant or WT. In addition to enumerating mutant versus WT, this method incorporates a reagent that binds to intracellular nucleic acids and permits the differentiation of immature erythrocytes (reticulocytes, RETs) from the more mature RBC population. This characteristic is important when considering the kinetics of response of *Pig-a* mutation following exposure. Current data support the characterization of the RET cohort as the "leading indicator" of mutation as these newly formed cells are recently derived from the bone marrow compartment and thus would reflect recent effects on the hematopoietic lineage.

By virtue of their longer lifespan in circulation, the more mature RBC cohort takes longer to turn over and reveal the impact of newly generated mutant cells coming from the bone marrow, and thus RBC have been called the "lagging indicator" of mutation. Based on results obtained from studies where rats were exposed for 3 consecutive days to the reference mutagen ethyl nitrosourea (ENU), mutant RET frequencies approached maximal values by 15 days after the start of treatment [15]. The mutant fraction of RBC, although significantly elevated at day 15, did not achieve maximal values until 6 weeks had elapsed. Certain experimental designs benefit from the analysis of both RET and RBC, as described in the next section.

Additional information about the basic biology that serves as the basis for the *Pig-a* assay can be obtained from kinetic studies performed with well-known mutagenic agents. The plateau in mutant RET frequency was maintained over time and has been observed as long as 6 months after the last exposure in other studies [16]. This stabilization of the response suggests that the mutation can be considered neutral in that the mutant progenitor cells and their progeny are not strongly selected for or against growth or survival advantage. This neutrality conveys additional information regarding how the assay would perform under a repeat-dose design, such that the effect of each dose should accumulate in a near-additive fashion. This was demonstrated experimentally by Miura et al. [17] when ENU was administered to rats either as a single bolus dose or as the same total dose but fractionated across several independent exposures; the resulting mutation frequencies were equivalent.

The fact that *Pig-a* mutation has been shown to accumulate over time suggests that this endpoint would benefit from experimental designs that call for multiple exposures over an extended period of time (e.g., 28-day studies). The long-term persistence of mutant RBC/RET in circulation also provides information about the target cells in the hematopoietic system that are affected via mutagen exposure. Recent studies examining *Pig-a* mutation in rats exposed to cisplatin showed a sustained presence of mutant phenotype RBC and continued output of mutant RET as long as 190 days after the start of

28 consecutive days of exposure [16]. This extended timeframe is sufficient for the turnover of the entire RBC pool, and is also consistent with timeframes established by studies that examined repopulation kinetics of the hematopoietic system following stem cell transplantation [18]. Thus, given an extended postexposure time period, any mutant cells in circulation would have to be derived from early pluripotent hematopoietic stem cells that experienced mutation of the *Pig-a* gene and passed this characteristic on to their progeny.

The final important aspect of the method described here is the use of immunomagnetic separation to specifically isolate mutant cells from the bulk of WT cells in the peripheral blood sample [19]. This is accomplished in conjunction with the Ab-based labeling that the flow cytometer uses to identify the populations of interest. Thus, the anti-CD59 Ab conjugated to the fluorescent protein phycoerythrin (PE) will bind to WT cells that express CD59 on their surface but will not label mutant cells. Staining a peripheral blood sample with this Ab and no additional processing will result in the resolution of two separate populations on the flow cytometer, the majority of which will be WT cells. Given the baseline frequency of approximately one mutant cell per million WT RBC, this would require significant time on the instrument to enumerate a sufficient number of cells such that one does not accumulate a predominance of zero mutant cells scored in the control samples. This would lead to reduced power of the assay to detect a response over baseline and limit the confidence one can place on the assignment of a negative response to a test article.

This limitation has been overcome by the application of superparamagnetic beads that bind specifically to the PE molecule found on the anti-CD59 Ab. This step then allows for the selective depletion of WT cells by applying the appropriately labeled sample to a column containing a ferrous matrix suspended on a strong magnetic field (Figure 11.2). The majority of WT cells are retained on the column and the unlabeled mutant population is washed and collected. As part of the protocol, a portion of the labeled sample is reserved prior to column separation and this is analyzed alongside the postcolumn sample. One additional component of the method makes it possible to directly compare the numbers obtained from the precolumn samples with those from the postcolumn sample. This component is a suspension of fluorescently labeled polystyrene beads that are delivered at a consistent density across precolumn and postcolumn samples. Based on the ratio of cells to a fixed number of beads in the precolumn sample, one can calculate a mutation frequency from the postcolumn sample. In a typical rat blood sample processed via immunomagnetic separation, mutant cell frequencies are obtained in approximately 4 min of flow cytometric analysis time. With this approach, one can typically evaluate more than 3 million RET and 150 million RBC equivalents per sample for the mutant phenotype, a throughput that is impossible without immunomagnetic separation. A spreadsheet formatted for the input of select data from the flow cytometer is used to provide information on %RET as well as mutant frequency in both the RET and RBC populations.

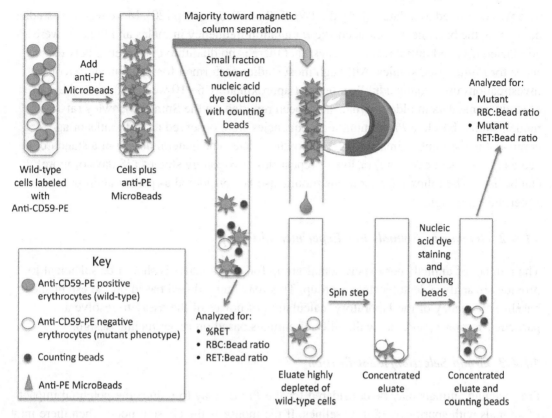

Figure 11.2
Diagram of Immunomagnetic Separation.

11.4 Study Design

Although there is no formal guidance document or other regulatory guideline specific to the *Pig-a* assay, the information provided in this chapter is intended to be in alignment with general practices for *in vivo* studies (e.g., OECD TG407, TG408, TG488, TG474) as well as consensus statements from expert working groups focused on the *Pig-a* assay [20].

11.4.1 Animal Species/Strain/Sex/Age

The *Pig-a* assay has been applied to both rat and mouse species and the breeds/strains investigated to date are Sprague-Dawley, Wistar, and F344 for rat and C57Bl/6, CD-1, and B6C3F1 for mouse. Several transgenic rat and mouse strains have also been investigated, including Big Blue® rat, Muta™ mouse, and *gpt*-delta mouse. The majority of studies in the literature used male rodents to study the *Pig-a* endpoint, and the scarcity of female rodent data was described as a data gap by the IWGT *Pig-a* Workgroup [20]. More recently, studies comparing the baseline and induced *Pig-a* mutation frequency in males and females were conducted [21] and initial results suggest that there is no qualitative difference between sexes for *Pig-a*-based studies. Although most studies performed for preclinical toxicology investigations use "young adult" animals of approximately 6−10 weeks of age at the start of study, some data in older animals have been reported. In the Sprague-Dawley rat model, similar baseline *Pig-a* mutation frequencies were observed at 10 months of age compared to the same animals at 1−1.5 months of age. The general design of a standard acute (1−3 days of exposure) or longer repeat-dose toxicology studies (28 days or more) can be used. The following conditions should also be considered as part of appropriate experimental design.

11.4.2 Number of Animals Per Experimental Group

The number of animals per experimental group for *Pig-a* analyses should be sufficient to provide six analyzable subjects per group. This may be modified based on the established baseline frequency of the laboratory, calculation of power of the assay to resolve a particular response, and the availability of animals based on experimental design.

11.4.3 Group Selection/Identification

Prescreening animals may be considered for the *Pig-a* assay to reduce the potential impact of animals with spuriously high baselines. If the mouse is the chosen model, then there may be merit to performing the prescreen at a time well before the start of exposure to test article (e.g., 2 weeks or more prior) to reduce the potential for stimulated erythropoiesis to impact the experiment.

11.4.4 Negative and Positive Controls

A positive control is not mandatory but should be considered based on the laboratory's demonstrated proficiency with the assay, historical controls, and/or expectation of a negative result with the test article. The use of a "mutant mimic" sample, described as the Instrument Calibration Standard (ICS), that is generated for each day of analysis is important for instrument set-up and provides verification that sample processing and analysis occurred appropriately.

11.4.5 Acute or Integrated Repeat-Dose Studies

Although it is possible to conduct *Pig-a* studies as standalone experiments, the current desire to align in-life work with the 3Rs concept encourages the combination of two or more endpoints together or direct integration of the *Pig-a* endpoint into other required studies such as a 28-day repeat-dose toxicology study. Additionally, based on the demonstrated accumulation of mutant cells with repeated exposures, the IWGT expert working group recommends integration of the *Pig-a* endpoint into repeat-dose studies such as the standard 28-day toxicology design [20]. The merit of acute study designs is acknowledged, and the decision to use these treatment schedules or combine endpoints/integrate with existing studies should be made based on multiple factors that factor in relevance of the study design and the intended use case of the test article (e.g., pharmaceutical safety assessment vs. industrial hygiene hazard identification).

11.4.5.1 Dose-range finding

Depending on the type of study under consideration (e.g., acute vs. short-term), standard dose-range—finding approaches, such as 14-day studies, can be useful for the determination of maximum tolerated dose (MTD).

11.4.5.2 Top dose and dose spacing

Three exposure levels with the highest dose being the MTD should be accommodated. If not limited by toxicity or when justified by practical considerations, the top dose should be 1000 mg/kg/day for studies of 14 days or more and 2000 mg/kg/day for acute designs. Most of the published *Pig-a* studies to date utilized a two-fold dose interval when conducting acute and subacute experiments.

11.4.5.3 Timing of sample collection

Whether using an acute study design of 3 days or less or investigating longer subchronic exposures, the kinetics of appearance of mutant RET and RBC must be taken into consideration. As described, the leading indicator of *Pig-a* gene mutation will be found in the RET cohort and can be observed as early as 15 days after the start of exposure. Observation of *Pig-a* mutation induction in the general RBC population can take even longer.

Generally, in a typical design such as a 28-day study, both the RET and RBC cohorts have experienced sufficient input from the bone marrow combined with turnover of the existing pools to yield a detectable response in peripheral blood at days 28–31. It should be noted that observations made from samples collected on days 28–31 will only reflect a portion of the entire 28 days of exposure. The examination of recovery groups or other such satellite animals that are not sacrificed at days 28–31 may be useful for studying longer expression times and allow the entire dosing period to elicit gene changes that are translated into *Pig-a* mutant phenotype erythrocytes.

11.4.5.4 Assay configurations

As described, the *Pig-a* assay can be performed in several species including those commonly used in laboratory studies (e.g., mouse and rat). This chapter specifically addresses the preparation, processing, and analysis of rat peripheral blood samples. It focuses on the 96-well plate-based methodology as opposed to a single tube per sample approach. Instructions and materials to perform these and other versions of the *Pig-a* assay are available from other sources including Litron Laboratories (www.litronlabs.com). Any updates or changes to the method will also be made available to kit users via communications from Litron Laboratories and posting of current manuals at www.litronlabs.com.

11.5 Equipment

The following is a list of equipment required for the method.

- 37°C incubator or water bath
- Micropipettes (adjustable, repeating, and positive displacement)
- An 8- or 12-channel micropipette
- Pipette aids
- Centrifuge with swinging bucket rotor
- 96-well plate carriers for centrifuge
- 2 to 8°C refrigerator
- Flow cytometer equipped with 488-nm laser; although samples can be processed in plates and transferred to flow cytometry tubes for analysis, the most efficient execution of this assay requires an instrument that is equipped with a high-throughput autosampler (HTS)
- −10 to −30°C freezer
- An eight-channel aspirator manifold with fixed bridge (V&P Scientific, VP 180B & VP 180S)
- MidiMACS™ Separator, Miltenyi Biotec 130-042-302 or QuadroMACS™ Separator, Miltenyi Biotec 130-090-976; the QuadroMACS Separator has the advantage of enabling four simultaneous separations
- Aspiration device (see Section 11.19)

Advance preparation of specific materials and equipment is advised to facilitate sample processing. Label all necessary tubes and vials with sample ID numbers prior to beginning sample processing. At least two flow cytometry tubes, three centrifuge tubes (15 mL), and two microcentrifuge tubes are required per sample.

Aspiration Device Preparation: It is very important to carefully control and standardize aspirations, especially the last aspiration (Section 11.12.2, step 2). To achieve this, fashion an aspirator with a bridge that controls the depth to which the tip can reach when aspirating from a standard 15 mL centrifuge tube (Section 11.19). With this bridge, the aspirator will leave a consistent and low volume of supernatant across all tubes and not contact the bottom of the tube or disturb the cell pellet. The goal for the volume of supernatant left after the final aspiration is a consistent volume within the range of 20 μL to 50 μL. This volume will be used to make mutant cell frequency calculations (Section 11.14).

11.6 Consumables

The following is a list of consumables required for this method (sterile where appropriate):

- Flaked/chipped ice
- 15 mL polypropylene centrifuge tubes
- Microcentrifuge tubes
- Disposable reagent reservoirs compatible with multichannel pipettes
- Flow cytometry tubes
- Small-volume 0.2 μm filters (e.g., Acrodisc, PALL Life Sciences 4192)
- Large-volume 0.2 μm filters (e.g., 250–1000 mL)
- 96-well round-bottom deep-well plates, 2 mL (e.g., Axygen Scientific 4192)
- 96-well round-bottom plates (e.g., Corning 3360 or 3799)
- Blood collection supplies, such as syringes, razor blades, lancets
- Heparin-coated capillary tubes (e.g., Fisher Scientific 22-260-950, depending on blood collection technique)
- K_2EDTA microtainer tubes (e.g., BD 365974, depending on the storage or shipping conditions)
- Heat-inactivated fetal bovine serum (FBS)
- Lympholyte®-Mammal, sterile liquid, Cedarlane Laboratories CL5110, CL5115, or CL 5120
- LS columns, Miltenyi Biotec 130-042-401
- Anti-PE MicroBeads, Miltenyi Biotec 130-048-801
- CountBright™ Absolute Counting Beads, Invitrogen C36950

11.7 Reagents and Recipes

As indicated, many of the reagents and materials described are provided with MutaFlow® kits available from Litron Laboratories (Rochester, NY). Additional materials and supplies that are required, but not supplied with the kits, are specifically noted in Section 11.6.

Individual reagents provided with the MutaFlow^{PLUS} kit:

> Anticoagulant solution
> Buffered salt solution
> Stock anti-CD59-PE solution
> Stock anti-CD61-PE solution
> Stock nucleic acid dye solution

11.7.1 Solution and Materials Preparation

The following solutions are made fresh daily under sterile conditions. When working with the bead stock or any solution containing beads, be sure to sufficiently suspend the beads prior to use via pipettor, but *do not vortex or sonicate*. The recipes here are based on the volumes required for one sample and should be scaled up appropriately. To ensure best performance and integrity of the stock reagents, it is recommended that all solutions should be prepared using aseptic conditions/practices.

11.7.1.1 Buffered salt solution plus 2% FBS

Combine 19.6 mL of buffered salt solution with 0.4 mL of FBS. Filter-sterilize with a 0.2 μm filter and store at 2 to 8°C.

11.7.1.2 Working nucleic acid dye plus counting beads solution

Add 45 μL of stock nucleic acid dye solution and 45 μL of CountBright™ Beads to 1.41 mL of buffered salt solution plus 2% FBS. Pipette to mix and store at room temperature, protected from light.

For each precolumn sample, transfer 990 μL of working nucleic acid dye plus counting beads solution to a single well of the 96-well plate. Periodically pipette the working nucleic acid dye plus counting beads solution up and down to ensure that the counting beads do not settle. Aseptically transfer 500 μL of working nucleic acid dye plus counting beads solution to an appropriate well for the generation of the Instrument Calibration Standard (ICS) sample (part A). Cover the vessel containing unused working nucleic acid dye plus counting beads Solution with foil and store at room temperature until needed again.

11.7.1.3 Working antibody solution

Combine 65 μL of buffered salt solution plus 2% FBS with 30 μL stock anti-CD59-PE solution and 5 μL stock anti-CD61-PE solution. Pipette to mix and store protected from light at 2 to 8°C. Using a reagent reservoir and a multichannel pipettor, aseptically transfer 100 μL of working antibody solution to wells of a 96-well round-bottom plate (one well for each sample).

11.7.1.4 Working anti-PE MicroBead suspension

Add 25 μL of anti-PE MicroBeads to 75 μL of buffered salt solution plus 2% FBS. Pipette to mix and store at 2 to 8°C, protected from light.

11.7.1.5 Aliquot anticoagulant solution and Lympholyte®-Mammal

Aliquot 100 μL anticoagulant solution into labeled microcentrifuge tubes (one for each blood sample). Refrigerate until use. This can be done prior to the day of blood collection.

On the morning of leukodepletion, gently shake the Lympholyte®-Mammal bottle and allow for air bubbles to disappear. For each blood sample, aliquot 1.5 mL into a deep-well 96-well plate. Protect from light and allow the plate to equilibrate to room temperature before use.

11.8 Method Overview

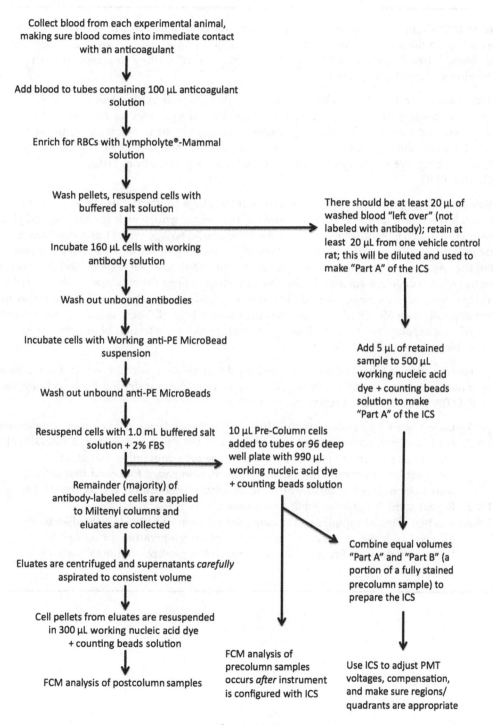

Collect blood from each experimental animal, making sure blood comes into immediate contact with an anticoagulant

↓

Add blood to tubes containing 100 μL anticoagulant solution

↓

Enrich for RBCs with Lympholyte®-Mammal solution

↓

Wash pellets, resuspend cells with buffered salt solution

↓

Incubate 160 μL cells with working antibody solution

↓

Wash out unbound antibodies

↓

Incubate cells with Working anti-PE MicroBead suspension

↓

Wash out unbound anti-PE MicroBeads

↓

Resuspend cells with 1.0 mL buffered salt solution + 2% FBS

↓

Remainder (majority) of antibody-labeled cells are applied to Miltenyi columns and eluates are collected

↓

Eluates are centrifuged and supernatants *carefully* aspirated to consistent volume

↓

Cell pellets from eluates are resuspended in 300 μL working nucleic acid dye + counting beads solution

↓

FCM analysis of postcolumn samples

There should be at least 20 μL of washed blood "left over" (not labeled with antibody); retain at least 20 μL from one vehicle control rat; this will be diluted and used to make "Part A" of the ICS

↓

Add 5 μL of retained sample to 500 μL working nucleic acid dye + counting beads solution to make "Part A" of the ICS

10 μL Pre-Column cells added to tubes or 96 deep well plate with 990 μL working nucleic acid dye + counting beads solution

Combine equal volumes "Part A" and "Part B" (a portion of a fully stained precolumn sample) to prepare the ICS

↓

FCM analysis of precolumn samples occurs *after* instrument is configured with ICS

Use ICS to adjust PMT voltages, compensation, and make sure regions/quadrants are appropriate

Figure 11.3
Overview of methodology.

11.9 Blood Collection

Use an IACUC-approved method to collect whole blood. As described, the volume collected is dependent on the method used. Whatever blood collection technique is used, it is essential that blood is free-flowing from an animal whose heart is still beating to prevent platelet activation and cellular aggregation.

If blood will be collected by nicking a tail vein with a surgical blade, then it is important to warm the animals under a heat lamp for several minutes to improve blood flow and achieve a free-flowing sample; this may not be necessary if sampling directly from a vein (e.g., use heparin-coated capillary tube(s) to collect approximately 120 µL/rodent). We recommend heparin-coated capillary tubes from Fisher Scientific (#22-260-950).

If you are collecting blood intravenously with a small-gauge (butterfly) needle and a 1 mL syringe, it is important to first coat the inside of the needle/syringe with several hundred µL of kit-supplied anticoagulant solution. Then, hold the needle/syringe upright and expel any air that may be in the barrel of the syringe. Proceed by discharging the anticoagulant solution from the syringe. For most needle and syringe combinations, this will leave behind the desired amount of anticoagulant solution in the so-called dead volume (approximately 50 to 60 µL). If using a fixed needle syringe with considerably less dead volume, then it will be necessary to leave approximately 50–60 µL of anticoagulant solution behind. Then, to achieve the proper ratio of anticoagulant solution to blood, your goal should be collection of approximately 300 µL blood from each rodent.

If you do not plan to label and analyze blood on the same day it is collected, or if you plan to ship blood samples to an off-site facility, then we recommend transferring the blood samples into K_2EDTA blood collection tubes.

11.9.1. Collect free-flowing blood sample based on notes and required volumes as indicated.
11.9.2. For blood that will be labeled and analyzed on the day it is collected, IMMEDIATELY transfer 80 µL into the labeled microcentrifuge tube containing 100 µL of anticoagulant solution. This transfer is not recommended for blood that will be stored overnight or shipped. For these alternative procedures, see Section 11.18.
11.9.3. Repeat steps 1 and 2 for additional animals.
11.9.4. It is best if blood samples in anticoagulant solution can be refrigerated as soon as possible; however, they can be stored at room temperature for up to 4 h before refrigeration. Process samples through Lympholyte®-Mammal within 8 h of collection.

11.10 Leukodepletion and Platelet Removal

The following steps should be performed at room temperature and all samples should be processed until all leukodepletion steps have been accomplished.

11.10.1 Process Blood Through Lympholyte-Mammal

11.10.1.1. Using a pipettor, gently transfer the entire contents of the microcentrifuge tube (80 μL blood plus 100 μL anticoagulant solution) onto the top of the prealiquoted room temperature Lympholyte®-Mammal in the deep 96-well plate. Repeat for the remaining samples.

11.10.1.2. Centrifuge at 800 × g for 20 min at room temperature. While samples are in the centrifuge, aliquot 1.5 mL buffered salt solution plus 2% FBS into the appropriate wells of a deep-well 96-well plate. Store at 2 to 8 °C until needed.

11.10.1.3. Carefully remove samples from centrifuge. Note that the resulting cell pellets will be loosely packed; therefore, avoid tapping or bumping the plates because this will cause the pellets to loosen or potentially become dislodged from the bottom of the well. Maintain plates at room temperature until further processing.

11.10.2 Wash Cell Pellets

11.10.2.1. While keeping the plate horizontal, use the multichannel aspirator with fixed bridge to carefully aspirate the supernatants, removing as much as possible without disturbing the loosely packed pellets.

11.10.2.2. Add 140 μL cold buffered salt solution (without FBS) directly to each pellet. Do not wash this down the side of the well, because that can reintroduce platelets and/or white blood cells that adhered to the side of the well. Gently pipette up and down to resuspend cells until there is no visual evidence of aggregation.

11.10.2.3. Transfer the entire contents of each well to the sample's corresponding deep-well plate containing 1.5 mL of cold prealiquoted buffered salt solution plus 2% FBS. Pipette at least 10 times to mix. Repeat for remaining samples.

11.10.2.4. Centrifuge at 235 × g for 10 min at room temperature. After centrifugation, aspirate as much of the supernatant as possible without aspirating the pellet.

11.10.2.5. Add 140 μL cold buffered salt solution (without FBS) directly to each pellet. Gently pipette up and down to resuspend cells

11.10.2.6. Proceed immediately to the next steps. Otherwise, store at 2 to 8°C for up to 24 h before proceeding.

11.11 Sample Labeling

Once samples are fully labeled, it is advisable to analyze them within 3 h. It is important to proceed through Sections 11.11–11.13 in sequence; therefore, careful timing of the steps described here and planning of the workday is critical. At least one of the wells (preferably from a vehicle control sample) from Section 11.11.1, step 5, will need to be saved. The cells remaining in this well will be used in Section 11.11.5, step 1, to make the part A portion of the ICS. These unstained cells will become the "mutant mimicking cells."

(Continued)

(Continued)

11.11.1 Label Leukodepleted Blood with Antibody Solution

11.11.1.1. Use a pipettor set to 160 μL to resuspend the first set of wells containing leukodepleted blood in buffered salt solution. Continue aspiration as necessary until there is no visual evidence of aggregation—10 times is usually sufficient. Note that steps 1 and 2 can be performed at room temperature if accomplished within 10 min. If more time is required, place the plates on wet ice for these steps.

11.11.1.2. Carefully transfer 160 μL of the resuspended cells directly into the corresponding sample's wells of the plate containing prealiquoted working antibody solution. Carefully pipette up and down to mix, taking care not to splash cells onto the side of the wells. Continue pipetting up and down to ensure adequate mixing—10 times is usually sufficient. Ensure that all the cells come into full contact with the working antibody solution.

11.11.1.3. Repeat steps 1 and 2 for the remaining samples. Use a new pipette tip for each sample. After all samples are labeled, use new pipette tips to move each sample to new wells of the same or a new round-bottom 96-well plate.

11.11.1.4. Incubate cells with working antibody solution for 30 min at 2 to 8°C, covered to protect from light.

11.11.1.5. As described, save at least one well and its remaining contents (preferably from a vehicle control) at 2 to 8°C. This will be used to make part A of the ICS sample. There should be approximately 20 to 30 μL remaining in the well after step 3. Add 200 μL of buffer plus 2% FBS to this sample before using it to make part A of the ICS sample as described.

11.11.1.6. During the incubation, aliquot 1.5 mL cold buffered salt solution plus 2% FBS into wells in a new deep-well plate or an unused portion of the same plate, one well for each sample. Store at 2 to 8°C or on ice until needed in Section 11.11.2.

11.11.2 Wash Labeled Samples out of Working Antibody Solution

11.11.2.1. After the incubation, resuspend the cells by gently pipetting the contents up and down and transfer directly into the cold prealiquoted buffered salt solution plus 2% FBS prepared in Section 11.11.1, step 6. Be sure to only transfer cells that have been in contact with working antibody solution for the entire incubation period. For instance, do not transfer blood that may have been on the side of the well. Carefully pipette up and down to mix. Continue pipetting up and down to ensure adequate mixing—10 times is usually sufficient.

11.11.2.2. Centrifuge at 340 × g for 5 min at room temperature.

11.11.2.3. After centrifugation, maintain the plate at room temperature. Aspirate supernatants using the multichannel aspirator with a fixed bridge, removing as much of the supernatant as possible without aspirating the pellet. The goal is to leave a minimal volume of supernatant behind.

11.11.3 Incubate Samples in Working Anti-PE MicroBead Suspension

11.11.3.1. Resuspend the working anti-PE MicroBead suspension and place into a reagent reservoir.

11.11.3.2. Using a multichannel pipettor, add 100 μL of the MicroBead suspension to each well of the first set of samples by washing it down the inside of the wells starting

(Continued)

(Continued)

approximately 0.5 cm above the pellet. Carefully pipette up and down to mix, making sure not to splash cells high onto the sides of the wells. Continue as necessary until there is no visual evidence of aggregated cells—10 times is usually sufficient. Change pipette tips and repeat for the remaining samples.

11.11.3.3. Incubate cells for 30 min at 2 to 8°C, covered to protect from light.

11.11.3.4. After incubation, add 1.5 mL of cold buffered salt solution plus 2% FBS to each well. Gently pipette to mix thoroughly—five times is usually sufficient.

11.11.3.5. Centrifuge at $340 \times g$ for 5 min at room temperature.

11.11.3.6. After centrifugation, keep at room temperature. Using a multichannel aspirator with fixed bridge, aspirate supernatants, removing as much of the liquid as possible without aspirating the pellet (Figure 11.4).

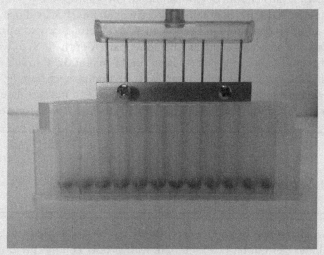

Figure 11.4
Multi-channel aspirator with fixed bridge and a 96 deep well plate.

11.11.4 Stain the Precolumn Samples

11.11.4.1. Using a multichannel pipettor, add 1.0 mL cold buffered salt solution plus 2% FBS directly to the first set of samples. Carefully pipette up and down to mix without splashing cells onto the sides of the wells. Continue as necessary until there is no visual evidence of aggregation—four times is usually sufficient.

11.11.4.2. Transfer exactly 10 μL of this suspension to the appropriate well of the 96-well deep-well plate containing 990 μL of room temperature working nucleic acid dye plus counting beads solution. Shake or pipette gently to mix. This dilution is critical in determining the final mutation frequencies, so be careful to transfer this exact amount.

11.11.4.3. Repeat steps 1 and 2 for the remaining samples. These samples represent the *precolumn* samples. Maintain the plate at room temperature until each sample has been processed to this point. They will be incubated after part A of the ICS is

(Continued)

(Continued)

prepared (Section 11.11.5). One of these samples, preferably from a vehicle control, will also be used as "part B" of the ICS (see Section 11.13.1, step 4).

11.11.4.4. The cells remaining in the plates will be processed further and are now referred to as *postcolumn* samples. Maintain these samples in the dark at 2 to 8°C or on ice until proceeding to Section 11.12.

11.11.5 Prepare Part A of the Instrument Calibration Standard (ICS) and Incubate the Precolumn Samples

11.11.5.1. Prepare part A of the ICS by retrieving the leukodepleted sample (preferably from a vehicle control animal) that was stored in Section 11.11.1 and had 200 μL of buffered salt solution plus 2% FBS added. Gently resuspend cells by pipetting up and down. Transfer 5 μL of this sample to the appropriate well of the 96-well plate containing 500 μL of room temperature working nucleic acid dye plus counting beads solution (prepared in Section 11.7.1). Pipette gently to mix.

11.11.5.2. Incubate the *precolumn* samples (including part A of the ICS) in working nucleic acid dye plus counting beads solution for 15 min at 37°C in the dark.

11.11.5.3. After incubation, transfer the samples to ice and protect from light. Ensure that the plates are surrounded by flaked/chipped ice and not resting on top. Store on ice for at least 5 min, but no more than 3 h, before flow cytometric analysis.

11.12 Column Separation and Sample Staining

Important Notes: Avoid creating bubbles when adding samples or buffered salt solution plus 2% FBS to the column. Air bubbles can interfere with proper column performance and prevent the eluate from passing through. Also, once the column has been "prewet" according to the directions, it should be used immediately. The entire elution process should occur by the force of gravity only; DO NOT force buffer or blood through the column with a plunger or other device. Depending on the number of samples being processed and the equipment being used, the actions described in this section can be performed with groups of up to eight samples (note that processing eight samples simultaneously requires two QuadroMACS™ separators).

11.12.1 Elute Samples through Immunomagnetic Columns

11.12.1.1. Insert the appropriate number of LS columns into either a MidiMACS™ or a QuadroMACS™ Separator. Place a reservoir under the columns to collect the "prewet" rinse of the columns.

11.12.1.2. Gently add 3 mL cold buffered salt solution plus 2% FBS to each column reservoir to prewet it. Be careful to avoid creating bubbles, and avoid disturbing the column matrix.

(Continued)

(Continued)

11.12.1.3. Once the prewet volume has stopped dripping from the column, remove the reservoir and discard the collected rinse. Place a clean, labeled 15 mL centrifuge tube under each column to collect the eluates for further processing. Ensure that the bottoms of the columns are inside the open tops of the centrifuge tubes (see Figure 11.5). Proceed immediately to the next step.

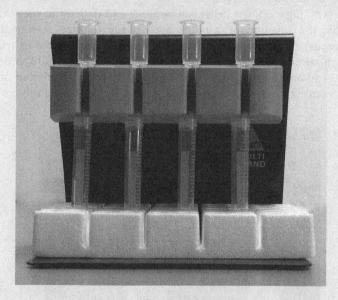

Figure 11.5
QuadroMACS™ Separator with LS Columns. Elution tubes placed directly underneath.

11.12.1.4. Take a sample (Section 11.11.4, step 4) and carefully pipette up and down to resuspend the cells and anti-PE MicroBeads without creating bubbles. Gently add the entire 1 mL of sample into the appropriate prewet LS column reservoir. Continue with additional samples, one per column.

11.12.1.5. When a sample has fully entered the column (e.g., when the sample cannot be seen above the column matrix), slowly add 5 mL cold buffered salt solution plus 2% FBS to the column reservoir as a column wash. Be careful to avoid creating bubbles, and avoid disturbing the column matrix. Continue with remaining samples/columns.

11.12.1.6. It takes approximately 5 min for the entire sample and wash to pass through the column and for the eluates to collect in the centrifuge tubes. The eluates will appear clear because the majority of the cells will be trapped in the column (see Figure 11.6).

11.12.1.7. Once eluates from this set are collected, store them in the dark at 2 to 8°C or on ice and repeat steps 1 through 5 until all *postcolumn* samples in the batch of eight

(Continued)

(Continued)

have been through the column. Discard each LS column after one use. DO NOT
reuse the columns.

11.12.2 Centrifuge and Stain Postcolumn Samples

11.12.2.1. Centrifuge a set of up to eight eluate tubes from Section 11.12.1 at $800 \times g$ for
5 min at room temperature.

11.12.2.2. After centrifugation, the pellet will be small and difficult to see—this is normal.
Holding the tube upright, carefully aspirate supernatants starting at the top
(meniscus) and working downward to prevent disturbing the pellet. It is critical
that all samples have the same volume, and it is important to understand the
average volume left in tubes. See Section 11.19 for a description of an apparatus
for consistent aspiration that guards against disturbing the cell pellets.

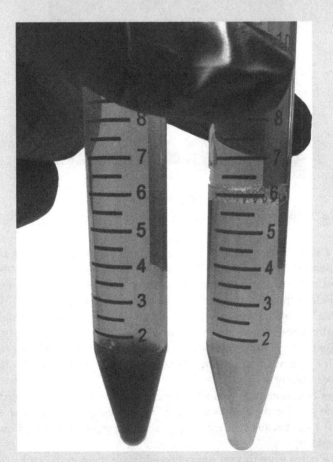

Figure 11.6
Pre-column sample on left, post-column sample on right.

(*Continued*)

(Continued)

11.12.2.3. Gently tap pellets loose. Be careful that supernatants are not splashed high onto the sides of the tubes, because this may result in cells that do not come into contact with working nucleic acid dye plus counting beads solution.

11.12.2.4. Resuspend working nucleic acid dye plus counting beads solution with a pipettor prior to adding to the first sample; to ensure a homogenous suspension of counting beads, resuspend after adding to every four or five samples.

11.12.2.5. Add 300 μL room temperature working nucleic acid dye plus counting beads solution to each *postcolumn* sample. Carefully pipette up and down to resuspend the cells and counting beads, taking care not to splash onto the side of the tubes.

11.12.2.6. Once a sample has been resuspended, cap the tubes and incubate in the dark at 37°C for 15 min.

11.12.2.7. After incubation, transfer the tubes to ice and protect from light. Ensure that the tubes are buried in the flaked/chipped ice and not resting on top. Store on ice at least 5 min, but no more than 3 h, before flow cytometric analysis.

11.12.2.8. Repeat Sections 11.12.1 and 11.12.2 with the remaining batches of up to eight samples.

11.13 Flow Cytometric Analysis: 96-Well Plate-Based Protocol

As described, part A of the ICS is prepared from a nonantibody-labeled leukodepleted blood sample, preferably from a negative control animal, in working nucleic acid dye plus counting beads solution. Part B of the ICS is part of an antibody-labeled and stained precolumn sample, preferably from a negative control animal. Once the complete ICS is made, it should be analyzed immediately.

Maintain a consistent fluidics rate throughout the analysis (for ICS and experimental samples). For digital instruments, such as a FACSCanto™, when analyzing ICS and precolumn samples in a 96-well plate, a sample flow rate of approximately 2000 to 3500 events per second is recommended. This is usually achieved by running samples at 1.0 μL/sec sample flow rate. Use a stop mode based on the length of time needed to acquire at least 1000 counting beads. Some initial experimentation may be required to determine the specific time for each flow cytometer, but 1 min is usually sufficient when using a 1.0 μL/sec sample flow rate on a FACSCanto™. The same loader settings used for the ICS should be used for experimental samples except: sample volume = 60 μL for precolumn and 180 μL for postcolumn when using 1.0 μL/sec.

It is important to *maintain the same fluidics rate* setting for *postcolumn* samples that was used for the ICS and *precolumn* samples, even though the *postcolumn* samples will have lower cell densities (and therefore lower events per second).

(Continued)

(Continued)

11.13.1 Instrument Calibration

11.13.1.1. Before analyzing samples, ensure that the flow cytometer is working properly. Follow the manufacturer's instructions for the appropriate setup and quality control procedures. Download the data acquisition template file from www.litronlabs.com/support.html or create your own using the instructions provided here.

11.13.1.2. Prepare the ICS by combining equal volumes (e.g., 150 µL) of part A (Section 11.11.1) and the retained experimental *precolumn* sample "part B" (preferably from a vehicle control animal, see Section 11.11.4, step 3) in a designated well in a 96-well plate. Pipette each part to resuspend before combining. Place the remaining part A sample back on ice in case you need to prepare another ICS sample. The remaining sample that part B was taken from should be placed with the other *precolumn* samples waiting for analysis. This ICS now consists of adequate numbers of anti-CD59-PE positive and negative events to guide selection of photomultiplier tube (PMT) voltages and compensation settings.

11.13.1.3. Immediately after creating the ICS, place it on the flow cytometer. The following loader settings are a good place to start:
   a. Throughput = standard
   b. Sample flow rate = typically 1.0 µL/sec
   c. Sample volume = 200 µL when using 1.0 µL/sec
   d. Mixing volume = 100 µL
   e. Mixing speed = 200 µL
   f. Number of mixes = 4
   g. Wash volume = 250 µL

11.13.1.4. Threshold on FSC so that any remaining platelets and other subcellular debris are eliminated. If your instrument is capable, then threshold on both FSC and SSC, but be careful not to set the values so high that counting beads are thresholded out. In plot A, adjust the "single cells" region so that it closely defines the major population of single, unaggregated erythrocytes. The resulting plot should look similar to the plot on the left in Figure 11.7.

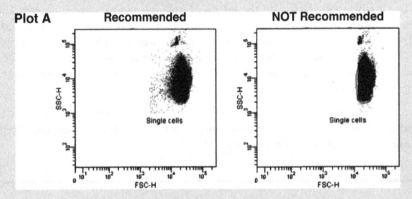

Figure 11.7

(Continued)

(Continued)

11.13.1.5. Viewing plot B, adjust the "total RBC" region to eliminate contaminating leukocytes (those cells with high nucleic acid dye fluorescence). Together with the "single cells" region, this region is used to eliminate leukocytes from RBC-based measurements. The resulting plot should look similar to the plot in Figure 11.8.

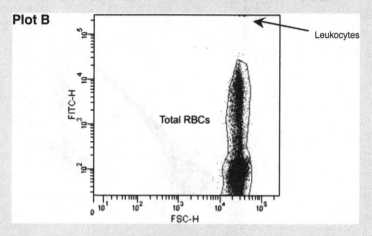

Figure 11.8

11.13.1.6. Viewing plot D, adjust the FL4 (or FL3) PMT voltage so that counting beads fall within the "beads" region. Adjust the position and size of the region as necessary, but do not change once formal analyses begin. The resulting plot should look similar to one of the plots in Figure 11.9.

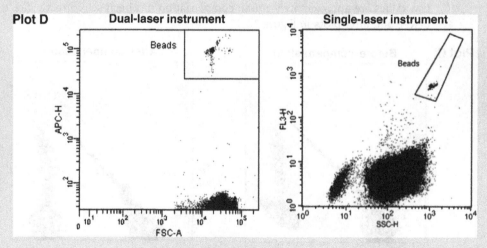

Figure 11.9

(Continued)

(Continued)

11.13.1.7. Viewing plot C, adjust PMT voltages so that mutant phenotype mature RBC (lower left quadrant (LL)) are in the first to second decade of FITC and PE fluorescence. The resulting plot should look similar to the plot in Figure 11.10.

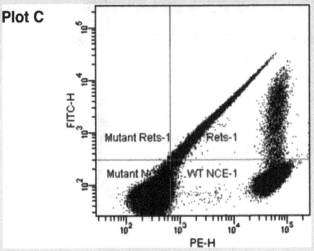

Figure 11.10

11.13.1.8. Viewing plot C, adjust compensation so that the green (FITC) component of the PE label is eliminated. This is evident when the WT phenotype mature RBC (lower right quadrant (LR)) are at the same FITC fluorescence intensity as the mutant phenotype mature RBC (LL). One way that you can determine this is by looking at the "Y Geo Mean" values for the LL and LR quadrants. When these two values are approximately equal, compensation has been set correctly. See the before and after plots in Figure 11.11.

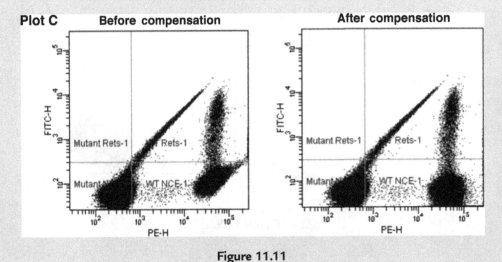

Figure 11.11

(Continued)

(Continued)

11.13.1.9. Viewing plot C, adjust compensation so that the orange (PE) component of the nucleic acid dye is eliminated. This is evident when the mutant phenotype RET (upper left quadrant (UL)) are positioned directly above the mutant phenotype mature RBC (LL). It is appropriate for the cells with the highest FITC fluorescence to lean slightly to the right, as shown in the center plot of Figure 11.12.

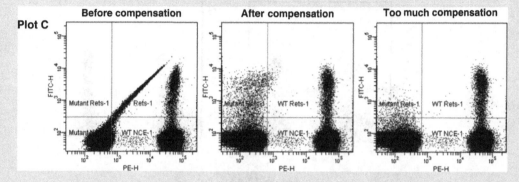

Figure 11.12

If using a digital instrument capable of biexponential scaling, it can be useful to temporarily view the PE fluorescence with biexponential scaling. This view can highlight overcompensation that may not be evident otherwise. The resulting plot should look similar to the one on the left in Figure 11.13.

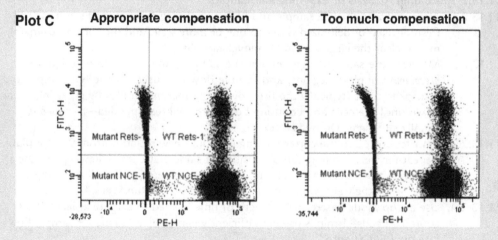

Figure 11.13

(Continued)

(Continued)

11.13.1.10. Viewing plot C, adjust the quadrant's position to ensure it is appropriate. Use a conservative approach for scoring cells as mutant phenotype RBC (i.e., these cells need to exhibit low PE fluorescence, similar to that of the mutant mimics). The resulting plot should look similar to the plot on the left in Figure 11.14.

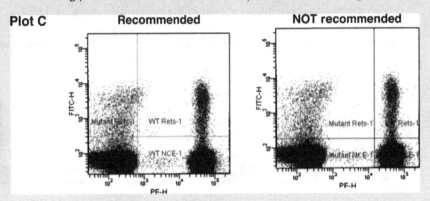

Figure 11.14

In the right plot, the horizontal demarcation line that distinguishes mature RBC from RET is too low. This can lead to subtle variations in staining intensity causing greatly overestimated %RET values. Additionally, the vertical demarcation line is positioned too far right. This can lead to subtle variations in staining intensity, causing greatly overestimated frequencies of mutant phenotype cells.

11.13.2 Precolumn Analysis of Experimental Samples

11.13.2.1. After analyzing the ICS sample and before analyzing experimental samples, add fresh distilled or deionized water to one or more wells and run for approximately 3 min to clear the lines of mutant-mimicking cells.

11.13.2.2. Maintain the same settings (except the sample volume should be 60 µL for *precolumn* samples), regions, and sample flow rate used for the ICS sample and resuspend a set (typically the first row) of *precolumn* samples by pipetting up and down until the cells and counting beads are well resuspended—10 times is usually sufficient. Do not vortex.

11.13.2.3. Transfer 200 µL to the corresponding wells in a new round-bottom 96-well plate. Repeat for the remaining samples using the same plate. Immediately place the plate with the *precolumn* samples on the flow cytometer, with well A1 at the top right. Select the wells you want to analyze and press "Run Wells."

11.13.2.4. Use a stop mode based on the length of time needed to acquire at least 1000 counting beads—1 min is usually sufficient when using a 1.0 µL/sec sample flow rate on a FACSCanto™.

11.13.2.5. Repeat until all *precolumn* samples have been analyzed

(Continued)

(Continued)

11.13.3 Postcolumn Analysis of Experimental Samples

11.13.3.1. After analyzing the *precolumn* samples and before analyzing the *postcolumn* samples, add fresh distilled or deionized water to one or more wells and run for approximately 3 min to clear the lines.

11.13.3.2. Maintain the same settings, regions, and fluidics rate setting used for the *precolumn* samples, although a sample volume of 180 μL should be used. Use a stop mode based on the length of time needed to analyze nearly the entire volume of cells and counting beads—3 min is usually sufficient when using a 1.0 μL/sec sample flow rate on a FACSCanto™.

11.13.3.3. Remove the first *postcolumn* sample tube from ice and pipette up and down until well suspended—four to five times is usually sufficient. Do not vortex. Transfer the entire content to the appropriate well of a new round-bottom 96-well plate. Repeat for the next five samples. Immediately place the plate with the *postcolumn* samples on the flow cytometer, with well A1 at the top right. Select the wells you want to analyze and begin acquiring data.

11.13.3.4. Repeat until all *postcolumn* samples have been analyzed.

11.14 Tabulating and Summarizing Results

11.14.1 Mutant Cell Frequency Calculations

The data used to calculate %RET and mutant phenotype cell frequencies are derived from both *precolumn* and *postcolumn* analyses.

Abbreviations

RET reticulocytes, RNA-positive fraction of total erythrocytes

Mature RBC RNA-negative fraction of total erythrocytes, or normochromatic erythrocytes (NCE)

RBC total erythrocytes, includes both RNA-positive and negative fractions

UL number of gated events occurring in plot C's upper left quadrant, that is, mutant RET

UR number of gated events occurring in plot C's upper right quadrant, that is, wild-type RET

LL number of gated events occurring in plot C's lower left quadrant, that is, mature mutant RBC

LR number of gated events occurring in plot C's lower right quadrant, that is, mature wild-type RBC

Counting beads number of events occurring in plot D's counting bead region

Sample volume variables

a starting volume of antibody-labeled blood and working nucleic acid dye plus beads (μL), Section 11.11.4, step 2; usually 1000

b volume of antibody-labeled blood added to working nucleic acid dye plus counting beads solution (μL), Section 11.11.4, step 2; usually 10

c volume of working nucleic acid dye plus counting beads solution used to prepare precolumn samples (μL), Section 11.7.1; usually 990

d LAB-SPECIFIC value: the supernatant volume remaining in postcolumn samples following the final centrifugation and aspiration (μL), Section 11.12.2, step 2; should be between 20 and 50

e volume of working nucleic acid dye plus counting beads solution added to each postcolumn sample (μL), Section 11.12.2, step 5; usually 300

(Continued)

(Continued)

Calculations based on sample volume and dilution variables
f cell dilution factor = (b + c)/b
g cell concentration factor = (a−b)/(d + e)
h bead dilution factor = (e*100)/(d + e)

Precolumn data
i UL
j UR
k LL
l LR
m counting beads

Calculations based on precolumn data:
n precolumn RBC to counting bead ratio = (i + j + k + l)/m
o precolumn RET to counting bead ratio = (i + j)/m
p %RET = (i + j)/(i + j + k + l)*100

Postcolumn data
q UL
r LL
s counting beads

Calculations based on precolumn and postcolumn data
t total RBC equivalents = n*s*f*g*100/h
u total RET equivalents = o*s*f*g*100/h
v number of mutant RBC per 106 total RBC = (q + r)/t*106
w number of mutant RET per 106 total RET = q/u*106

An Excel spreadsheet can be obtained from Litron (download from http://www.litronlabs.com/support.html or e-mail pigatechsupport@litronlabs.com). This spreadsheet can be used to make these calculations and also provides examples of actual flow cytometric data.

11.15 Evaluation and Interpretation of Results

11.15.1 Statistics

The application of standard parametric tests such as ANOVA with pairwise comparisons using a significance level of 0.05 to determine differences between specific treatment groups is well established. Frequently, data must be log(10) transformed to meet the normality assumptions required by ANOVA. Because the *Pig-a* endpoint measures an induced frequency, the analyses may be one-tailed to provide more power to detect an increase from baseline. It may also be necessary to apply an off-set of 0.1 to all reticulocyte mutation values to accommodate the transformation of zero values that can occur for baseline/negative samples.

11.15.2 Criteria for a Valid Assay

Assay validity can be judged based on several factors including the assessment of instrument performance provided by ICS samples, comparison of the control baseline, and/or positive control *Pig-a* mutant frequencies with respective historical data. Additional considerations like demonstration of systemic exposure and/or specific analysis of the test substance and related metabolites in the bone marrow can be especially important if negative results are obtained. Finally, proof of laboratory proficiency in the standard conduct of the assay may be advisable as a part of a regulatory submission package.

11.15.3 Comparison to Historical Controls

Generation of historical controls should be guided by standard practice for *in vivo* genotoxicity assays as described in related guidelines and the literature [22]. Laboratories should develop their own historical control databases that cover the necessary species and experimental designs they use as a part of a functioning safety assessment program. Baseline values from vehicle control-treated groups in individual studies should be compared to the historical baseline and contribute to assay validity as described.

As an example, data from more than 700 naïve male Sprague-Dawley rats approximately 7 weeks old reveal an upper bound 95% tolerance interval (at alpha 0.05) of 2.9×10^{-6} for both mutant RET and mutant RBC. Positive (genotoxic response) calls generally require several predefined criteria to be met. One that can be useful is that at least one dose group mean mutant cell frequency exceeds such an upper bounds value. This number, 2.9×10^{-6}, is provided for general guidance only, and it is recommended that each laboratory should generate its own historical controls and calculate acceptable tolerance intervals to establish its own positive call (and assay validity) criteria.

11.15.4 Biological Relevance

Existing OECD TGs for genotoxicity assays have formulated strategies and standards for the assessment of a positive response. The statistics described will be valuable for determining the required effect size to achieve dose-dependent increases and/ or increases seen for at least one concentration studied. Once these data are established, the interpretation of biological relevance is an additional important consideration.

Because the *Pig-a* mutation endpoint can be assessed in both RET and RBC, it should be appreciated that the observation of a positive response in both cell types can strengthen conclusions relating to biological relevance. Depending on the study design, additional information from more than one time point can also factor into the determination of relevance. Thus, one would expect to see an elevation in the RET cohort at an earlier time point, such as Day 15, when compared to the RBC population.

11.16 Flow Cytometric Template Preparation

Data acquisition template files are available from Litron (download from www.litronlabs.com/
support.html or e-mail pigatechsupport@litronlabs.com) but are specific to CellQuest™ or
FACSDiva™ software. The next pages show actual screen images of the CellQuest™ and
FACSDiva™ template graphs. Flow cytometry operators who are not using CellQuest™ or
FACSDiva™ software should find these pages valuable for constructing their own data
acquisition and analysis template.

We recommend that if you are using FACSDiva™ software, you should set the fluorescence
parameter to "Height" rather than "Area." The ICS may be run using Single-Color Compensation
controls and auto-compensation if available with your software package.

1. Defining Gates:
   a. G1 = R1 = "Single Cells"
   b. G2 = R2 = "Total RBCs"
   c. G3 = R3 = "Beads"
   d. G4 = R1 and R2 and NOT R3 = "Single Cells" and "Total RBCs"
      and NOT "Beads"
2. Gate and parameters for each Plot:

Plot A	No Gate	SSC-H vs. FSC-H
Plot B	G1	FL1-H vs. FSC-H
Plot C	G4	FL1-H vs. FL2-H
Plot D[a]	No Gate	FL4-H vs. FSC-A or FL3-H vs. SSC-H

[a]If you have a second red diode laser, use FL4 and either FSC or SSC for plot D. Otherwise,
use FL3. SSC is needed for single-laser analysis to provide optimal resolution when not using
a red diode laser.

3. Quadrant Key for Plot C:
   a. UL = mutant RET
   b. UR = wild-type RET
   c. LL = mutant mature RBC (i.e., mutant normochromatic erythrocytes (NCE))
   d. LR = wild-type mature RBC (i.e., wild-type normochromatic erythrocytes (NCE))
4. Alternate names for detectors:

Green	FL1	FITC
Orange	FL2	PE
Red	FL3	PerCP-Cy5.5
Far Red	FL4	APC

Save the template file. This template file should be suitable for all analyses. To ensure
consistency of data, it is preferable that no changes are made to the location and size of the
regions between samples (Figure 11.15).

(Continued)

(Continued)

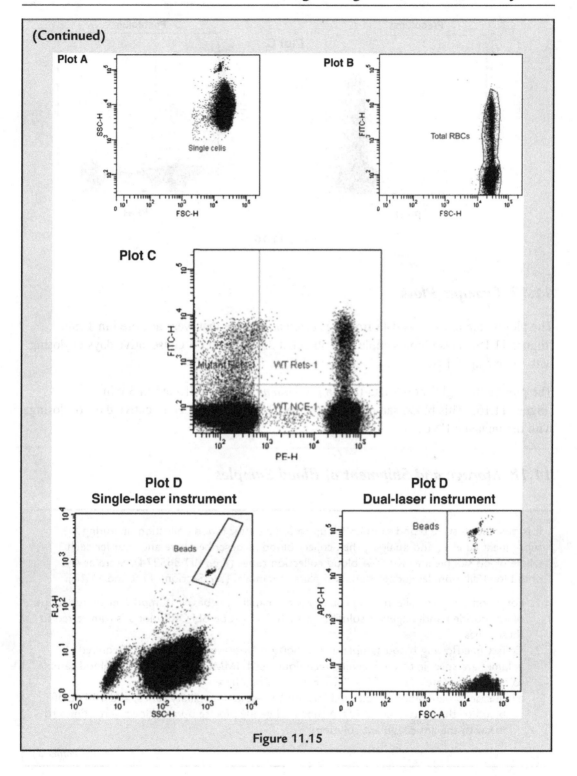

Figure 11.15

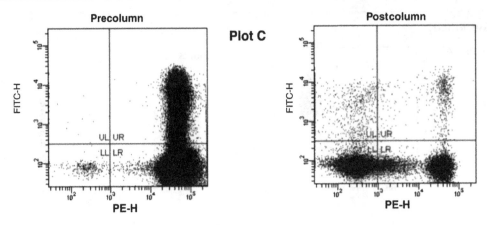

Figure 11.16

11.17 Example Plots

The plot on the left shows data from a *precolumn* sample that were acquired in 1 min (Figure 11.16). This blood sample was obtained 25 days after 3 consecutive days of dosing with the mutagen ENU.

The plot on the right shows data from a *postcolumn* sample collected in 3 min (Figure 11.16). This blood sample was obtained 25 days after 3 consecutive days of dosing with the mutagen ENU.

11.18 Storage and Shipment of Blood Samples

It is possible to store blood samples for up to 3 days after blood collection. If storing for subsequent labeling and analysis, then collect blood as described here and transfer each whole blood sample into K_2EDTA blood collection tubes (e.g., BD 365974). Store at 4°C until blood dilution, leukodepletion, and platelet removal (see Sections 11.9 and 11.10).

1. For blood samples collected in heparin-coated capillary tubes, it is important to add 20 μL of kit-provided anticoagulant solution to each EDTA tube BEFORE blood is transferred to these tubes.
2. Collect free-flowing blood sample (see Important Notes in Section 11.9). Required volumes are specific to the bleeding technique used. IMMEDIATELY transfer blood sample to the appropriately labeled EDTA tube as described here:
   a. In cases where blood is collected into heparin-coated capillary tubes, add 100 μL of blood to the bottom of an EDTA tube and gently pipette up and down three times to mix with the anticoagulant solution.

(Continued)

(Continued)

    b. In cases when blood is collected in an anticoagulant solution—coated needle/syringe, transfer the entire volume of blood (approximately 300 μL) into the bottom of an EDTA tube (prealiquoted anticoagulant solution is not necessary in this case). It is important to open the caps on the EDTA tubes as opposed to puncturing the septum with the needle. Once blood is added to a tube, make sure the tube is tightly recapped for transport.

3. Repeat step 2 for each rodent. Blood can be maintained in EDTA tubes at ambient temperature for up to 2 h. For longer periods of time up to 3 days, maintain EDTA tubes at 4°C.

    a. It is also possible to transport EDTA blood samples for off-site labeling and analysis. Samples in the K_2EDTA tubes can be shipped overnight, but they must be kept cold, not frozen. Litron recommends using Exakt-Pak® shipping containers (e.g., MD8204V20) and cold packs (e.g., Cold Chain Technologies 306F Koolit® Foam Brick) frozen at −20°C. To prevent freezing of the blood samples, make sure ice packs do not come into direct contact with the storage tubes (see schematic) (Figure 11.17).

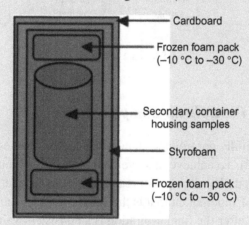

Figure 11.17

    b. For both cases described here, it is advisable for each laboratory to generate its own data to support these storage and/or shipping strategies. This is most readily done by splitting samples between same-day collection and analysis versus stored or shipped conditions and comparing the resulting data.

4. After storage or shipment, transfer 80 μL into the labeled microcentrifuge tube containing 100 μL of anticoagulant solution.

5. Refrigerate blood samples in anticoagulant solution as soon as possible, although they can be stored at room temperature for up to 4 h before refrigeration. Process samples through Lympholyte®-Mammal (Section 11.10).

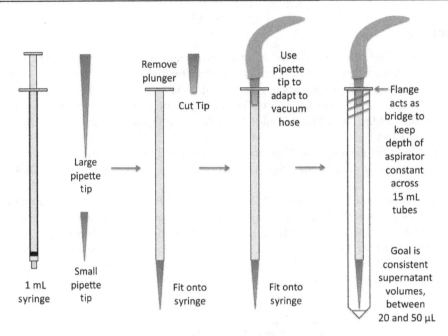

Figure 11.18

11.19 Aspiration of Postcolumn Samples

It is very important to carefully control and standardize aspirations, especially the last aspiration (Section 11.12.2). To achieve this, we recommend fashioning an aspirator with a bridge that controls the depth that the tip will reach. With this bridge, the aspirator will leave a consistent, low volume of supernatant that is the same across all tubes. The goal for the volume of supernatant left after the final aspiration is a consistent value within the range of 20 μL to 50 μL in each tube. Note that a consistent volume that ensures cells are not aspirated off is required to make accurate mutant cell frequency calculations (Figure 11.18).

References

[1]   Dertinger SD, Phonethepswath S, Avlasevich SL, Torous DK, Mereness J, Bryce SM, et al. Efficient monitoring of *in vivo* Pig-a gene mutation and chromosomal damage: summary of 7 published studies and results from 11 new reference compounds. Toxicol Sci 2012;130:328−48.

[2]   Miura D, Dobrovolsky VN, Kasahara Y, Katsuura Y, Heflich RH. Development of an *in vivo* gene mutation assay using the endogenous *Pig-a* gene: I. Flow cytometric detection of CD59-negative peripheral red blood cells and CD48-negative spleen T-cells from the rat. Environ Molec Mutagen 2008;49:614−21.

[3]   Casciano DA, Aidoo A, Chen T, Mittelstaedt RA, Manjanatha MG, Heflich RH. HPRT mutant frequency and molecular analysis of HPRT mutations in rats treated with mutagenic carcinogens. Mutat Res 1999;431:389−95.

[4] Myers NT, Grant SG. The blood-based glycophorin A (GPA) human *in vivo* somatic mutation assay. Methods Mol Biol 2014;1105:223−44.

[5] Swiger RR. Quantifying *in vivo* somatic mutations using transgenic mouse model systems. Methods Mol Biol 2014;1105:271−82.

[6] Phonethepswath S, Bryce SM, Bemis JC, Dertinger SD. Erythrocyte-based *Pig-a* gene mutation assay: demonstration of cross-species potential. Mutat Res 2008;657:122−6.

[7] Dobrovolsky VN, Miura D, Heflich RH, Dertinger SD. The *in vivo* Pig-a gene mutation assay, a potential tool for regulatory safety assessment. Environ Mol Mutagen 2010;51:825−35.

[8] Borowitz MJ, Craig FE, Digiuseppe JA, Illingworth AJ, Rosse W, Sutherland DR, et al. Guidelines for the diagnosis and monitoring of paroxysmal nocturnal hemoglobinuria and related disorders by flow cytometry. Cytometry B Clin Cytom 2010;78(4):211−30.

[9] Nishimura J, Murakami Y, Kinoshita T. Paroxysmal nocturnal hemoglobinuria: an acquired genetic disease. Am J Hematol 1999;62(3):175−82.

[10] Araten DJ, Nafa K, Pakdeesuwan K, Luzzatto L. Clonal populations of hematopoietic cells with paroxysmal nocturnal hemoglobinuria genotype and phenotype are present in normal individuals. Proc Natl Acad Sci U S A 1999;96(9):5209−14.

[11] Peruzzi B, Araten DJ, Notaro R, Luzzatto L. The use of *PIG-A* as a sentinel gene for the study of the somatic mutation rate and of mutagenic agents *in vivo*. Mutat Res 2010;705(1):3−10.

[12] Chen R, Eshleman JR, Brodsky RA, Medof ME. Glycophosphatidylinositol-anchored protein deficiency as a marker of mutator phenotypes in cancer. Cancer Res 2001;61(2):654−8.

[13] Rondelli T, Berardi M, Peruzzi B, Boni L, Caporale R, Dolara P, et al. The frequency of granulocytes with spontaneous somatic mutations: a wide distribution in a normal human population. PLoS One 2013;8 (1):e54046.

[14] Kawagoe K, Takeda J, Endo Y, Kinoshita T. Molecular cloning of murine *pig-a*, a gene for GPI-anchor biosynthesis, and demonstration of interspecies conservation of its structure, function, and genetic locus. Genomics 1994;23(3):566−74.

[15] Dertinger SD, Phonethepswath S, Franklin D, Weller P, Torous DK, Bryce SM, et al. Integration of mutation and chromosomal damage endpoints into 28-day repeat dose toxicology studies. Toxicol Sci 2010;115:401−11.

[16] Dertinger SD, Avlasevich SL, Torous DK, Bemis JC, Phonethepswath S, Labash C, et al. Persistence of cisplatin-induced mutagenicity in hematopoietic stem cells: implications for secondary cancer risk following chemotherapy. Toxicol Sci 2014;140(2):307−14.

[17] Miura D, Dobrovolsky VN, Kimoto T, Kasahara Y, Heflich RH. Accumulation and persistence of *Pig-a* mutant peripheral red blood cells following treatment of rats with single and split doses of N-ethyl-N-nitrosourea. Mutat Res 2009;677:86−92.

[18] Janczewska S, Ziolkowska A, Durlik M, Olszewski WL, Lukomska B. Fast lymphoid reconstitution after vascularized bone marrow transplantation in lethally irradiated rats. Transplantation 1999;68(2):201−9.

[19] Dertinger SD, Bryce SM, Phonethepswath S, Avlasevich SL. When pigs fly: immunomagnetic separation facilitates rapid determination of *Pig-a* mutant frequency by flow cytometric analysis. Mutat Res 2011;721:163−70.

[20] Gollapudi BB, Lynch AM, Heflich RH, Dertinger SD, Dobrovolsky VN, Froetschl R. et al. The *in vivo* Pig-a assay: a report of the International Workshop On Genotoxicity Testing (IWGT) Workgroup. Mutat Res Genet Toxicol Environ Mutagen <http://dx.doi.org/10.1016/j.mrgentox.2014.09.007>.

[21] Labash C, Avlasevich SA, Carlson K, Torous DK, Berg A, Bemis JC, et al. Comparison of male versus female responses in the *Pig-a* mutation assay. Mutagenesis 2014. Available from: http://dx.doi.org/ 10.1093/mutagen/geu055.

[22] Hayashi M, Dearfield K, Kasper P, Lovell D, Martus HJ, Thybaud V. Compilation and use of genetic toxicity historical control data. Mutat Res 2011;723(2):87−90.

Index

Note: Page numbers followed by "*f*" and "*t*" refer to figures and tables, respectively.

A

AAALAC, 274–275
Aberrant cell, 336–337
Absolute counting bead, 194
Access controls and hierarchy, 14
Acclimation period, 329
Acridine orange (AO), 282
  blood smear stained with, 287*f*
  bone marrow smear stained
    with, 287*f*
  staining, 285–286
Acrylonitrile, 349–350
Acute studies, 390–392
Acute toxicology test, 22
Agarose layers, for comet slide
    preparation, 364*f*
Aliquot anticoagulant solution and
    Lympholyte®-Mammal,
    394
Alkali-labile sites, 346
Alkaline electrophoresis, 365–367
Alkaline *in vivo* comet assay, 346
AMES assay, 348–350
Ames test, 12, 43–45, 126–127
9-Aminoacridine, 83, 113
2-Aminoanthracene, 113
Ampicillin discs, 87
Analytical method, 59, 74–75
Andor Technology Komet™
    software, 367
Aneugenic agents
  identification of, 291
  treatment with, 273
Aneugenicity, 174
Aneugens, 166*t*, 202, 273, 324
Aneuploidy-inducing agents, 164
Animal euthanasia, 329–330

Animal observations, 329
ANOVA, 410
Antibacterial agents, 107
Anti-CD59 Ab, 388
Anticoagulant/diluent vials,
    298
Antimicrobial and antifungal
    agents, 145
Apurinic/apyrimidinic sites, 346
Aqueous solvents, 109, 227
Aqueous suspending agents,
    61–62, 71–72
Aqueous vehicles, 148, 326
Aroclor 1254, 167
Asbestos, 346
Aspiration device preparation,
    392
Aspiration of postcolumn samples,
    416
Assay acceptability, criteria for, 11
Assay configurations, 391–392
Assay Stocks, 146–147
Attachment cell protocol, for flow
    cytometric method,
    188–189
  cell harvest, 188
  complete nucleic acid dye A
    staining, 189
  simultaneous cell lysis and
    nucleic acid dye B staining,
    189
  treatment, preliminary
    assessments, 187
Attachment cells, 201
Autoclave, 86, 88, 212, 217–218
Automated plate scoring systems,
    152

Automatic (computerized robotic)
    metaphase finder systems,
    264
Automatic colony counter,
    118–119
Automation, 264

B

B6C3F1, 389–390
Background lawns, 83, 110–111,
    111*f*, 119
Bacteria, growth characteristics of
    determination of, 131
Bacterial counting chamber grid,
    133*f*
Bacterial DNA repair tests, 127
Bacterial genetic toxicity tests, 80
Bacterial mutagen, 83
Bacterial mutation, 2, 17
Bacterial mutation test, 62, 68, 94,
    218–219
Bacterial reverse mutation
    test, 79
  bacterial strains, 94–105
    diagnostic mutagen test,
      101–105
    freezing of selected isolates,
      100–101
    genotypes of routinely used
      strains, 95
    phenotyping of new isolates,
      98–100
    receipt of, 96–98
    tester strains, obtaining,
      95–96
  consumables, 85
  equipment, 84–85

Bacterial reverse mutation
    test (*Continued*)
fundamentals, 83—84
history, 80—83
reagents and recipes, 86—93
    ampicillin discs, 87
    biotin, 87
    crystal violet, 87
    glucose, 87
    glucose-6-Phosphate, 88
    HBT solution, 88
    histidine, 88
    KMg, 88
    minimal glucose agar (MGA)
        plates, 88—89
    NADP, 90
    nutrient agar plates, 90
    nutrient broth, 90
    phosphate buffer, 90
    positive control and
        diagnostic mutagen
        solutions, 90—91
    S9 fraction, 91
    S9 mix, 91—92
    tetracycline disc, 92
    top agar complete, 92
    top agar incomplete, 92
    tryptophan, 93
    Vogel-Bonner salts, 93
routine testing, 105—113
    designing a study, 105—106
    positive controls, 113
    test article considerations,
        106—113
screening tests, 126—130
    reduced format tests using
        standard tester strains,
        129—130
    simplified test systems,
        126—127
    using standard tester strains,
        127—129
standard test procedures,
    114—126
    examination of the plates,
        118—119
    interpretation of results,
        119—121
    plate incorporation method,
        114—115

preincubation method,
    115—116
presentation of results,
    121—125
standard study design,
    116—117
testing of volatile and gaseous
    compounds, 125—126
suggested phases in
    development of the test,
    93—94
suspension cultures, growing
    and monitoring, 130—134
Bacterial strains, 94—105
    diagnostic mutagen test,
        101—105
    freezing of selected isolates,
        100—101
    genotypes of routinely used
        strains, 95
    phenotyping of new isolates,
        98—100
    receipt of, 96—98
    tester strains, obtaining, 95—96
Base analog bromodeoxyuridine
    (BUDR), 325—326
BD-brand HTS systems, 190
Binocular light microscope,
    212—213, 330—331
Binuclear assay
    analysis of slides, 179—180
    coding of slides, 179
    criteria for valid assay, 180
    donors, 178
    evaluation of data, 180—181
    evaluation of results, 180
    human peripheral blood
        lymphocytes, 178
    lymphocyte culture, 178—179
    materials, 172
    methods, 169
    staining and analysis, 179
    treatment schedules, 177
BioLum method, 128
Biotin, 87
Blood and bone marrow samples,
    fixation of, 300—302
Blood collection, 299
    for *Pig-a* endogenous gene
        mutation assay, 396

Blood donors, 178
Blood samples, storage and
    shipment of, 414
Blood smears, 283
Blood/plasma toxicokinetic data,
    328
Bluescreen, 127
Boilerplate protocol, standardized,
    28—29
Boilerplate reports, 35
Bone marrow cell-cycle time, 329
Bone marrow collection, 332—333
    and processing, 299—300
Bone marrow samples
    collecting and fractionating, 300
    fixation of, 300—302
5-Bromo-2'-deoxyuridine (BUDR),
    224—225, 325—326
Buffered salt solution plus 2%
    FBS, 394
Bulk formulations, formulation of,
    71

C

C57Bl/6, 389—390
Calibrated peristaltic pump, 86
Carcinogenicity, 361—362
CCD camera, 367—368
CD-1, 389—390
CD71 antigen, 271—272
CE. *See* Cloning efficiency (CE)
Cell characterization, 221—225
    cell-cycle time, 224—225
    modal chromosome number,
        222—223
    mycoplasma, 224
Cell culture, 146—147
Cell density, 6—7, 37
Cell harvesting, 220
Cell lines, 210, 221—222,
    242—243
Cell maintenance log, 231—233
Cell pellets, washing, 397
Cell-cycle progression, 254, 257,
    337
Cell-cycle time, 224—225,
    230—231
CellQuest software, 306, 312
CellQuest™ Pro, 189
    version 5.2, 195—198

Cellulose columns, preparing, 299–300
Centrifuge, 213, 402–403
Centromere, 164, 245–246
Centromere-positive micronuclei, 273
Centromere-specific probes, 170, 171*f*, 172, 183
Centromeric disruption, 244, 251*f*
Centromeric labeling
  alterative protocol for FISH, 182
  FISH using programmable hotplate such as HYBrite™/ Thermobrite™, 181–182
  materials, 172
  methods, 169–170
  slide checking, 182
  slide scoring, 183
Centromeric staining, using FISH, 291–294
  alterative protocol for FISH, 293
  materials, 292
  programmable hotplate, FISH method using, 292–293
  slide checking, 293
  slide scoring, 294
Certificate of analysis (COA), 23–24, 59, 147
Chemical analysis and stability, 74–76
Chemical mutagens and cytotoxic drugs, 52
Chinese hamsters (*Cricetulus griseus*), 324
Chlorambucil, 346, 347*f*
CHO cells, 225–226, 263
  routine maintenance, 231–233
  test procedures, 233–237
CHO-K1 cells, 194, 222
  medium for, 186
Chromatid break, 244–245, 251*f*
Chromatid exchange, 248, 251*f*
Chromatids, 244–246, 325–326, 334
Chromosome 11b structure, 140
Chromosome aberration scoring sheet, 252*f*

Chromosome aberration test, 7–8, 12, 38, 40, 66–67, 208–209, 317–318, 324, 339. *See also* In vitro chromosome aberration test
Chromosome aberrations, 208–209
Chromosome break, 212*f*, 248, 251*f*
Chromosome breakage, 209, 211–212, 273, 324
Chromosome fragments, 273
Chromosome paints, 164, 181, 248, 292
Chromosome-damaging agent, 270–271
Cisplatin, 346, 347*f*, 387–388
Class II safety cabinets, 145
Clastogenicity, 142, 257–258, 261
Clastogens, 202
  with and without metabolic activation, 166*t*
Cloning efficiency (CE), 146, 154–155
CMC. *See* Sodium carboxymethylcellulose (CMC)
COA. *See* Certificate of analysis (COA)
Co-factor-supplemented postmitochondrial fraction (S9), 167
Colcemid in PBS, 216
Colchicine, 216, 219–220, 278–279, 325–326, 329, 339
Colony counting (agar version), 153
Colony counting (microtiter version), 152
Colony counts, 118–119
Comet assay test, *in vivo*, 345
  consumables, 354
  data and reporting, 369–377
    statistical analysis, 369–372
  equipment and nondisposable supplies, 352–353
  evaluating unclear results, 378–381
  equivocal results, 379

  negative results, 380–381
  positive results, 379–380
  fundamentals, 351–352
  reagents, 354
  in regulatory safety testing, 348–351
    negative *in vitro* standard battery tests, 351
    positive *in vitro* standard battery tests, 350
  solutions, 355–356
    alkaline electrophoresis buffer, 356
    EDTA, adding, pH 10, 356
    low melting point agarose, adding, 355
    lysing stock solution, 355
    mincing buffer, 355
    NaOH, adding, 356
    normal melting agarose, adding, 355
    Trizma base, adding, 356
    working lysing solution, 356
  standard test procedures, 362–369
    alkaline electrophoresis, 365–367
    comet slide preparation, 364–365
    image analysis scoring, 367–369
    preliminary procedures, 362–363
    sample collection, 363–364
    slide staining, 367
  study design considerations, 357–362
    dose selection and cytotoxicity, 361
    number of animals, 359
    positive control, 359
    route of exposure, 359–360
    test article, 357
    tissue selection, 361–362
    treatment schedule/sample time, 360–361
    vehicle selection, 357–359
  test system, 356–357
Comet slides
  example labeling for, 363*f*
  preparation, 364–365

Commercial system, validation of, 14
Complete lysis solution 1, 186
Complete lysis solution 2, 186
Complete nucleic acid dye A staining, 187, 189
Computer systems, use of, 13–15
Consumables, 57
  bacterial reverse mutation test, 85
  in vitro chromosome aberration test, 214–215
  in vitro micronucleus assay, 185
  in vivo comet assay test, 354
  in vivo rodent micronucleus assay, 282
  Pig-a endogenous gene mutation assay, 393
  rodent bone marrow chromosomal aberration test, 331
Contract laboratory, qualifying, 47–48
Contract Research Organization (CRO), 116
Coplin jar, 181–182
Costs reduction, 44–45
Coulter counter, 131–132, 236
CountBright™ Beads, 394
Covalent binding, 273
CREST staining, 273
Cricetulus griseus, 324
Criteria for interpretation of results, 18–19
Criteria for negative/positive/ equivocal outcome, 253–256
CRO. *See* Contract Research Organization (CRO)
Crystal violet, 87
Culture medium, 214
Culture number identification, 231
Culture vessels, 214
Culture-to-culture variation, 20
Cyclophosphamide, 278
Cyclophosphamide monohydrate (CP), 218
Cytochalasin-B, 163–164, 170, 178
Cytogenetic analysis, 251

Cytogenetic assay, 36–37
Cytogenetic examination and statistical analysis, 338*t*
Cytokinesis-block method, 163–164
Cytonucleus test, 317–318, 339
Cytostatic substances, 278–279, 328
Cytotoxic chemicals, 278–279
Cytotoxicity, 361, 373–375
Cytotoxicity measures, 167–168, 174, 180, 194–195
  in absence of cytochalasin B, 168
  in presence of cytochalasin B, 168

D

Data tabulation, 30
Deionized reverse-osmosis purified water, 86, 216
Deoxythymidylate (dTMP), 139–140, 144–145
Design and development history file, 15
Development and validation strategy, 14
Diagnostic mutagen test, 101–105, 101*t*, 102*t*
1,2-Dibromoethane, 349–350
1,2-Dichloroethane, 349–350
Dichloromethane, 61–62
Dimethyl sulfoxide (DMSO), 60, 62–63, 66, 103, 215–216, 218, 354–355
Dimethylhydrazine, 278–279
Direct data capture systems, 13–14, 30
Direct data entry, 13–14, 29–31
Disodium hydrogen phosphate, 218
DMSO. *See* Dimethyl sulfoxide (DMSO)
DNA damage, 346, 351–352, 360–361, 364
  expression of, 347*f*
  types of, 347*f*
DNA migration, 346, 347*f*, 351–352, 357–358, 358*f*
DNA of mycoplasma, 224
DNA repair deficiency systems, 80

DNA staining solution, 299
DNA-damaging activity, 351
Donor horse serum, 146
Dose levels, 109–113, 151
  selection, 16*t*, 227–230
Dose regimens, 225–226
Dose solutions, formulation of, 68–70
Dose volume, 109, 227, 281
Dose-range finding, 391
Dose-response curve, 16–17
Double-strand breakage, 244–245
Double-stranded break (DSB), 208–209, 244–245
Doubling time, 224
Drosophila, 80–81, 209–210
DSB. *See* Double-stranded break (DSB)
DTMP (deoxythymidylate), 144–145
Dulbecco's phosphate-buffered saline (DPBS), 214, 234–238
DUMP (deoxyuridylate), 144–145
Dunnett multiple comparison test, 371

E

Eagle's minimum essential medium, 216
Early pluripotent hematopoietic stem cells, 387–388
Efficient air-flow system design, 54
Electronic cell counter, 213
Electronic signature and management systems, 15
EMA-positive events, 194
Emulsions, formulation of, 71
Endogenous mutation assays, 384
Endonuclease DNA digestion, 373–374
Endoplasmic reticulum, 286–288
Endoreduplication, 245, 251*f*
Environmental and Molecular Mutagenesis (EMM), 37
Environmental Mutagenesis and Genomics Society (EMGS), 37
Epoxy flooring, 54

Equipment
 bacterial reverse mutation test,
  84–85
 in vitro chromosome aberration
  test, 212–214
 in vitro micronucleus assay,
  184–185
 in vivo comet assay test,
  352–353
 in vivo rodent micronucleus
  assay, 282
 Pig-a endogenous gene mutation
  assay, 392
 rodent bone marrow
  chromosomal aberration
  test, 330–331
Error-prone translesion synthesis,
 81–82
E-rule, 14–15
Erythrocyte micronucleus test, 271,
 326
Erythropoiesis, 273, 290, 390
Escherichia coli mutation system,
 80–81
Escherichia coli WP2 uvrA strain,
 113
Etching machine, 45
Ethyl methanesulfonate (EMS),
 141–142, 359
Ethyl nitrosourea (ENU), 387
European Collection of Animal
 Cell Cultures (ECACC),
 143, 146
Evaluation and interpretation of
 results, 335–337, 410–411
 biological relevance, 411
 comparison to historical
  controls, 411
 statistics, 410
 valid assay, criteria for, 411
Evaluation criteria, 17–20, 262,
 335–336
 criteria for interpretation of
  results, 18–19
 general recommendations,
  17–20
 mouse lymphoma TK assay,
  155–156
 statistical analysis, 19–20
 valid assay, 17–18

Exogenous metabolic activation
 system (S9), 209, 211
Exogenous metabolizing system,
 147
Experimental completion date,
 258–259
Experimental design, for *in vitro*
 assays, 167
Experimental design spreadsheet,
 231–233, 232*t*
 CHO cells: routine maintenance,
  231–233
Experimental samples, analysis of,
 311
Expiry dates, 216
Exposure conditions, 225
Extra-low-dispersion (ED) glass
 lenses, 330–331

F
F-12 complete, 216
F344, 389–390
FACSCanto™, 403, 409
FACSDiva™, 189–190, 312, 412
 version 6.1, 195–198
False-positive calls, 336–337
False-positive claim, 19–20
False-positive rate, 156–157
FASCDiva software, 306, 312
FDA e-rule, 14
Fetal bovine serum (FBS), 214
Fetal calf serum (FCS), 214, 282
Feulgen staining technique, 325
Filter paper discs, 86–87
Filter-sterilization, 216
Fischer's medium, 145
FISH. *See* Fluorescent *in situ*
 hybridization (FISH)
Fisher exact test, 254, 255*t*
Fixative tubes, 298
Fixed samples, storage of,
 303–304
 washing samples out of fixative,
  303–304
Flow analysis
 labelling washed samples for,
  305–306
Flow cytometer calibration with
 biological standards,
 306–311

Flow cytometric analysis,
 306–311, 403–409
 experimental samples
 postcolumn analysis
  of, 409
 precolumn analysis of, 408
 instrument calibration, 404–408
 template preparation for,
  312–313
Flow cytometric data analysis,
 193–195
 criteria for positive/negative
  outcomes, 194–195
 criteria for valid assay, 194
 independent cytotoxicity
  assessment, 194
Flow cytometric method,
 184–203, 299
 advice for test article exposure,
  200–202
 analysis template, creation,
  195–198
 attachment cell protocol,
  188–189
 consumables, 185
 equipment, 184–185
 example plate layout, 198
 example results table, 199
 flow cytometric data acquisition,
  189–193
 flow cytometric data analysis,
  193–195
 multichannel aspirator with
  bridge, use of, 202
 nucleic acid dye B
  photoactivation, plate
  placement during, 203
 reagents and recipes, 185–186
 suspension cell protocol,
  187–189
 updates and future work, 203
Flow cytometric template
 preparation, 412–411
Fluctuation test, 128–129
Fluorescent *in situ* hybridization
 (FISH), 169–170, 170*f*,
 273, 292
 alterative protocol for, 182
 centromeric staining using,
  292–294

Fluorescent *in situ* hybridization
    (FISH) (*Continued*)
    alterative protocol for FISH,
        293
    materials, 292
    programmable hotplate, FISH
        method using, 292–293
    slide checking, 293
    slide scoring, 294
    for nondisjunction assay,
        183
    using programmable hotplate,
        181–182
Fluorescent staining with Hoescht,
    224
5-Fluorouracil resistance,
    126–127
Follow-up *in vivo* testing,
    257–258
Formulation constraints, 23
Formulation Instruction/Record
    Sheet, 70
Formulation of test articles, 51
    bulk formulations, 71
    chemical analysis and stability,
        74–76
    dose solutions, 68–70
    formulation laboratories, 53–57
        genetic toxicology
            formulation area, designing
            and equipping, 53–56
        personal protective clothing,
            56–57
    formulation types and planning,
        59–60
    receipt of test article, 59
    safety, 52
    safety data sheets (SDS), 57–59
    selection of appropriate
        formulation, 52–53
    solubility and *in vitro*
        compatibility testing,
        60–67
    choice of solvent, 61–62
    compatibility of formulation
        with culture medium,
        65–67
    small-volume (*in vitro*)
        assays, 64–65
    solubility testing, 62–64

suspensions, 71–74
    aqueous suspending agents,
        71–72
    large volume suspensions, 73
    small volume suspensions, 74
Formulation stability data, 22
Formulation types and planning,
    59–60
Forward mutation, 80, 126–127,
    139–140, 142
Frameshift mutation, 81–82
Free-flowing blood, 396, 414–415
Freezing and diagnostic mutagen
    testing, 98–100
Freezing medium, 216
Fume hoods, 54–55

G
G6P 1M: glucose-6-phosphate, 217
G6P cofactors, 226
Gaps, 245, 247
Gaseous compounds, testing of,
    125–126
Gaussian (normal) distribution, 13,
    336
G-banding, 221
Gene mutation tests, 349–350
General recommendations, 5
    computer systems, use of,
        13–15
    contract laboratory, qualifying,
        47–48
    evaluation criteria, 17–20
        criteria for interpretation of
            results, 18–19
        statistical analysis, 19–20
        valid assay, 17–18
    improving quality and
        efficiency, 37–45
        accommodating repeat or
            supplementary tests, 40
        potential problems,
            minimizing, 38–39
        reducing costs/labor
            requirement, 44–45
        reducing the effort needed to
            perform the study, 43–44
        reducing the effort needed to
            prepare protocols, tables,
            and reports, 43

reducing the need for
    repetition of parts of study,
        39–40
running more studies in given
    timeframe, 40–41
timeframe for routine studies,
    41–42
laboratory historical control
    databases, 11–13
    positive control database, 13
    spreadsheet calculations, 13
    vehicle/negative control
        database, 11–13
new assay, establishing, 6–10
    method set-up, 6–8
    method validation, 8–10
planning a study, 22
preparing a protocol complying
    with GLP, 23–29
    standardized boilerplate
        protocols, 28–29
QA, 45–46
reports, 31–35
results, collecting, 29–31
    data tabulation, 30
    presentation of report tables,
        30–31
SOPs, organization of, 20–22
spreadsheets and manipulation
    of results, 10–11
study design, 15–17
study monitor, responsibilities
    of, 48
training, 36–37
General test conditions, 148–150
Genetic Toxicology Association
    (GTA), 37
Genetic Toxicology Department at
    Charles River Laboratories
    (CTBR), 2
Genetic Toxicology Group, 37
Genetic toxicology staff, 46
Genetic Toxicology Testing
    Committee (GTTC) project,
    143
Genotoxic agents, 271, 339
Genotoxicity, 209, 254, 261
Genotoxicity assays, 19–20
Genotoxicity testing, 346–348,
    351

Genotoxins, 208–209, 273
Giemsa stain, 283
Giemsa stain Gurr solution, 215, 241
Giemsa staining, 284–285
Giemsa-type stains, 275
Glass microscope slides, 283
Global Evaluation Factor (GEF), 142–143
Globally Harmonized System, 57–58
GLP study protocols, 23
GLP toxicology test programs, 53, 59
 chemical analysis, 59
GLP-compliant report, 31
Glucose, 87
Glucose-6-phosphate, 88
Glycosylphosphatidylinositol (GPI) anchors, 384–387
Good laboratory practice (GLP), 1–2
 environment, 10, 14, 95–96
 in vitro micronucleus assay, 165
 preparing protocol complying with, 23–29
  standardized boilerplate protocols, 28–29
 regulations, guidelines, and related documents, 27*t*
GPI anchors. *See* Glycosyl-phosphatidylinositol (GPI) anchors
Greenscreen, 127
Growth medium, 145–146
Guide for the Care and Use of Laboratory Animals, 274–275
Gurr's improved R66, 283

H
(Ham's) F-12 medium, 214, 216
Hanks' balanced salt solution (HBSS), 331–332, 354
 preparation, 331–332
Harvest, 235–236
HBSS. *See* Hanks' balanced salt solution (HBSS)
HBT (histidine, biotin and tryptophan) solution, 88

Hedgehog comets, 375, 375*f*
Helminthosporium dematioideum, 163–164
Hematopoiesis/hemolysis, 23–24
Hematopoietic cells, 348–349
Hemocytometer, 131–132, 236
Hemolysis, 324
Heparin sodium, 217
High-sensitivity methods, 385
Histidine HCl.H2O, 88
Historical control databases, 11–13, 276
Historical control results, 262
Historical controls, for *in vitro* assays, 169
Historical negative/vehicle control results, 124*f*
Historical positive control data, 277, 327
Historical positive control results, 125*t*, 277
Homeostasis perturbations, 373–374, 379–380
Hormone-regulating tissues, 362
Howell-Jolly bodies.
 See Micronuclei
HPMC. *See* Hydroxy-propylmethylcellulose (HPMC)
HPRT (hypoxanthine-guanine phosphoribosyl transferase) locus, 141
hprt gene, 141
Human centromeric-specific chromosomes (light-sensitive) probes, 172
Human lymphocytes, 169–170, 172, 178, 221
 binuclear assay, 172
 structural aberrations and other lesions in, 251*f*
Human peripheral blood lymphocytes (HPBL), 169, 211, 218–220, 225–226, 243–244, 262–263
 selection of slides for provisional detailed examination, 243
 test procedures, 238–241

Humidified atmosphere, 181
Hybrid animal, 275
HYBrite programmable hotplate, 292–293
HYBrite™ machine, 293
HYBrite™/Thermobrite™, for FISH method, 181–182
Hydrogen peroxide, 346
Hydroxypropylmethylcellulose (HPMC), 71–72
Hypotonic solution, 217

I
IACUC. *See* Institutional animal care and use committee (IACUC)
ICH S2R1 guidelines, 184, 326, 348–350, 349*f*
IEs. *See* Immature erythrocytes (IEs)
Image analysis scoring, 367–369
 CCD camera, 368
 microscope, 367–368
 software, 368
Image analysis systems, 13–14, 129, 153, 367–368
Immature erythrocytes (IEs), 271–272
 proportion of, 316–317
In vitro chromosome aberration test, 207, 324, 334
 automation, 264
 cell characterization, 221–225
  cell-cycle time, 224–225
  modal chromosome number, 222–223
  mycoplasma, 224
 consumables and reagents, 214–215
 equipment, 212–214
 fundamentals, 211–212
 history, 209–211
 interpretation of results, 253–263
  criteria for negative/positive/equivocal outcome, 253–256
  follow-up *in vivo* testing, 257–258
  historical control results, 262

In vitro chromosome aberration test (*Continued*)
  interpretation of numerical aberrations, 257
  reporting, 258–261
  toxicity, evaluation of, 253
  unexpected and borderline results, 257
  validity of study, 253
  volatile and gaseous compounds, testing of, 262–263
phases in development of, 219–221
reagents and recipes, 215–219
  colcemid 10 μg/ml in PBS, 216
  F-12 complete, 216
  fix, 216
  freezing Medium 10% (CHO cells), 216
  G6P 1M: glucose-6-phosphate, 217
  heparin sodium 1000 U/mL, 217
  hypotonic solution (0.075 M KCl), 217
  KMg, 217
  phosphate buffer 0.2 M, pH 7.4, 218
  phytohemagglutinin (PHA) M form, 217
  positive control solutions, 218
  RPMI complete, 218
  S9 fraction, 218–219
  S9 mix, 219
  β-nicotinamide adenine dinucleotide phosphate (NADP) 0.1 M, 217
routine testing, 225–230
  dose level selection, 227–230
  dose regimens, 225–226
  general considerations of, 225
  metabolic activation system, 226
  positive controls, 230
  test substance considerations, 226–227
  vehicle selection and dose volume, 227

screening versions of test, 263
standard test procedures, 230–252
  CHO cells: test procedures, 233–237
  experimental design spreadsheet, 231–233
  human peripheral blood lymphocyte (HPBL) test procedures, 238–241
  preliminary slide reading, 243–244
  selection of slides for detailed examination, 242–243
  slide coding, 243
  slide scoring, 244–252
  slide staining: all cell types, 241
In vitro compatibility testing, 60–67
In vitro cytogenetics, 2–3
In vitro mammalian cell assay, 348–350
In vitro mammalian cell genotoxicity assays, 156, 158f
In vitro mammalian cell tests, 17, 19, 40, 348–349
In vitro MicroFlow® kit, 185–186
In vitro micronucleus assay, 161
  flow cytometric method, 184–203
    advice for test article exposure, 200–202
    analysis template, creation, 195–198
    attachment cell protocol, 188–189
    consumables, 185
    equipment, 184–185
    example plate layout, 198
    example results table, 199
    flow cytometric data acquisition, 189–193
    flow cytometric data analysis, 193–195
    multichannel aspirator with bridge, use of, 202

    nucleic acid dye B photoactivation, plate placement during, 203
    reagents and recipes, 185–186
    suspension cell protocol, 187–189
    updates and future work, 203
  materials, 171–172
    binuclear assay, 172
    centromeric labeling, 172
    mononuclear assay, 171
    nondisjunction assay, 172
  methods, 169–170, 172–183
    binuclear assay, 169, 177–181
    centromeric labeling, 169–170, 181–183
    mononuclear assay, 169, 173–177
    nondisjunction assay, 170
    S9 mix, 172–173
  practical considerations, 165–169
    cell types, 166
    controls, 166–167
    cytotoxicity measures, 167–168
    experimental design, 167
    good laboratory practice (GLP), 165
    historical controls, 169
    laboratory proficiency, 166
    metabolic activation, 167
    regulatory guidelines, 165
    S9 rat liver homogenate, 167
In vitro micronucleus formation, 184
In vitro micronucleus testing, 166
In vitro studies, 9, 17, 38–39, 42t, 45–46
In vitro testing, 2–3, 10, 15, 17, 20
In vivo chromosome aberration, 335–336
In vivo comet assay, 346
In vivo cytogenetics, 2–3
In vivo genotoxicity assays, 349–350, 411

In vivo genotoxicity tests, 328, 335–336
In vivo hematopoietic cell micronucleus assay, 156
In vivo micronucleus test, 22–24, 38, 57
In vivo studies, 9, 23
In vivo systems, 2–3, 9, 15–17
Inbred animal, 275
Independent cytotoxicity assessment, 194
Industrial Genotoxicology Group (IGG), 37
Infinity-corrected extra-low dispersion glass lenses, 212–213
Institutional animal care and use committee (IACUC), 356–357
Instrument Calibration Standard (ICS), 390, 411
  part B of, 403–404
  sample (part A), 394, 403
Integrated repeat-dose studies, 390–392
  assay configurations, 391–392
  dose-range finding, 391
  timing of sample collection, 391
  top dose and dose spacing, 391
Intercalating agents, 113
Intercalation, 273, 324
Interference with DNA metabolism, 273
International Conference on Harmonisation (ICH), 6, 142, 228–229
International Life Sciences Institute/Health and Environmental Sciences Institute (ILSI/HESI), 143
International System for Chromosome Aberration Nomenclature, 248
International Workgroup on Genotoxicity Tests for the MLA (IWGT-ML), 142–143
International Workshop on Genotoxicity Testing (IWGT), 11, 346–348

Interpretation of numerical aberrations, 257
ISO 10993 series of standards, 60
ISO standards, 26–28
IWGT *Pig-a* Workgroup, 389–391
IWGT. *See* International Workshop on Genotoxicity Testing (IWGT)

J

Japanese Collection of Research Bioresources Cell Bank (JCRB), 143, 146
Japanese Environmental Mutagenesis Society (JEMS), 37

K

K_2EDTA tubes, 414–415
Kendall rank correlation test, 369–371
Kimwipes, 215
Kineotochore labeling, 294–296
  materials, 294
  methods, 294–296
    analysis of slides, 296
    assessment of results, 296
    phase 1, 295
    phase 2, 295
    slide checking, 295
    slide coding, 295–296
Kinetochore proteins, 294
KMg, 88, 217
Köhler illumination, 212–213

L

L-5178 cells, 141–142
Labeling solution, 298–299
  bone marrow, 298
  whole blood, 298
Labeling washed samples for flow analysis, 305–306
Labor requirement, 44–45
Laboratory historical control databases, 10–13
  positive control database, 13
  spreadsheet calculations, 13
  vehicle/negative control database, 11–13

Laboratory proficiency, 166, 166t, 411
Lagging chromosomes, 273, 291
Large volume suspensions, 73
Leukodepletion, 394
Leukodepletion and platelet removal, in *Pig-a* endogenous gene mutation assay, 397
  cell pellets, washing, 397
  processing of blood through Lympholyte-Mammal, 397
Limit of toxicity, 19–20, 228, 236
Linear regression test, 371
Liquid nitrogen, 233
Liver comet, 377t
LMP. *See* Low melting point agarose (LMP)
Long-term storage solution (LTSS)
  transferring samples to, 304–305
  washing samples out of, 304–305
  washing solution for samples in, 298
Low melting point agarose (LMP), 355
Lower-dose formulations, 69
Low-molecular-weight (LMW) DNA diffusion assay, 373–374
Luer-Lok syringe-fitting, 214
Lymphocyte culture, 178–179, 208–209, 220
Lymphocytes, 178, 214, 220, 224
  mitotic activity of, 220
  structural aberrations in, 251f
Lympholyte®-Mammal, 397, 415

M

Main mutation test, 151–155
  acceptance criteria, 155
  expression period, 151–152
    Day 1, 151–152
    Day 2, 152
  posttreatment procedures, 151
  results, analysis of, 153–155
    mutant frequency assessment (agar version), 154–155

Main mutation test (*Continued*)
  mutant frequency assessment
    (microtiter version), 154
  relative suspension growth
    (RSG), 153
  toxicity assessment, 154
  viability assessment and mutant
    selection (agar version),
    152–153
  colony counting, 153
  viability assessment and mutant
    selection (microtiter
    version), 152
  colony counting, 152
Main test, standard study design,
  112*t*
Malling's metabolic system,
  82–83
Mammalian cell mutation test, 17,
  139–140, 142
Mammalian cell test, 9, 60–62,
  210–211
Mammalian erythroblasts,
  271–272
Mammalian erythrocyte
  micronucleus test, 271
Mann-Whitney tests, 371
Manual counting, 118
Master frozen permanents,
  221–222
Master permanents, 94, 105
Master stock, 94, 146–147
Mature erythrocytes (ME),
  270–272
Maximum tolerated dose (MTD),
  15–17, 279, 281, 391
MC. *See* Methylcellulose (MC)
ME. *See* Mature erythrocytes (ME)
Mean colony counts, 122
Measures to ensure safety, 54
Medical devices, 26–28, 60, 106,
  226, 230
Megafunnel™, 174
Metabolic activation, 83, 106, 147,
  202, 226
  in vitro assays and, 167
Metafer, 176, 177*f*
Metaphase, 219–220, 245–247,
  325–326
  classification, 248–252

identification criteria, 247
preparations, 339
Metaphase test. *See* Rodent bone
  marrow chromosomal
  aberration test
MetaSystems, 176
Metered agar pump, 45
Methemoglobinemia, 324
Method set-up, 6–8
Method validation, 8–10
Methotrexate resistance, 144–145
Methyl methane sulfonate (MMS),
  148
Methylcellulose (MC), 71–72
3-Methylcholanthrene, 141–142
MF. *See* Mutant frequency (MF)
Microbial contamination, 40
Microbial load, 108
Micronucleated erythrocytes,
  272–273
  nongenotoxic mechanisms of
    induction of, 317–318
  avoiding and recognizing
    irrelevant positives,
    317–318
  causes, 317
Micronucleated immature
  erythrocytes (MIE),
  270–271, 276–277
Micronucleated type I
  reticulocytes, 272
Micronuclei, 163–164, 175, 177,
  270–271
  identification of, 290
Micronucleus frequency, 178
Micronucleus test, 314, 324, 328
MicroNuc™ module, 174–176
Microscope, 85, 118, 367–368
Microscopic methods, 283–290
  acridine orange staining,
    285–286
  blood smears, 283
  Giemsa staining, 285
  identification of micronuclei,
    290
  microscopic evaluation,
    288–290
  mouse bone marrow smears,
    284
  rat bone marrow smears, 284

smear fixation and staining,
    284–285
  supravital staining of blood,
    286–288
Microsuspension assay, 128
Microtiter fluctuation test
  technique, 141–142
Microtiter mouse lymphoma assay,
  149*f*
MIE values, 314–316
MIE. *See* Micronucleated
  immature erythrocytes
  (MIE)
Millex®, 214
Minimal glucose agar (MGA)
  plates, 88–89
Misclassification, 245
Mitogen-stimulated lymphocytes,
  208–209
Mitomycin C (MMC), 81–82, 99,
  210, 218, 278–279
Mitotic index (MI), 219–220, 228,
  241, 243–244, 328,
  334–336
MN frequency, 194–197
Modal chromosome number,
  221–223
  scoring sheet, 223*f*
Moltox, 86, 95–96, 215, 219
Monocrotaline, 278–279
Mononuclear assay, 173–177
  analysis of slides (microscope),
    175–176
  analysis of slides
    (semiautomated scoring),
    176–177
  cell culture and treatment, 174
  coding of slides, 175
  materials, 171
  methods, 169
  slide preparation, 174–175
  treatment schedules, 173–174
Mouse bone marrow smears, 284
Mouse lymphoma L5178Y cell
  line clone 3.7.2C, 166, 169
Mouse lymphoma L5178Y tk$^{+/}$
  $^{-}$assay (MLA), 139–140
  evaluation criteria, 155–156
  history of, 141–143
  materials, 145–148

cell culture, 146—147
growth medium, 145—146
metabolic activation, 147
positive controls, 148
safety, 145
test item, 148
vehicle, 148
predictivity of, 156—158
provenance of cells, 143—144
spontaneous mutant frequency, 144—145
study design, 148—155
general test conditions, 148—150, 149*f*
main mutation test, 151—155
preliminary toxicity test, 150
MTD. *See* Maximum tolerated dose (MTD)
Multichannel aspirator, 202
MutaFlow^{PLUS} kit, 393
Mutagenesis (journal), 37
Mutagenesis assay, 142
Mutagenicity, 82—83, 94, 349—350
Mutant cell frequency calculations, 409—410, 416
Mutant frequency (MF), 144—145, 154—156
Mutant frequency assessment
agar version, 154—155
microtiter version, 154
Mutant mimic sample, 390
Mutant mimicking cells, 397
Mutant offspring, 385
Mutation frequency
calculating, 388
estimating, 139—140
Mycoplasma, 224
contamination, 221
infection, 224

N
Negative control animals, 277
Negative control data, 11, 220—221
Negative control database, 10, 220—221
Negative *in vitro* standard battery tests, follow-up of, 351
New assay, establishing, 6—10

method set-up, 6—8
method validation, 8—10
Nicotinamide adenine dinucleotide phosphate (NADP), 90, 217, 226
4-Nitroquinoline-1-oxide (NQO), 148
NMA. *See* Normal melting agarose (NMA)
NOEL (no observable effect level), 291
Nondisjunction assay
FISH method, 183
materials, 172
methods, 170
slide checking, 183
slide scoring, 183
Non-GLP preliminary work, 23
Non-GLP-screening tests, 113
Nonhazardous reagents, 56
Nonparametric methods, 336
Normal melting agarose (NMA), 355
NORMINV function, 276
Nuclear anomalies, 271
Nucleic acid dye A working solution, 186
Nucleic acid dye B
photoactivation, plate placement during, 203
Nuclei-to-bead ratios, 193, 196
Nutrient agar plates, 90
Nutrient broth, 90

O
OECD 475, 326
OECD GLP, 45—46
OECD guideline 471, 82—83, 105—106, 110—111
OECD guideline 487, 165, 184
OECD guidelines, 210—211, 225, 228, 242
OECD international guideline, 325, 338—339
OECD Test Guideline 476, 142
OECD TG473, 221, 230, 238, 253—254, 258—259, 262
OECD TG 489, 348—349, 357, 359—361, 372—373, 375—376

Oil immersion lens, 212—213
Olive tail moment (OTM), 351—352
One-tailed Fisher exact test, 254
1X Buffer Solution, 186
OOS. *See* Out of Specification (OOS)
Open source programs, 108
Organization of Economic Cooperation and Development (OECD), 6—8, 11, 14—16, 19—20, 28
e-rule requirements, 14—15
OSHA, principles of, 54
Osmolality, 66, 150, 210—211
Out of Specification (OOS), 75
Outbred animal, 275

P
P (petite) arm, 245—246
Pan-centromeric paint, 172, 181
Paroxysmal nocturnal hemoglobinurea (PNH), 385
PBS. *See* Phosphate-buffered saline (PBS)
PERCENTILE function, 276
Personal protective clothing, 56—57
capital equipment, 56—57
consumables, 57
standard, 56
Personal protective equipment, 52
Petroff-Hausser bacterial counting chamber, 131—132, 132*f*
pH of culture medium, 150
Pharmacy, 53, 55
Phase contrast microscope, 110—111, 132
Phases, of multiple studies, 42*t*
Phosphate buffer 0.2 M, pH 7.4, 90, 218
Phosphate-buffered saline (PBS), 294, 354
Phosphatidylinositol glycan complement class A (*Pig-a*) gene, 384—385
Photomultiplier tube (PMT), 404—406

Phycoerythrin (PE), 388
Phytohemagglutinin (PHA), 178, 210, 217
Pig-a endogenous gene mutation assay, 383–384, 387–390
aspiration of postcolumn samples, 416
blood collection, 396
column separation and sample staining, 400–403
  eluting samples through immunomagnetic columns, 400–402
  postcolumn samples, centrifugation and staining, 402–403
consumables, 393
equipment, 392
example plots, 414
flow cytometric analysis, 403–409
  instrument calibration, 404–408
  postcolumn analysis of experimental samples, 409
  precolumn analysis of experimental samples, 408
flow cytometric template preparation, 412–411
fundamentals, 385–388
history, 384–385
leukodepletion and platelet removal, 397
  process blood through Lympholyte-Mammal, 397
  wash cell pellets, 397
method overview, 395
reagents and recipes, 393–394
  solution and materials preparation, 393–394
results, evaluation and interpretation of, 410–411
  biological relevance, 411
  comparison to historical controls, 411
  statistics, 410
  valid assay, criteria for, 411
results, tabulating and summarizing, 409–410

mutant cell frequency calculations, 409–410
sample labeling, 397–400
  labeling leukodepleted blood with antibody solution, 398
  part A of the Instrument Calibration Standard (ICS), preparation of, 400
  precolumn samples, incubating, 400
  precolumn samples, staining, 399–400
  samples incubation in working anti-PE microbead suspension, 398–399
  washing labeled samples out of working antibody solution, 398
storage and shipment of blood samples, 414
study design, 389–392
  acute or integrated repeat-dose studies, 390–392
  animal species/strain/sex/age, 389–390
  group selection/identification, 390
  negative and positive controls, 390
  number of animals per experimental group, 390
Plan fluorite, 212–213, 330–331
Plate incorporation method, 83–84, 114–115
Plate incorporation test, 123*t*
Plate-based flow cytometric assay, 198
Platelet activation, 396
PNH. *See* Paroxysmal nocturnal hemoglobinurea (PNH)
Poisson distribution, 154
Polyploidy, 209, 245
Population doubling, 164, 174, 194
Positive controls, 44, 56, 113, 148, 202, 230, 390
  and cytotoxic agents, 56
  database, 13
  and diagnostic mutagen solutions, 90–91
  group, 327

for plate incorporation assay, 124*t*
solutions, 218
substance, 278
Positive *in vitro* standard battery tests, follow-up of, 350
Postcolumn samples, 388, 402–403
aspiration of, 416
Powder containment cabinet, 54, 68
Practical guide to genetic toxicology testing, 1
Precipitation, 65–66, 110–111
Preincubation assay, 125–126
Preincubation method, 83–84, 108, 115–116
Preliminary slide reading, 243–244
Preliminary testing and records, 15
Preliminary toxicity test, 16–17, 149–150
Premutagenic lesions, 350
Preparation artifact, 244, 247, 334
Pricing, 48
Process-based scheme, 45–46
Programmable hotplate, FISH method using, 292–293
Proliferative index (PI), 224
Purged Cell Assay Stocks, 147
Purging, of tk$^{-/-}$ mutants (cleansing), 146–147

Q

Q arm, 245–246
QA, 45–46
QuadroMACS™ separator, 400
Quality and efficiency, improving, 37–45
  accommodating repeat or supplementary tests, 40
  minimizing the potential problems on studies, 38–39
  reducing costs/labor requirement, 44–45
  reducing the effort needed to perform the study, 43–44
  reducing the effort needed to prepare protocols, tables, and reports, 43

reducing the need for repetition of parts of study, 39–40

running more studies in given timeframe, 40–41

timeframe for routine studies, 41–42

Quebec counter illumination system, 118, 129

R

Radiation-induced chromosome exchange, 244–245

Rat bone marrow smears, 284

Rat peripheral blood samples, 391–392

RCC. *See* Relative cell counts (RCC)

Reagents and recipes
bacterial reverse mutation test, 86–93
in vitro chromosome aberration test, 215–219
in vitro micronucleus assay, 185–186
Pig-a endogenous gene mutation assay, 393–394

Receipt of test article, 59

Red blood cells (RBC), 385, 387, 391, 407, 409

Reduced format tests using standard tester strains, 129–130

Region of interest (ROI), 368

Regulatory guidelines
in vitro micronucleus assay, 165

Regulatory safety testing, *in vivo* comet assay in, 348–351
negative *in vitro* standard battery tests, 351
positive *in vitro* standard battery tests, 350

Relative cell counts (RCC), 167–168

Relative increase in cell count (RICC), 167–168, 194, 228, 242–243, 253

Relative population doubling (RPD), 167–168, 194, 228, 242–243, 253

Relative suspension growth (RSG), 153

Relative total growth (RTG), 142–143, 151, 154–156

Repeat/supplementary tests, accommodating, 40

Repeat-dose design, 387

Replication index (RI), 167–168, 179–180

Report tables, presentation of, 30–31

Reticulocytes (RETs), 286–288, 387, 391, 407, 409

Revertants, dose-related increase in, 84*f*

RI. *See* Replication index (RI)

RICC. *See* Relative increase in cell count (RICC)

Rimonabant, 348–349

RMI, 260–261

Rodent bone marrow chromosomal aberration test, 323–324
history, 324–325
related methods, 325–326
study design and performance, 326–330
animal euthanasia, 329–330
animal observations, 329
dose administration, 328
dose selection, 328
number of groups, 327
positive control group, 327
sex and group size, 327
target organ exposure, evidence of, 328
treatment schedule, 329
vehicle/negative control and formulation, 326
terminal procedures, 330–339
acceptability of study, 335
advance preparation, 331–332
bone marrow collection, 332–333
calculations and reporting of results, 334–335
consumables, 331
cytonucleus test, 339
equipment, 330–331

evaluation and interpretation of results, 335–337
integration into other studies, 339
slide examination, 334
slide preparation, 333
slide staining, 333
test report, 337–339

Rodent erythrocyte micronucleus test
equipments for, 330–331
limitations of, 318

Rodent micronucleus assay, 257–258, 269
automated analysis and flow cytometry, 297–313
analysis of experimental samples, 311
blood and bone marrow samples, fixation of, 300–302
blood collection, 299
bone marrow collection and processing, 299–300
bone marrow samples, collecting and fractionating, 300
flow cytometric analysis, 306–311
flow cytometry method, 299
individual reagents, 297
labelling washed samples for flow analysis, 305–306
solution and material preparation, 297–299
storage of fixed samples, 303–304
template preparation for flow cytometric analyses, 312–313
transferring samples to LTSS, 304–305
fundamentals, 271–273
history, 271
manual methods, 282–296
centromeric staining using FISH, 292–294
equipment and consumables, 282

Rodent micronucleus assay
      (*Continued*)
   identification of aneugenic
         agents, 291
   kinetochore labelling, 294—296
   microscopic methods, 283—290
   reagent preparation, 282—283
   records, 290—291
   sample preparation, 283
micronucleated erythrocytes,
      nongenotoxic mechanisms
      of induction of, 317—318
   avoiding and recognizing
         irrelevant positives,
         317—318
   causes, 317
results and statistical analysis,
      interpretation of, 315—317
   immature erythrocytes,
         proportion of, 316—317
   MIE values, 315—316
rodent erythrocyte micronucleus
      test, limitations of, 318
study design, 273—281
   acute and repeat-dose
         schedules, 278—279
   animal source, housing,
         maintenance, and
         identification, 274—275
   animal species, strain, age,
         and sex, 275—276
   dose administration, 281
   dose level selection, 279—280
   dose range-finding
         experiment, 280—281
   dose volume, 281
   historical negative/vehicle and
         positive control data,
         276—277
   number and size of treatment
         groups, 277—278
   study validity, 314
   test substance considerations,
         273
ROI. *See* Region of interest (ROI)
Roswell Park Memorial Institute
      (RPMI) 1640 medium,
      145—146
Route of exposure, for comet
      assay, 359—360
Routine scoring, 247

Routine testing, 8, 11, 21—22
   bacterial reverse mutation test,
         105—113
   in vitro chromosome aberration
         test, 225—230
      dose level selection, 227—230
      dose regimens, 225—226
      general considerations of, 225
      metabolic activation system,
            226
      positive controls, 230
      test substance considerations,
            226—227
      vehicle selection and dose
            volume, 227
RPD. *See* Relative population
      doubling (RPD)
RPMI 1640 medium, 145—146,
      214
RPMI 20 medium, 152—153
RPMI complete, 218
RTG. *See* Relative total growth
      (RTG)

S

S9 fraction, 91, 147, 218—219
S9 mix, 38—40, 83—84, 91—92,
      147, 219, 230
   in *in vitro* micronucleus assay,
         172—173
S9 rat liver homogenate, 167
Safety data sheets (SDS), 57—59
Salmonella enterica, 81—82
Salmonella histidine, 81—82
Salmonella strain TA1530, 82—83
Salmonella tester strains, 81
Salmonella typhimurium, 81—82
Salmonella typhimurium strain
      TA102, 108
Sample collection
   for *in vivo* comet assay test,
         363—364
   timing of, 391
Screening tests, 126—130
   reduced format tests using
         standard tester strains,
         129—130
   simplified test systems,
         126—127
   using standard tester strains,
         127—129

Screening versions, of *in vitro*
      chromosome aberration
      test, 263
SDS. *See* Safety data sheets (SDS)
Selection of slides for detailed
      examination, 242—243
   cell lines, 242—243
   human peripheral blood
         lymphocyte (HPBL), 243
SG. *See* Specific gravity (SG)
Shapiro-Wilk test, 370
Simplified test systems, 126—127
Single cells region, 306, 404
Sister chromatid exchanges
      (SCEs), 325—326
Skin sensitization, 56
Slide checking, 295
   centromeric labeling, 182
   nondisjunction assay, 183
Slide code, 243, 295—296, 331
Slide code labels, 43
Slide code numbers, 243
Slide examination, 248
   rodent bone marrow
         chromosomal aberration
         test, 334
Slide labeling, 45
Slide preparation
   for CHO cells: test procedures,
         237
   for HPBL test procedures,
         238—241
   for *in vitro* micronucleus assay,
         174—175
   rodent bone marrow
         chromosomal aberration
         test, 333
Slide quality, 19
Slide reading, 42
Slide scoring, 244—252
   basics, 244—245
   centromeric labeling, 183
   classification, 248—252
   nondisjunction assay, 183
   normal karyotype,
         understanding, 245—247
   routine scoring, 247
Slide staining, 367
   all cell types, 241
   rodent bone marrow chromosomal
         aberration test, 333

Slide storage system, 213
Sloped (gradient) plate method, 128
Small-volume assays, 64–65
Small volume suspensions, 74
Smear fixation and staining, 284–285
Sodium carboxymethylcellulose (CMC), 71–72
Sodium dihydrogen phosphate, 218
Solubility and and *in vitro* compatibility testing, 60–67
   choice of solvent, 61–62
   compatibility of formulation with culture medium, 65–67
   small-volume (*in vitro*) assays, 64–65
   solubility testing, 62–64
Solubility testing, 22, 60–64
SOPs, 22
   maintenance, 15
   organization of, 20–22
   typical list of, in genetic toxicology laboratory, 21*t*
Specific gravity (SG), 64
Spermatogonial chromosomal aberration test, 325
S-phases, 224, 244–245
Spontaneous mutant frequency, 144–145
Spontaneous revertant colony counts, 99, 120
Sprague-Dawley, 389–390
Spreadsheet
   calculations, 13
   and manipulation of results, 10–11
Staff training, 21–22
Staining methods and terminology, 272*t*
Standard 24-well plate format, comparison of, 130*f*
Standard battery genotoxicity tests, 351
Standard deviations, 30–31
Standard plate incorporation assay, 125–126
Standard study design, 116–117, 117*t*
Standard test procedures
   bacterial reverse mutation test, 114–126

in vitro chromosome aberration test, 230–252
in vivo comet assay test, 362–369
Standard tester strains
   reduced format tests using, 129–130
   screening tests using, 127–129
Standardized boilerplate protocols, 28–29
Statistical analysis, general recommendations for, 19–20
Statistical analysis, *in vivo* comet assay test, 369–372
   normality test, 370
   pairwise comparisons, 371
      nonparametric tests, 371
      parametric tests, 371
   trend tests, 371–372
      cytotoxicity, 373–375
      nonparametric test, 371–372
      parametric test, 371
      positive response criteria, 372–373
      reporting results, 376–377
      validity of a test, 372
Steel multiple comparison test, 371
Stock formulation, 68–69
Storage and shipment of blood samples, 414
Structural aberrant cell frequency, 334–335
Structural aberrations, 209, 212, 222, 244–245, 247–248, 251*f*
Structural chromosomal aberrations, 334–336
Study design
   bacterial reverse mutation test, 116–117
   general recommendations, 15–17
   in vivo comet assay test, 357–362
   in vivo rodent micronucleus assay, 273–281
   mouse lymphoma TK assay, 148–155
   Pig-a endogenous gene mutation assay, 389–392
   rodent bone marrow chromosomal aberration test, 326–330

Study plan/protocol, 9, 22
Study set-up, 42
Supravital staining of blood, 286–288
Surfactant, 145
Suspending agents, 71–72
Suspension cell protocol, for flow cytometric method, 187–189
   cell harvest, 187
   complete nucleic acid dye A staining, 187
   simultaneous cell lysis and nucleic acid dye B staining, 188
   treatment, preliminary assessments, 187
Suspension cells, 200–201
Suspension cultures, growing and monitoring, 130–134
Suspension growth (SG), 153
   relative, 153–154
Suspensions, formulation of, 71–74
   aqueous suspending agents, 71–72
   large volume suspensions, 73
   small volume suspensions, 74
System change control, 15
System Manager, designation of, 15
System operation, 15

T
TAC. *See* Top agar complete (TAC)
TAI. *See* Top agar incomplete (TAI)
Tail length (TL), 351–352
Tail moment (TM), 351–352
Target organ, 361–362, 373, 380–381
Target organ exposure, evidence of, 328
Tedlar gas sampling bags, 125–126
Template preparation for flow cytometric analyses, 312–313

Template protocol, 41
Terminal Procedures, 330–339
Terminal procedures, of rodent
    bone marrow chromosomal
    aberration test, 330–339
  acceptability of study, 335
  advance preparation, 331–332
  bone marrow collection,
    332–333
  calculations and reporting of
    results, 334–335
  consumables, 331
  cytonucleus test, 339
  equipment, 330–331
  evaluation and interpretation of
    results, 335–337
  integration into other studies,
    339
  slide examination, 334
  slide preparation, 333
  slide staining, 333
  test report, 337–339
Test article considerations,
    106–113
Test article exposure, advice for,
    200–202
  attachment cells, 201
  metabolic activation, 202
  positive controls, 202
  suspension cells, 200–201
Test batch frozen permanents,
    221–222
Test reliability, 9–10
Test report, 337–339
Test robustness, 9–10
Test sensitivity, 9
Test substance considerations,
    226–227
Test system maintenance log, 7, 15
Tetracycline disc, 92
Tetrahydrofolate, 144–145
Thymidine deoxyriboside (dThd),
    139–140
Thymidine kinase, 139–142, 151
Tissue repair timeline, 360*f*
Tissue-specific follow-up testing,
    351
TK6 cells, medium for, 186
Top agar complete (TAC), 92
Top agar incomplete (TAI), 92

Top dose and dose spacing, 391
Total RBC region, 405
Toxicity, evaluation of, 253
Toxicity assessment, 154
Toxicity tests, 20, 53
  preliminary, 150
Training, 36–37
Transgenic mutation assay in
    rodents (TGR), 349–350
Travel sickness, 334
"Treat and Plate" modification,
    107
Trend tests, 371–372
  cytotoxicity, 373–375
  dose-response curves with linear
    elements detected
    by, 372*f*
  nonparametric test, 371–372
  parametric test, 371
  positive response criteria,
    372–373
  reporting results, 376–377
  validity of a test, 372
Trenimon, 271
Trifluorothymidine (TFT),
    139–140, 151–152
Trituration, 73
Trypsin, 231–238
Tryptophan, 93
Tween 20, 294

U
UDS tests, 2
UK Environmental Mutagenesis
    Society, 1–2
Umu test, 127
Unexpected and borderline results,
    121, 257
Unexplainable positive rate,
    156–157
United Kingdom Environmental
    Mutagenesis Society
    (UKEMS), 37
US EPA, 32–35

V
Valid assay, 17–18
  criteria for, 180, 194, 411
Validation plan protocol, 15
Validation testing, 15

VEGA program, 108
Vegetable oils, 326
Vehicle selection
  in vitro chromosome aberration
    test, 227
  in vivo comet assay test,
    357–359
Vehicle/negative control database,
    10–13
Viability assessment and mutant
    selection (agar version),
    152–153
  colony counting (agar version),
    153
Viability assessment and mutant
    selection (microtiter
    version), 152
  colony counting (microtiter
    version), 152
Vinblastine, 278
Vogel-Bonner (VB) salts, 93
Volatile and gaseous compounds,
    testing of, 125–126,
    262–263
Volatile solvents, 62–63

W
Washing solution for samples in
    LTSS, 298
Water-miscible organic solvents,
    61–62
96-Well plate–based protocol,
    403–409
Whole blood cultures, 179
Wider spacing, 30–31
Wild-type (WT) cells, 387
Wistar, 389–390
Working antibody solution, 394
Working anti-PE microbead
    suspension, 394
Working nucleic acid dye plus
    counting beads solution,
    394

X
Xenobiotic metabolic systems,
    82–83
Xenobiotic metabolizing enzymes,
    218